SURGERY SECRETS

HRATCH L. KARAMANOUKIAN, M.D.
Associate Director
Center for Less Invasive Cardiac Surgery
and Robotic Heart Surgery
Kaleida Health–Buffalo General Hospital
Buffalo, New York

PAULO R. SOLTOSKI, M.D.
Attending Thoracic and Cardiovascular Surgeon
Hospital Santa Cruz
Curitiba, Parana, Brazil

TOMAS A. SALERNO, M.D., FRCS(C), FACS, FCCP (Surgery)
Professor of Surgery
University of Miami School of Medicine
Chief, Division of Cardiothoracic Surgery
Jackson Memorial Hospital
Miami, Florida

HANLEY & BELFUS, INC./Philadelphia

Publisher: HANLEY & BELFUS, INC.
               Medical Publishers
               210 South 13th Street
               Philadelphia, PA 19107
               (215) 546-7293; 800-962-1892
               FAX (215) 790-9330
               Web site: http://www.hanleyandbelfus.com

Library of Congress Cataloging-in-Publication Data

Karamanoukian, Hratch L., 1964–
    Thoracic Surgery Secrets / edited by Hratch L. Karamanoukian,
Paulo R. Soltoski, Tomas A. Salerno.
        p. ; cm. — (The Secrets Series®)
    Includes bibliographical references and index.
    ISBN 1-56053-373-0 (alk. paper)
        1. Chest—Surgery—Examinations, questions, etc.   I. Soltoski,
Paulo R., 1964–   II. Salerno, Tomas A.   III. Title.   IV. Series.
        [DNLM: 1. Thoracic Surgical Procedures—Examination Questions.
    WF 18.2 K18t 2000]
    RD536.K38 2000
    617.5′4059′076—dc21

                                                    00-037579

THORACIC SURGERY SECRETS   ISBN 1-56053-373-0

Last digit is the print number: 9 8 7 6 5 4 3 2 1

CONTENTS

I. PRINCIPLES OF GENERAL THORACIC SURGERY

II. THE ESOPHAGUS

Contents

VIII. MINIMALLY INVASIVE THORACIC SURGERY

CONTRIBUTORS

Reginald G. M. Abraham, M.D.
Fellow and Instructor, Division of Cardiothoracic Surgery, Department of Surgery, State University of New York at Buffalo School of Medicine and Biomedical Sciences; Kaleida Health-Buffalo General Hospital, Millard Filmore Hospital, Buffalo Children's Hospital, Veterans Administration Medical Center, Buffalo, New York

Mark S. Allen, M.D.
Associate Professor, Department of Surgery, Mayo Medical School, and Chair, Division of General Thoracic Surgery, Mayo Clinic, Rochester, Minnesota

Kathryn D. Anderson, M.D.
Professor, Department of Surgery, University of Southern California School of Medicine, Surgeon-in-Chief and Vice President of Surgery, Children's Hospital of Los Angeles, Los Angeles, California

Timothy M. Anderson, M.D.
Assistant Professor, Department of Surgery, State University of New York at Buffalo, Attending Thoracic Surgeon, Division of Thoracic Surgical Oncology, Roswell Park Cancer Institute, Buffalo, New York

Lisa Apfel, M.D.
Department of Surgery, University of California at San Diego, San Diego, California

Jacob Bergsland, M.D.
Assistant Professor and Director, Center for Less Invasive Cardiac Surgery, Department of Medicine, State University of New York at Buffalo School of Medicine and Biomedical Sciences, Kaleida Health-Buffalo General Hospital, Buffalo, New York

Scott C. Boulanger, M.D., Ph.D.
Department of Pediatric Surgery, State University of New York at Buffalo, Buffalo, New York

Kevin Broder, M.D.
Resident, Department of Surgery, State University of New York at Buffalo, Buffalo, New York

Marcio P. T. Cartacho, M.D.
Attending Physician, Anesthesiology and Intensive Care Medicine, Clinica Santa Helena, Cabo Frio, Rio de Janeiro, Brazil

Michael G. Caty, M.D.
Associate Professor of Surgery and Pediatrics, Division of Pediatric Surgery, State University of New York at Buffalo, Buffalo Children's Hospital, Buffalo, New York

Jacob DeLaRosa, M.D.
Chief Resident, General Surgery, Department of Surgery, University of California at San Diego, San Diego, California

Timothy G. DeZastro, M.D.
Assistant Clinical Director, Department of Radiology, Kaleida Health System, Site Director, Radiology, Millard Filmore Hospital, Buffalo, New York

Harry W. Donias, M.D.
Department of Surgery, State University of New York at Buffalo School of Medicine and
Biomedical Sciences, Buffalo, New York

Mohammad H. Eslami, M.D.
Department of Surgery, State University of New York at Stony Brook Health Sciences Center
School of Medicine, Stony Brook, New York

Paula Michele Flummerfelt, M.D.
Clinical Instructor and Fellow, Division of Cardiothoracic Surgery, State University of New York
at Buffalo, Kaleida Health-Buffalo General Hospital, Buffalo, New York

William J. Flynn, M.D.
Associate Professor, Department of Surgery, State University of New York at Buffalo, Director,
Trauma Intensive Care Unit, Erie County Medical Center, Buffalo, New York

William J. Gibbons, M.D., FCCP
Assistant Professor, Division of Pulmonary and Critical Care Medicine, Department of Medicine,
State University of New York at Buffalo, Kaleida Health-Buffalo General Hospital, Buffalo, New
York

Philip L. Glick, M.D.
Professor of Surgery, Pediatrics, and Obstetrics/Gynecology, State University of New York at Buf-
falo School of Medicine and Biomedical Sciences, Surgeon-in-Chief, Department of Pediatric
Surgery, Children's Hospital of Buffalo, Buffalo, New York

George Golightly, M.D.
Chief Resident, Department of Surgery, State University of New York at Buffalo, Buffalo, New
York

Marcos R. Gunther, M.D.
Attending Physician, Pulmonary Care and Intensive Care Medicine, Hospital Santa Cruz and
Santa Casa de Misericordia de Curitiba, Parana, Brazil

Eddie L. Hoover, M.D.
Professor and Chairman, Department of Surgery, Chief of Cardiothoracic Surgery, State
University of New York at Buffalo, Buffalo, New York

Mark R. Jajkowski, M.D.
Administrative Chief Resident, Department of Surgery, State University of New York at
Buffalo School of Medicine and Biomedical Sciences, Buffalo, New York

Constantine P. Karakousis, M.D., Ph.D.
Professor, Department of Surgery, State University of New York at Buffalo, Millard Filmore Hospital, Buffalo, New York

Hratch L. Karamanoukian, M.D.
Associate Director, Center for Less Invasive Cardiac Surgery and Robotic Heart Surgery, Kaleida
Health-Buffalo General Hospital, Buffalo, New York

Raffy L. Karamanoukian, M.D.
Resident, Department of Surgery, University of California at San Diego, San Diego, California

Paul C. Kerr, D.O.
Clinical Instructor, Division of Cardiothoracic Surgery, State University of New York at Buffalo, Buffalo, New York

Jennifer I. Lin, M.D.
Resident, Department of Surgery, University of North Carolina, Chapel Hill, North Carolina

Vivian Lindfield, M.D.
Resident, Department of Surgery, State University of New York at Buffalo, Buffalo, New York

Kamal A. Mansour, M.D.
Professor, Division of Cardiothoracic Surgery, Emory University School of Medicine, Atlanta, Georgia

Asif Muhammad, M.D.
Pulmonary Fellow, Division of Pulmonary and Critical Care Medicine, Department of Medicine, State University of New York at Buffalo, Buffalo, New York

Chukwumere E. Nwogu, M.D.
Assistant Professor, Division of Cardiothoracic Surgery, State University of New York at Buffalo, Attending Thoracic Surgeon, Roswell Park Cancer Institute, Buffalo, New York

Mohammad Pourshahmir, M.D.
Chief Resident in General Surgery, State University of New York at Buffalo, Buffalo, New York

Colin J. Powers, M.D.
Resident, Department of Surgery, State University of New York at Buffalo, Buffalo, New York

John P. Pryor, M.D.
Instructor in Surgery, Division of Trauma and Surgical Critical Care, Department of Surgery, University of Pennsylvania School of Medicine, Philadelphia, Pennsylvania

Marco Ricci, M.D., Ph.D.
Resident, Division of Cardiothoracic Surgery, University of Miami College of Medicine, Jackson Memorial Hospital, Miami, Florida

John J. Ricotta, M.D., FACS
Professor and Chief, Department of Surgery, State University of New York at Stony Brook Health Sciences Center School of Medicine, Chief of Surgery, University Hospital and Medical Center, Stony Brook, New York

Eliot R. Rosenkranz, M.D.
Division of Cardiothoracic Surgery, University of Miami College of Medicine, Jackson Memorial Hospital, Miami, Florida

Paul G. Ruff IV, M.D.
Resident, Division of Plastic Surgery, University of California at San Diego, San Diego, California

Paulo R. Soltoski, M.D.
Attending Thoracic and Cardiovascular Surgeon, Hospital Santa Cruz, Curitiba, Parana, Brazil

Monica B. Spaulding, M.D.
Professor, Department of Medicine, State University of New York at Buffalo, Western New York
VA Health Care System, Buffalo, New York

Lynn M. Steinbrenner, M.D.
Associate Professor, Department of Medicine, State University of New York at Buffalo, Western
New York VA Health Care System, Buffalo, New York

Hiroshi Takita, M.D., D.Sc.
Clinical Associate Professor of Surgery, State University of New York at Buffalo, Millard
Filmore Hospital, Buffalo, New York

Burke Thompson, M.D.
Resident, Department of Surgery, State University of New York at Buffalo, Buffalo, New York

John D. Urschel, M.D., FRCSC, FACS, FRCSEd
Associate Professor, Department of Surgery, Faculty of Health Sciences, McMaster University,
Chief of Surgery, St. Joseph's Hospital, Hamilton, Ontario, Canada

Jeffrey Visco, M.D.
Resident, Department of Surgery, State University of New York at Buffalo, Buffalo, New York

Carmine M. Volpe, M.D., FACS
Assistant Professor, Division of Surgical Oncology, Department of Surgery, University of Maryland Medical Systems, Baltimore, Maryland

Kurt VonFricken, M.D.
Clinical Assistant Professor, Division of Cardiothoracic Surgery, State University of New York
at Buffalo, Buffalo, New York

Jennifer Wingate, M.D.
Chief Resident, Department of Otolaryngology, State University of New York at Buffalo,
Buffalo, New York

Sung W. Yoon, M.D.
Resident, Department of Surgery, State University of New York at Buffalo, Buffalo, New York

PREFACE

The purpose of *Thoracic Surgery Secrets* is to provide medical students, surgical and cardiothoracic residents, pulmonary specialists, and practicing surgeons an opportunity to review the field of thoracic surgery in preparation for varied examinations. The questions were written by authorities in the field and the answers provided in a succint and thorough manner. Medical students will find the breadth of topics more than appropriate for written examinations and oral questioning on the wards. Surgical and cardiothoracic residents will find this book a great source to study for their in-training examinations and both qualifying and certifying board examinations. Busy practicing surgeons will find it useful in preparing for recertification in cardiothoracic surgery.

Our goal of "taming" the complex field of thoracic surgery into questions and answers was made possible by contributions from national and international authorities as well as the hard work of Natasha Andjelkovic and William Lamsback, our editors at Hanley & Belfus. Their tireless contributions made the task of editing *Thoracic Surgery Secrets* a pleasure. As we stated in the preface to *Cardiac Surgery Secrets,* "if one of our readers becomes passionate about [cardiothoracic surgery] after reading [Thoracic Surgery Secrets], then this book will have served its purpose, and we will have served ours."

Hratch L. Karamanoukian, MD
Paulo R. Soltoski, MD
Tomas A. Salerno, MD

DEDICATION

To our medical students, residents, and fellows who have inspired us to continue teaching future generations of cardiothoracic surgeons. We are forever indebted to our families for their continued support.

Hratch L. Karamanoukian, MD
Paulo R. Soltoski, MD
Tomas A. Salerno, MD

I. Principles of General Thoracic Surgery

1. GAS EXCHANGE, PULMONARY MECHANICS, AND MECHANICAL VENTILATION

Marcio P.T. Cartacho, M.D., Marcos R. Gunther, M.D., and Paulo R. Soltoski, M.D.

1. What is the total alveolar surface area of the lungs?
Approximately 100 m^2.

2. What is the thickness of the air–blood interface?
About 0.5 μm.

3. What layers separate air from blood in the lungs?
- Alveolar epithelium (type I and II pneumocytes)
- Alveolar basement membrane
- Interstitial space
- Capillary basement membrane
- Capillary endothelium

4. What determines gas exchange in the lungs?
The solubility coefficient of the gas in any particular phase of the alveolar-capillary membrane, and the partial pressure gradient of the gas between these phases.

5. How does diffusion occur?
Diffusion is the spontaneous movement of a gas from a higher to a lower partial pressure environment. Its force is determined by the pressure gradient, the thickness of the alveolo-capillary membrane, and the properties of the gas itself.

6. Why do abnormalities of the alveolo-capillary membrane affect O$_2$ diffusion earlier than CO$_2$ diffusion?
Because while O$_2$ is nearly 14-fold more difusible, CO$_2$ is 20-fold more soluble in blood, and the combination of these variables results in CO$_2$ diffusing nearly twice as fast as O$_2$.

7. What is the oxygen-carrying capacity of hemoglobin in normal conditions?
One gram of hemoglobin (Hb) carries 1,34 ml of O$_2$.

8. Which factors determine the oxygen-carrying capacity of the blood?
- Hemoglobin level
- O$_2$ saturation of the hemoglobin
- Minimal amount of dissolved O$_2$

9. How can we quickly determine the blood O$_2$ content?

$$\text{Blood O}_2 = [\text{Hb} \times (\text{SpO}_2/100) \times 1{,}34] + [\text{PaO}_2 \times 0{,}0031]$$

The fist part of the equation refers to the oxygen bound to hemoglobin. The second part refers to the oxygen dissolved in the blood.

10. What is the O_2–Hb dissociation curve?

It represents the changes in the hemoglobin affinity for oxygen under several different conditions.

11. What is the meaning of a right shift in the O_2–Hb dissociation curve?

It indicates that there is less hemoglobin affinity for oxygen in certain conditions, such as a rise in H^+ ions, acidosis, elevation of the 2,3-DPG, high levels of CO_2, and elevated temperature. These conditions stimulate O_2 release from hemoglobin to the tissues as part of normal metabolism.

12. What is the right shift of the O_2–Hb dissociation curve due to an acidic environment called?

Bohr effect.

13. What happens to poorly ventilated areas in the lung?

Hypoxemia and, more importantly, local acidosis cause pulmonary arterial constriction, which in turn limits blood flow to poorly ventilated alveoli, optimizing gas exchange.

14. What are the three lung zones of West?

The perfusion pressure of the pulmonary arteries is relatively low, ranging from 10 to 20 mmHg. With such low pressures, the upper third of the normal adult lung in the upright position, **zone I**, is well ventilated but poorly perfused. In this case PA > Pa > Pv, where PA is the gas pressure in the alveolus, Pa is the pulmonary arterial pressure, and Pv the pulmonary venous pressure. In **zone II**, the middle third of the lung, Pa > PA > Pv, therefore blood flow occurs when the intravascular pressure exceeds the alveolar pressure, i.e., during inspiration. In **zone III**, Pa > Pv > PA, and blood flows throughout the respiratory cycle.

15. What is the most important role of the surfactant?

The reduction of the alveolar wall tension, which keeps the smallest alveoli open, maintaining lung stability.

16. What happens when there is too much surfactant?

Bronchiolar plugs may form, requiring aggressive treatment for removal of the excessive surfactant. This condition is called alveolar proteinosis.

17. What is lung compliance?

It corresponds to change in volume divided by change in pressure. It is inversely related to lung volume, decreasing at end-inspiration. Emphysema, due to its lung destruction, increases compliance, whereas pulmonary fibrosis decreases it.

18. What is the closing volume of the lungs?

It is the residual volume trapped in the alveoli secondary to closure of small airways at the end of expiration. It increases with age.

19. Can we easily measure the total amount of air contained in the lungs?

No, because we are unable to measure the residual volume of the lungs with simple spirometry. Constant-volume plethysmography can measure all gas within the thoracic cavity, but it is cumbersome and it may measure intra-abdominal gas as well.

20. What are the static lung volumes?

The total lung capacity (TLC) is the total amount of air in the lungs after a maximal inspiration. It corresponds to the vital capacity (VC) plus the residual volume (RV). The VC is further divided into inspiratory reserve volume (IRV), tidal volume (TV), and expiratory reserve volume (ERV).

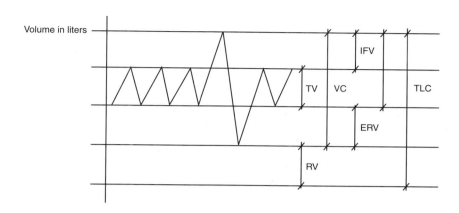

Static lung volumes. RV, residual volume; TV, tidal volume; VC, vital capacity; IRV, inspiratory reserve volume; ERV, expiratory reserve volume; TLC, total lung capacity.

21. How do changes in pH, PO_2, and PCO_2 interfere with the mechanism of breathing?

Peripheral chemoreceptors located in the aorta and carotid bodies, the latter extremely sensitive to changes in PO_2, and central chemoreceptors located in the medulla, which are sensitive to the H^+ concentrations in the CSF, determine changes in ventilation to correct hypoxia and acidosis.

22. How do central chemoreceptors work?

They respond to changes in the H^+ concentration of the cerebrospinal fluid (CSF). High levels of H^+ stimulate the work of breathing. Since neither bicarbonate nor hydrogen can cross the blood–brain barrier, CO_2 must diffuse into the CSF to correct the acidosis. This explains why the correction of metabolic acidosis takes longer than respiratory acidosis.

23. What are the respiratory centers?

Respiratory centers are groups of specialized cells located in the brain stem that are responsible for the automatic breathing: The respiratory centers are (1) **pneumotaxic center** (upper pons), which inhibits inspiration; (2) **apneustic center** (lower pons), which stimulates inspiration; and (3) **medullary centers** (medulla), two groups of cells cycling periods of inspiration and expiration.

24. What is the hypoxic ventilatory drive?

Although not very important for normal individuals, in the presence of chronically elevated PCO_2 such as found in COPD patients, the ventilatory response to PCO_2 is blunted because the metabolic alkalosis in the CSF makes the pH of the CSF much less responsive to changes in PCO_2. In these situations, the hypoxic drive over the chemoreceptors becomes extremely important, and the elevation of the PO_2 may severely depress respiration.

25. Where does most of the airway resistance occur within the respiratory tree?

In the trachea and major bronchi, where the gas flow is turbulent and the cross-sectional area is relatively small.

26. How is helium useful in airway obstructive problems?

The turbulence caused by a partial airway obstruction can be minimized by a reduction in the density of the gas flowing across the lesion, such as Heliox (80% helium and 20% oxygen), which has 1/3 of the density of air.

27. What is the respiratory quotient (RQ)?

The CO_2 production is a function of the substrate used for energy, and it is usually related to the amount of O_2 consumed. If the CO_2 production equals the O_2 consumption, normally observed with carbohydrate as a substrate, the RQ equals 1. For fat the RQ is 0.7, and for protein 0.8. The normal fasting adult has an RQ near 0.8.

28. What is the alveolar–arterial oxygen gradient [P (A–a) O_2]?

It is a useful method of assessing the gas exchange in the lung. In ideal situations the alveolar PO_2 (PAO_2) should be equal to the arterial PO_2 (PaO_2). Normal values range from 2–16 mmHg at room air to 25–65 mmHg at 100% O_2. The following factors increase the A–a gradient: diffusion defects, right-to-left shunt, and V/Q mismatch.

29. What are the indications for starting mechanical ventilation?

- Acute respiratory failure secondary to alveolar hypoventilation
- Increased respiratory work
- To provide pulmonary support while the underlying cause of respiratory failure is investigated

30. What are the basic ventilator settings?

- FiO_2: ideally 50% or less
- Tidal volume: 6–10 ml/kg in adults
- Respiratory rate: 10–12 breaths per minute in adults.
- PEEP: optional

31. When should we use positive end-expiratory pressure (PEEP) or continuous positive airway pressure (CPAP)?

If an acute parenchymal disease process reduces the resting lung volume or there is loss of negative intrathoracic pressure, use of PEEP or CPAP may improve the ventilation-perfusion (V/Q) mismatches and the mechanical characteristics of the respiratory system. This will allow a decrease in inspired O_2 concentration. PEEP and CPAP are essentially the same mode of therapy applied to mechanical ventilation and spontaneous breathing, respectively.

32. What are the two basic modes of mechanical ventilation?

Total and partial ventilatory support, each one set either by pressure- or volume-control devices.

33. Describe some of the most frequently used modes of mechanical ventilation.

Controlled mechanical ventilation (CMV)	This mode delivers a preselected ventilatory rate independent of the patient's spontaneous effort, providing complete control over respiration. This is one of the modes used during general anesthesia, and since it does not allow the patient to participate in the work of breathing, it is a poor choice for prolonged ventilation.
Assist-control ventilation (ACV)	The patient or a timing device, whichever comes first, will trigger the ventilator.
Intermittent mandatory ventilation (IMV)	It allows the patient to breathe spontaneously, adding ventilator-triggered breaths at preset intervals. No support is provided to any of the patient's own respiratory efforts. This is a frequently used ventilation mode.
Synchronized intermittent mandatory ventilation (SIMV)	A small variation of the IMV, this technique allows spontaneous breaths between mechanically delivered breaths.
Pressure support ventilation (PSV)	This mode is used to decrease the work of breathing of patients with decreased lung-thorax compliance and increased airway resistance. In the PSV mode, after selection of the airway pressure level, the patient controls all other parameters of ventilation. This is a frequently used mode of weaning.

34. Describe one scenario in which PEEP may actually worsen V/Q relationships and cause overinflation of unaffected regions of the lung.

In severe localized parenchymal disease, PEEP may actually worsen arterial blood oxygenation.

35. What is the ideal ventilatory support?

Controlled ventilation should only be used if absolutely necessary, and progression to modes that allow spontaneous breathing should be encouraged. Spontaneous breathing maintains muscle strength and coordination, but excessive workload may actually decrease muscle strength. Therefore, equilibrium of ventilatory support and spontaneous breathing appears to be ideal.

36. Name a few variables used to wean patients from mechanical ventilation.
- $PaO_2 > 60$ mmHg
- $FiO_2 < 40\%$
- A–a PO_2 gradient < 350 mmHg
- VC > 10 ml/kg
- NIF < -30 cm H_2O
- Minute ventilation < 10 L/min

37. Name four commonly used weaning techniques.
- T-piece trial
- Continuous positive airway pressure (CPAP) trial
- Intermittent mandatory ventilation (IMV) trial
- Pressure support ventilation (PSV) trial

38. Describe jet ventilation.

High-frequency ventilation is defined by frequencies higher than 60/min, ranging from 60–3,000 breaths per minute, with tidal volumes sometimes lower than the patient's anatomic dead space. There are several theories attempting to explain the adequate mixing of gas in the conductance airways, but at the level of the alveoli, diffusion is the most important mechanism.

39. Name a few clinical applications of high-frequency jet ventilation.
- Difficult airway management
- Bronchopleural fistula
- Tracheal and thoracic surgery

BIBLIOGRAPHY

1. Amdekar YK, Ugra D : Pulmonary function tests. Indian J Pediatr 63:149–152, 1996.
2. Civetta JM, Taylor RW, Kirby RR (eds): Critical Care, 3rd ed. Philadelphia, Lippincott-Raven, 1997.
3. Ferguson MK, Little L, Rizzo L, et al: Diffusing capacity predicts morbidity and mortality after pulmonary resection. J Thorac Cardiovasc Surg 96:894–900, 1988.
4. Ferguson MK, Reeder LB, Mick R: Optimizing selection of patients for major lung resection. J Thorac Cardiovasc Surg 109:275–281, 1995.
5. Kearney DJ, Lee TH, Reilly JJ, et al: Assessment of operative risk in patients undergoing lung resection. Importance of predicted pulmonary function. Chest 105:753–759, 1994.
6. O'Leary JP (ed): The Physiologic Basis of Surgery, 2nd ed. Baltimore, Williams & Wilkins, 1996.
7. Pearson FG, Deslauriers J, Ginsberg RJ, et al (eds): Thoracic Surgery. New York, Churchill-Livingstone, 1995.
8. Reilly JJ Jr: Evidence-based preoperative evaluation of candidates for thoracotomy. Chest 116(Suppl 6):474S–476S, 1999.
9. Sabiston DC, Spencer FC (eds): Surgery of the Chest, 6th ed. Philadelphia, W.B. Saunders, 1995.
10. Shoemaker WC, Ayres SM, Grenvik A, Holbrook PR (eds): Textbook of Critical Care, 3rd ed. Philadelphia, W.B. Saunders, 1995.
11. Wang J, Olak J, Ferguson MK. Diffusing capacity predicts operative mortality but not long-term survival after resection for lung cancer. J Thorac Cardiovasc Surg 117:581–586, 1999.
12. Zeiher BG, Gross TJ, Kern JA, et al: Predicting postoperative pulmonary function in patients undergoing lung resection. Chest 108:68–72, 1995.

2. ANESTHESIA AND PREOPERATIVE PULMONARY FUNCTION TESTING

Marcio P.T. Cartacho, M.D., Marcos R. Gunther, M.D., and Paulo R. Soltoski, M.D.

1. What is the most important risk factor for pulmonary complications in thoracic surgery?
Preexisting lung disease.

2. How much lung function is lost with thoracic or upper abdominal incisions?
In 1927, Churchill and McNeil observed a 75% decrease in vital capacity (VC) in the first 24 hours after a cholecystectomy. The values returned to preoperative levels after 2 weeks, clearly demonstrating the negative effects of such incisions.

3. What is the most frequently found easily treatable preoperative problem often responsible for serious morbidity and mortality in the perioperative period?
Uncontrolled and untreated preoperative hypertension.

4. What is the mortality rate associated with perioperative myocardial infarction?
From 28 to 68%.

5. What is the worst combination of hemodynamic abnormalities in patients with ischemic myocardial disease?
Tachycardia associated with hypotension, because the poor diastolic myocardial perfusion that results from tachycardia is further complicated by hypotension.

6. What defines optimal anesthetic management of patients with ischemic heart disease?
The maintenance of appropriate oxygen delivery to the increased myocardial demand during and especially after the surgical procedure. These patients must have taken all their appropriate antianginal and antihypertensive medications, and extreme care must be taken to avoid tachycardia and hypotension throughout this period. At completion of anesthesia, pain, agitation, and other physiologic imbalances may increase O_2 consumption, making the immediate postoperative period a danger zone for myocardial infarction.

7. What are the components of the preoperative pulmonary function testing?
- Spirometry
- Diffusing capacity
- Blood gas analysis
- Chronic hemoglobin level
- Activity level
- Exercise testing
- Chest x-ray

8. What is the importance of spirometry?
Spirometry is an inexpensive technique for evaluation of static lung volumes and the flow-volume curves. It is used for identification of clinically important pulmonary abnormalities.

9. Why is spirometry performed with and without bronchodilators?
Because reduced FEV values reflect obstructive airway disease. If the small airways are compromised, bronchodilators may improve such values, suggesting that appropriate treatment may improve the perioperative course.

6

10. What important data are derived from spirometry?

FVC	The forced vital capacity (FVC) is a highly reproducible parameter. If decreased, it suggests a restrictive ventilatory defect. FVC < 50% or FVC < 2 L indicates a higher risk of postoperative pulmonary complications.
FEV_1	The forced expiratory volume in one second (FEV_1) is a direct measurement of airflow obstruction. Predicted FEV_1 values lower than 0.8 L indicate very high risk.
FEV_1/FVC	This ratio is diagnostic of obstructive lung disease.
MVV	Maximal voluntary ventilation (MVV) is a nonspecific parameter, but it has a good prognostic value. Preoperative MVV lower than 50% indicates moderate risk.

11. Can spirometry be performed in children?

Yes. It is an excellent aid in the diagnosis of hyperreactive airways and asthma.

12. How can spirometry assist in the diagnoses of various types of lung and airway diseases?

If the patterns of lung volume during maximal inspiration and expiration are plotted into a graph, they generate a flow-volume curve. The inspiratory portion of the curve, at the bottom of the chart, has a symmetric round shape, whereas the expiratory curve has a triangular shape. The shape of the flow-curve loop is dependent on the elasticity of the lung, its volume, and the quality of the airways.

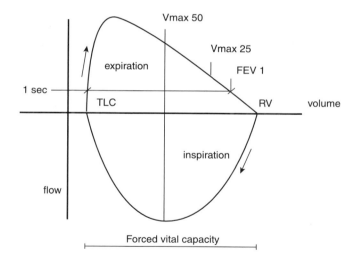

Spirometry. This curve represents the flow-volume chart observed in a normal individual. Small airway obstructive disease is best represented in the interval FEF 25% to 75% of the forced vital capacity. The FEV_1 is the residual volume of air in the lungs exhaled after one second of expiration.

13. Describe the appearance of the following diseases in a flow-volume chart: restrictive lung disease, obstructive lung disease, and upper airway obstruction.

In restrictive lung disease the FEV_1/FVC ratio is increased and VC is decreased. In obstructive lung disease FEV_1/FVC is decreased and FEV_1 is decreased. In upper airway obstruction FEV_1/FVC ratio is decreased.

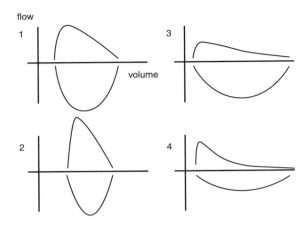

Flow-volume curves. 1, normal curve; 2, restrictive lung disease; 3, upper airway obstruction; 4, obstructive lung disease.

14. How can we evaluate a patient's diffusing capacity in our practice?

Using the carbon monoxide (CO) diffusing capacity test. The CO used as a tracer has a very strong affinity for hemoglobin, and at low concentrations it causes no harm. The diffusing capacity of CO (D_{LCO}), is defined as the volume of CO transferred into the blood per minute per mmHg of PaCO. A reduction of the diffusing capacity may be secondary to increased thickness or reduced area of the alveolo-capillary membrane. Pulmonary edema, pulmonary fibrosis, and interstitial lung disease are a few examples of increased thickness of the alveolo-capillary membrane. Surgical resection and emphysema are good examples of a decreased exchange area. Diffusing capacity may be elevated in diseases that increase the amount of circulating hemoglobin.

15. Name a few elements of pulmonary function tests used to estimate risk for lung resection.

Forced vital capacity (FVC)	< 50% predicted
Forced expiratory volume in 1 second (FEV_1)	< 2 L
FVC_1/FVC	< 50%
Maximum voluntary ventilation (MVV)	< 50% predicted
Residual volume (RV)/ total lung capacity (TLC) ratio	> 50%
$PaCO_2$	> 45 mmHg
Diffusion capacity (D_{LCO})	< 50% predicted
MVO_2	< 15 ml/kg/min

16. How accurate is the predicted FEV_1 in the risk assessment of patients undergoing lobectomy and pneumonectomy?

It is very accurate for patients undergoing lobectomy, but it usually underestimates the postoperative FEV_1 for patients undergoing pneumonectomy.

17. Which elements of the preoperative pulmonary testing battery are strong predictors of risk of complication and mortality after lung resection?

A low predicted postoperative D_{LCO} (less than 50% predicted) and a low predicted postoperative FEV_1 (less than 0.8 L).

18. If a patient is considered a poor candidate for surgery on the basis of FEV$_1$, what test could be performed to determine inoperability?

An exercise test. A predicted maximal oxygen consumption (MVO$_2$ < 10 ml/kg/min) identifies a patient at prohibitive risk for complications and death. Conversely, when the MVO$_2$ exceeds 20 ml/kg/min, most patients tolerate surgery without incidents. Another technique is the functional exclusion of the affected pulmonary arterial system with a pulmonary artery catheter. A mean Pa of 35 mmHg or higher and a PO$_2$ bellow 45 mmHg are indicators of poor outcome.

BIBLIOGRAPHY

1. Amdekar YK, Ugra D : Pulmonary function tests. Indian J Pediatr 63:149–152, 1996.
2. Civetta JM, Taylor RW, Kirby RR (eds): Critical Care, 3rd ed. Philadelphia, Lippincott-Raven, 1997.
3. Ferguson MK, Little L, Rizzo L, et al: Diffusing capacity predicts morbidity and mortality after pulmonary resection. J Thorac Cardiovasc Surg 96:894–900, 1988.
4. Ferguson MK, Reeder LB, Mick R: Optimizing selection of patients for major lung resection. J Thorac Cardiovasc Surg 109:275–281, 1995.
5. Kearney DJ, Lee TH, Reilly JJ, et al: Assessment of operative risk in patients undergoing lung resection: Importance of predicted pulmonary function. Chest 105:753–759, 1994.
6. Pearson FG, Deslauriers J, Ginsberg RJ, et al (eds): Thoracic Surgery. New York, Churchill Livingstone, 1995.
7. Sabiston DC, Spencer FC (eds): Surgery of the Chest, 6th ed. Philadelphia, W.B. Saunders, 1995.
8. Shoemaker WC, Ayres SM, Grenvik A, Holbrook PR (eds): Textbook of Critical Care, 3rd ed. Philadelphia, W.B. Saunders, 1995.
9. Reilly JJ Jr: Evidence-based preoperative evaluation of candidates for thoracotomy. Chest 116(Suppl 6):474S–476S, 1999.
10. Wang J, Olak J, Ferguson MK: Diffusing capacity predicts operative mortality but not long-term survival after resection for lung cancer. J Thorac Cardiovasc Surg 117:581–586, 1999.
11. Zeiher BG, Gross TJ, Kern JA, et al: Predicting postoperative pulmonary function in patients undergoing lung resection. Chest 108:68–72, 1995.

II. The Esophagus

3. EMBRYOLOGY AND SURGICAL ANATOMY OF THE ESOPHAGUS

Scott C. Boulanger, M.D., Ph.D., Vivian Lindfield, M.D., and Philip L. Glick, M.D.

1. When does the esophagus first appear embryologically?

The esophagus first appears at about 3–4 weeks of gestation as a ventral diverticulum, along with the trachea. This diverticulum (the respiratory or tracheobronchial diverticulum) is gradually partitioned into dorsal and ventral portions. The dorsal portion becomes the esophagus, whereas the ventral portion becomes the respiratory primordium.

2. At what point during gestation do the esophagus and trachea become completely separated?

By day 26 of gestation.

3. What are the two muscle layers of the esophagus?

The inner, circular layer and the outer, longitudinal layer.

4. Which appears first, the circular or longitudinal muscle layer of the esophagus?

The circular layer (by about 6 weeks of gestation), followed by the vagus nerves shortly thereafter.

5. When does the longitudinal muscle layer develop?

By the 9th week of gestation.

6. Is the musculature of the esophagus smooth muscle or striated?

Both. The upper third contains only striated muscle. From there on, the esophagus contains progressively more smooth muscle.

7. How does the epithelium of the esophagus develop?

The esophageal epithelium initially is a stratified columna. By week 8, the epithelium has occluded the esophagus. Vacuoles then form in the esophageal tube and start to coalesce. This eventually leads to recannulation, and at this point the epithelium is ciliated. It is subsequently replaced by squamous epithelium by the 20th week of gestation.

8. Name the two main developmental anomalies of the esophagus.

Tracheoesophageal fistula (TEF) with esophageal atresia (EA), and isolated esophageal atresia. These anomalies are related and are life-threatening.

9. Relate the most likely explanation for the formation of a TEF and EA.

TEFs probably result from an interruption of the process involved in separating the ventral diverticulum into ventral and dorsal portions. The EA is thought to be a result of the fistula in most cases. The rapid caudal development of the trachea may result in EA if there is a fistulous attachment between the two structures. The presence of the fistula may draw the esophagus forward and downward to be incorporated into the tracheal wall, resulting in EA. Isolated EA requires another explanation, perhaps a vascular accident.

10. Describe the various anatomic patterns of EA and TEF and their relative incidence.

The most common form is a proximal EA with distal TEF, present in 85–90% of all cases. EA with proximal TEF and EA with proximal and distal TEF are quite rare, each occuring in about 1% of cases.

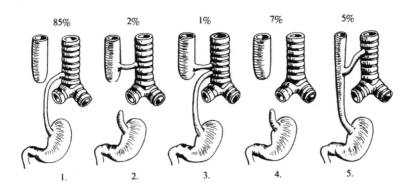

Types and relative incidence of esophageal atresia/tracheoesophageal fistula. (Modified from Myers MA, Aberdeen E: The esophagus. In Ravitch MM, Welch KJ, Benson CD, et al (eds): Pediatric Surgery, Vol. 1. Chicago, Year Book, 1979, p 450.)

11. What is the average length of the esophagus in adults?

The esophagus begins as continuation of the pharynx and ends as the cardia of the stomach. The **cervical** portion of the esophagus is approximately 5 cm long, whereas the **thoracic** and **abdominal** portions measure 20 cm and 2 cm, respectively. When measured endoscopically, the end of the esophagus is about 40 cm from the incisors in men and 37 cm from the incisors in women.

12. List the three normal areas of esophageal narrowing.

1. The entrance of the esophagus, caused by the cricopharyngeus muscle (see figure below).

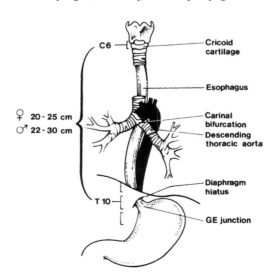

Anatomy of the esophagus. (From James EC, Schuchmann GF, Pansegrau DF: The esophagus. In James EC, Corry RJ, Perry JF Jr (eds): Basic Surgical Practice. Philadelphia, Hanley & Belfus, 1987, p 201, with permission.)

The lumen at this point is only 1.5 cm, representing the narrowest portion of the esophagus. This area is a common place for foreign bodies to lodge.

2. The middle esophagus, caused by crossing of the left main stem bronchus and the aortic arch.
3. The diaphragmatic hiatus, caused by the lower esophageal sphincter.

13. Describe the anatomic relationship of the thoracic duct to the esophagus.

In the chest, the thoracic duct lies dorsal to the esophagus and between the descending aorta on the left and the azygos vein on the right. It courses from right to left posteriorly around the upper third of the esophagus and enters the neck posterior to the left subclavian vein. Operations on the esophagus, especially after previous surgery or radiation therapy, may result in chylothorax from thoracic duct injury.

14. Describe the blood supply to the different portions of the esophagus.

* The cervical esophagus is supplied by the inferior thyroid artery.
* The thoracic esophagus is supplied by the bronchial arteries. About 75% of individuals have one right-sided branch and two left-sided branches; these branches arise directly from the aorta. There are several esophageal arteries that also come directly from the aorta.
* The abdominal esophagus is supplied by the left gastric and inferior phrenic arteries.

15. Why is devascularization of the esophagus during mobilization not as concerning as originally thought?

Although blood supply to the esophagus is segmental, on entering the wall of the esophagus, arteries assume a t-shaped form and course longitudinally in the submucosal and muscular layers. This intramural plexus provides a more extensively overlapping vascular network than was originally thought. The cervical vessels alone are capable of supplying most of the esophagus. Anastomotic failures are rarely the result of poor blood supply.

16. What is the relationship of the vagus nerve to the esophagus?

The vagus nerve lies on either side of the esophagus, forming a plexus. A little above the hiatus, the plexi coalesce into two trunks: the right posterior and the left anterior.

17. Which layer does the esophagus lack?

The esophagus has no serosa.

18. Why is the lack of a serosal layer of surgical importance?

The serosal layer in the GI tract contributes considerable strength. The lack of a serosal layer in the esophagus may contribute to the decreased rate of healing after injury compared with other regions of the GI tract. It also may be responsible for the increased rate of anastomotic leakage after esophageal resection or repair.

19. What is Belsey's artery?

A communicating artery between the left gastric and inferior phrenic arteries. It is variably present.

20. Describe the venous drainage of various portions of the esophagus.

The cervical esophagus drains through the brachiocephalic vein via the inferior thyroidal vein. Venous drainage of the thoracic esophagus is primarily through the azygos vein and, to a lesser extent, through the hemiazygos and intercostal veins. The abdominal portion drains via the left gastric vein.

21. What is the Z line?

The point in the esophagus where the stratified epithelium becomes columnar epithelium. It generally lies approximately 1–2 cm above the gastroesophageal junction.

22. What is its clinical significance of the Z line?

A Z line higher than 3 cm represents abnormal extension of the columnar epithelium (i.e., Barrett's esophagus). Barrett's esophagus is considered to be a dysplastic change of the normal epithelium and is premalignant.

23. The phrenoesophageal membrane is a continuation of which structure?

The **transversalis fascia.** Integrity of the phrenoesophageal membrane may be important for the prevention of gastric reflux.

24. What about the anatomy of esophageal lymphatics explains why it is difficult to obtain free margins when resecting esophageal carcinomas?

Lymphatic drainage of the esophagus is extremely rich. The lymphatics form a **submucosal plexus** that allows lymph to flow longitudinally for long distances. Tumor cells may take advantage of this to disperse widely.

25. Describe the innervation of the esophagus.

The esophagus receives sympathetic and parasympathetic innervation. The cervical esophagus receives innervation from branches of the superior laryngeal nerve as well as the recurrent laryngeal nerve. The recurrent laryngeal nerve supplies motor innervation to the upper esophageal sphincter and injury to this nerve may cause aspiration as well as hoarseness. The body and distal esophagus are innervated by the vagus nerve, which has extensive cross-links between the right and left side. As the right vagus nerve crosses over the right subclavian artery, it gives off the recurrent laryngeal nerve, which innervates the upper esophagus. The left vagus nerve continues down the side of the esophagus until the aortic arch, where the left recurrent nerve branches off. Vagal innervation controls motor and secretory function. The esophagus also receives sympathetic innervation from mediastinal branches of the thoracic sympathetic chain as well as recurrent branches of the celiac plexus.

26. What is the intrinsic innervation of the esophagus?

Branches of the parasympathetic, sympathetic, and paraesophageal nerves enter the wall of the esophagus and form ganglia. The two major ganglia are the **myenteric (Auerbach's) plexus,** located between the longitudinal and circular muscle layers, and the **submucosal (Meissner's) plexus,** located in the submucosal layers.

27. What is the function of the intrinsic innervation of the esophagus?

The myenteric plexus controls muscle contraction or peristalsis, whereas the submucosal plexus controls secretory function.

28. Describe the connective tissue surrounding the esophagus.

The esophagus and trachea are embedded in an envelope of connective tissue that consists of the pretracheal (previsceral) fascia anteriorly and the prevertebral (retrovisceral) fascia posteriorly. Both fasciae fuse in the upper chest to form the carotid sheath. The trachea, pleura, and retrovisceral fascia are connected to the esophagus via fine tissue strands composed of elastin and/or collagen fibers.

29. Why is the position of the esophagus within a well-defined fascial compartment clinically important?

Infection may spread from anterior lesions of the esophagus and follow the pretracheal space down to the pericardium. More important is the retrovisceral space. Most iatrogenic perforations of the esophagus are contained because they generally occur in the posterior hypopharynx above the upper esophageal sphincter. Below this, where most noniatrogenic or spontaneous perforations occur, there is no barrier to the spread of infection to the mediastinum. This may result in disastrous dissemination of sepsis.

BIBLIOGRAPHY

1. Liebermann-Meffert D: Anatomy, embryology and histology. In Pearson FG, et al (eds): Esophageal Surgery. New York, Churchill-Livingstone, 1995.
2. Pelligrini CA, Way LW: Esophagus and diaphragm. In Way LW (ed): Current Surgical Diagnosis and Treatment, 10th ed. Stamford, CT, Appleton & Lange, 1994.
3. Peters JH, DeMeester TR: Esophagus and diaphragmatic hernia. In Schwartz SI, Shires GT, Spencer FC, et al (eds): Principles of Surgery. New York, McGraw-Hill, 1994.
4. Sadler TW (ed): Langman's Medical Embryology, 6th ed. Baltimore, Williams & Wilkins, 1990.
5. Skinner DB, Belsey RHR: Management of Esophageal Disease. Philadelphia, W.B. Saunders, 1988.

4. ESOPHAGEAL IMAGING AND ENDOSCOPY

Vivian Lindfield, M.D., and Hratch L. Karamanoukian, M.D.

1. How are the many different tests available for studying the esophagus categorized?

Noninvasive (Radiographic)
Provide:
  Anatomic information
  Qualitative information

Invasive
Provide:
  Functional information
  Quantitative information

2. What type of tests are usually the first obtained in patients with esophageal complaints?
Radiographic.

3. List some advantages to radiographic tests.
- They are noninvasive.
- They can be performed easily in an ambulatory setting.
- They usually are inexpensive in comparison to more invasive tests.
- They are widely available at most facilities with little variation in interpretation of results.

4. List some of the more commonly used radiographic studies available today for patients with esophageal complaints.
- **Barium esophagram** or **barium swallow** (most common).
- Cinematographic esophagram, which is a videotaped contrast study.
- Nuclear esophageal and gastric emptying studies.

5. How is the barium esophagram different from an upper GI series?
The **upper GI series** focuses mainly on the stomach and the proximal small bowel, whereas the **barium swallow (esophagram)** focuses mostly on the esophagus and the proximal stomach.

6. For what type of disorders should an esophagram be performed?
- This is the test of choice for evaluating symptoms of chest pain of a noncardiac origin and symptoms of dysphagia.
- It is used to evaluate the anatomy of the esophagus and should be done before surgical intervention is attempted in this region for any cause.
- It is sensitive in detecting structural changes, such as luminal dilation, webs, strictures, rings, masses, fistulae, and diverticula.

7. How is a barium esophagram performed?
The standard examination consists of three different techniques, which provide a comprehensive look at the esophageal anatomy: a full column view, a mucosal relief maneuver, and an air/contrast interface.

For the **full column view,** the patient drinks about 250 mL of barium solution. Images of the full column are obtained. The esophagus should be dilated fully with barium for these images. Any constricting lesions or masses in the lumen can be identified easily at this time. The gastroesophageal junction also is examined to rule out any gastric pathology that may be present. The images are obtained with the patient in the upright position, which is good for revealing obstructions, and the supine position, which is better for revealing motor dysfunction.

Mucosal relief images are taken once the contrast material passes completely into the stomach, while the walls of the esophagus are collapsing to their normal shape. The walls still are coated with a thin layer of contrast material. Any mucosal defects, such as ulcers, inflammation, varices, and Barrett's esophagus, may be detected at this time.

Air/contrast interface images are obtained to detect more subtle changes that may occur in the mucosa. Gas-producing granules are added to the barium and ingested. This creates an interface of air and contrast material. If there are subtle areas of narrowing or changes noted and the patient has esophageal complaints, especially for dysphagia, a radiopaque food bolus is ingested by the patient. Serial spot films are obtained and can be used to follow the course of the food through the esophagus. Any areas that produce the same symptoms that the patient experiences can be detected.

8. Is the esophagram a good tool for investigating motor disorders of the esophagus?

It is a sensitive tool for identifying disorders such as achalasia and diffuse esophageal spasm. It is not good for examining nonspecific motor dysfunction disorders, such as scleroderma or nutcracker esophagus. Other tests must be used in combination to identify these disorders with accuracy.

9. What are some of the limitations of the barium esophagram?

- It has limited usefulness in detecting Barrett's disease or esophagitis.
- It can detect reflux in only approximately 40% of patients with complaints of gastroesophageal reflux disease (GERD).
- Although the esophagram should be the first test used in a patient suspected of having carcinoma, it is limited in its ability to detect early-stage tumors.

10. What is a cinematographic esophagram?

A videotaped contrast study. This is a dynamic study and differs from a standard barium swallow in that smaller boluses of contrast material are swallowed in repetition. The examination is videotaped, and intermittent static films are taken.

11. For what disorder is a cinematographic esophagram most commonly used?

Dysphagia, especially in patients who present with atypical symptoms or who have had a previously negative barium swallow. During the study, the examiner looks at the ease of flow of contrast from the oral cavity to the stomach. Areas of slowing are noted. Aspiration of contents is identified easily. Coordination of movements as the contrast material is transferred from the oral cavity to the pharynx, past the epiglottis, and through the upper esophageal sphincter is examined.

12. What are the advantages of cinematographic esophagram over the barium swallow?

- It allows for review of the videotape in slow motion. This allows examination of events that may occur too quickly in real time to be seen on a standard esophagram.
- It is one of the only good studies for looking at the oropharynx because manometry is difficult to assess in this region. Motility disorders, which may not be identified with a standard esophagram, may be identified without the need for manometry.
- It allows different swallowing maneuvers to be attempted and videotaped throughout the study to optimize passage of contents through the esophagus. This can then be reviewed later with the tape at different speeds for a more accurate examination.

13. List some disadvantages of cinematographic esophagram.

- Low sensitivity for detecting mucosal abnormalities.
- High cost compared with a barium swallow. (The cost can be justified because the need for manometry may be decreased.)
- Interpretation dependent on experience of radiologist.
- Limited availability.

14. When is it necessary to use a nuclear scintigraphic study?

When qualitative and quantitative information is needed for the esophagus and the stomach. When barium swallow and manometry have failed to provide a definite abnormality, these tests can be used. The lower esophageal sphincter can be assessed easily with nuclear studies. Similar to the other tests, different maneuvers are used to promote passage of contents from the esophagus into the stomach. Observations of peristalsis, dynamics, and function of the lower esophageal sphincter are considered qualitative. Calculations are made based on objective measurements of transit time and are classified as slow or rapid.

15. List disorders for which nuclear scintigraphic studies are appropriate.
- Motility disorders, such as achalasia
- Diffuse esophageal spasm
- GERD

16. What are some disadvantages of nuclear scintigraphic studies?
- Limited availability
- High cost compared with other tests

17. What is the purpose of esophageal manometry?
It is a relatively easy, short outpatient-based test used to assess the function of the sphincters at rest and during swallowing. It also provides information about the function of the esophageal body. Upper and lower sphincters can be assessed accurately.

18. When is esophageal manometry used?
- It is the definitive test for diagnosing achalasia, diffuse esophageal spasm, hypertensive lower esophageal sphincter, and nutcracker esophagus.
- It is used for patients with GERD who must undergo surgery to determine if an antireflux procedure needs to be performed.
- It can be used safely to evaluate chest pain that is thought to be noncardiac in nature.
- It can be used to help clarify symptoms of nonobstructive dysphagia when other tests have failed.

19. How is manometry performed?
This test is usually 2–3 hours long. Several devices are available; water-perfused catheters with an external pressure transducer are currently the most popular system in use. The catheter is advanced into the stomach. Pressures are measured as the catheter is pulled back up the esophagus. Propagation of contractions usually is in an orderly fashion from proximal to distal esophagus. Having the patient swallow a wet bolus can assess motility of the esophagus. Propagation of contractions is characterized as simultaneous, retrograde, or nonconducted.

20. How are the lower esophageal sphincter and upper esophageal sphincter assessed?
Three components of the **lower esophageal sphincter** are examined: (1) the overall length of the sphincter, (2) the resting pressures of the sphincters, and (3) the abdominal length of the sphincters. The values for each of the three components normally are 2 cm for overall length, 6 mmHg of pressure at rest, and an intraabdominal length of 1 cm.

The **upper esophageal sphincter** and pharyngeal area are more difficult to assess. They are last to be seen as the catheter is removed from the esophagus. Quick pressure changes occur in this region, making it difficult to evaluate. There are no real standardized values available for comparison in this region.

21. List the disadvantages of manometry.
- It is not as good as cine esophagram for evaluating the oropharynx.
- It is not reliable for providing information about sphincter relaxation, progression of food through the esophagus, and pharyngoesophageal emptying.
- It is not a good choice for evaluating GERD.
- The relationship between symptoms and motility disorders may not be documented easily with this study.

22. What is one advantage of manometry?

The cost is reasonable compared with other tests available.

23. Patients rarely have symptoms at the time of their tests. Also, tests may identify disorders in a completely asymptomatic patient. What can be done in an effort to establish a true cause in either case?

When test results do not provide an answer, **provocative tests** are available. These were developed to reproduce the symptoms that the patient may usually experience. Currently the drug of choice to induce symptoms is **edrophonium (Tensilon)**. This drug is safe and has few side effects. Edrophonium produces prolonged esophageal contractions, allowing for reliable tests. The endpoint of this test is chest pain with a wet swallow. Edrophonium and a placebo are administered consecutively followed by water swallows over a 5-minute period. If the presenting symptom results within 5 minutes, the test is considered positive.

Another provocative test is the **acid perfusion** test. A catheter is inserted into the esophagus. Hydrochloric acid and saline are alternatively injected into the esophagus. When the patient's symptoms are reproduced with acid and decreased with saline, the test is considered positive.

Both of these tests are easy to perform and have relatively low cost. A subjective perception of pain is the end result, however, which may vary from test to test or patient to patient. Placebo trials are necessary.

24. List the side effects of edrophonium.
- Nausea
- Dizziness
- Abdominal cramps

25. The diagnosis of GERD can be difficult to establish, and none of the tests mentioned previously are adequate for establishing this diagnosis. pH probe monitoring has become the most useful test for evaluating GERD. What are the indications for using this study?

1. In patients who have normal endoscopy but present with atypical symptoms or in patients with esophageal spasm symptoms
2. In patients who do not respond to medical therapy but present with typical symptoms
3. In patients to follow up the treatment of GERD with medical therapy
4. In all patients who may need surgery

Although no "gold standard" exists for the diagnosis of GERD, the pH probe monitoring sensitivity and specificity is 95% and 85%, respectively.

26. What are the sensitivity and specificity of pH probe monitoring for diagnosis of GERD?
- Sensitivity, 95%
- Specificity, 85%

27. Describe how pH probe monitoring is performed.

This is an ambulatory test performed over a 24-hour period. The probe is placed at the lower esophageal sphincter, which is determined with manometry. The patient carries a portable data recorder throughout the test. The patient is asked to perform normal daily activities. Alcohol, tobacco, and strenuous activity are to be avoided during the test. A journal is kept documenting symptoms of pain or reflux. Sleep and meal times are recorded. All of these data are then analyzed, calculated, and plotted on charts.

28. What are some of the advantages and disadvantages of pH probe monitoring?
- **Advantages** include low cost and ability to provide results that can exclude or confirm the diagnosis of GERD. Because the patient continues with normal activities, the results should provide a more accurate diagnosis of any symptoms.

- **Disadvantages** are that this is the longest test to perform, and day-to-day variations occur in acid reflux disease, which can affect the test results. If the probe is not positioned properly, inaccurate data and results can occur.

29. Discuss the uses of upper endoscopy.
- It is good for examining the whole esophagus by direct visualization.
- Several pathologic processes can be identified easily, including **strictures, tumors, ulcers, esophagitis,** and **diverticula.**
- It is the most sensitive test for detecting mucosal defects, especially **esophagitis** and **Barrett's disease.**
- **Brushings** and **biopsy specimens** can be obtained for cytology with relative ease.
- It can be used for **therapeutic measures,** such as dilation of obstructive lesions or strictures, placement of stents, and injection of medications (i.e., botulinum toxin for achalasia).

30. What are the advantages and disadvantages of upper endoscopy?
Advantages
- Available at most centers
- Cost comparable to several other tests

Disadvantages
- Motility disorder difficult to identify
- Low risk of esophageal perforation

BIBLIOGRAPHY

1. Fennessy JJ, Jokich PM: Radiologic investigation: Scanning techniques. In Skinner DB, Belsey RHR (eds): Management of Esophageal Disease. Philadelphia, W.B. Saunders, 1988, pp 40–47.
2. Miller LS: Endoscopy of the esophagus. In Castell DO (ed): The Esophagus. Boston, Little, Brown, 1992, pp 89–93.
3. Ott DJ: Radiology of the oropharynx and esophagus. In Castell DO (ed): The Esophagus. Boston, Little, Brown, 1992, pp 41–88.
4. Yang SC: Esophageal function tests. In Cameron JL (ed): Current Surgical Therapy, 5th ed. St. Louis, Mosby, 1995, pp 1–8.

5. ESOPHAGEAL MANOMETRY

George Golightly, M.D.

1. What is esophageal manometry?

An invasive method used to measure the amplitude, organization, and rate of progression of esophageal contraction. It allows for identification of the upper and lower esophageal sphincters (UES, LES) and can identify abnormalities in esophageal function.

2. Describe the types of esophageal manometry available.

Stationary manometers use a five-channel water-perfused catheter system to evaluate esophageal function. **Ambulatory manometers** use three microelectrodes and a data storage system to evaluate esophageal function over a 24-hour period.

3. List the indications for use of esophageal manometry.

- To evaluate patients with dysphagia that is not clearly defined by contrast studies or endoscopy
- To evaluate esophageal motility before antireflux procedures
- To evaluate noncardiac chest pain (used selectively)

4. List the functional zones of the esophagus.

The esophagus has three functional zones. The upper esophageal sphincter (UES) (cricopharyngeus muscle), the esophageal body, and the lower esophageal sphincter (LES).

5. How is stationary manometry performed?

A multichannel probe is placed through the nares and passed into the esophagus. Water is perfused through the channel of the catheter at low rates (0.6 mL/min), and pressure changes are recorded. The LES is defined using the pull-through technique. The lower orifice is positioned at the LES, and the remaining channels are located at the UES and throughout the esophageal body. The responses of the UES, LES, and esophageal body to wet and dry swallows are recorded.

6. What is the LES?

The high-pressure zone that separates the esophagus from the stomach. The LES is 3–5 cm long and has a resting pressure of 10–20 mm Hg. The LES is located at the diaphragmatic hiatus. The distal segment of the LES is located within the abdomen and is subject to pressure changes with respiration. The LES relaxes as the pressure wave pushes a bolus of food down the esophagus and into the stomach. There is no absolute length or pressure of the LES that defines incompetence; however, a resting pressure of <6 mm Hg and a length <2.0 cm are more likely to be associated with incompetence of the LES.

7. What is the function of the LES?

To prevent reflex of stomach contents into the esophagus.

8. Describe normal esophageal manometric findings.

Normal stationary esophageal manometric findings consist of UES relaxation in response to pharyngeal swallowing, followed by aboral contraction of the esophageal body. The pressure generated by this organized esophageal contraction increases from 25 to 35 mm Hg as it travels toward the stomach. The LES relaxes as the contractile wave moves the food bolus from the esophagus into the stomach.

9. Describe the esophageal manometric findings associated with achalasia.

Achalasia is characterized by failure of the LES to relax. There is poor contraction with poor peristalsis of the esophageal body. Resting LES pressure is elevated (>35 mm Hg). The LES may exhibit spontaneous pressure variations.

10. List the manometric characteristics of diffuse esophageal spasm.

- Esophageal body contractions that are multifocal and of elevated pressure
- Contractions that do not result in peristalsis
- Contractions that may be multiple in response to a single swallow or occur spontaneously
- Contractions with multiple peaks
- Intermittent episodes of normal peristalsis

11. What are the manometric findings in nutcracker esophagus?

A greatly elevated contractile force, prolonged contraction time, and normal peristaltic pattern. Peak pressure can reach 400 mm Hg. Pain is typically associated with these high-amplitude contractions.

12. What are the manometric findings in LES hypertension?

An increased resting pressure of the LES (>26 mm Hg). The remainder of the esophagus functions normally, and the LES relaxes in response to bolus propulsion.

13. List the manometric findings in nonspecific esophageal motility disorder.

- Failure of peristalsis
- Weak, disorganized esophageal body contractions
- Contractions in the distal esophagus
- Normal resting pressure and relaxation pattern of LES

14. What information is gained from ambulatory esophageal manometry?

A 24-hour picture of esophageal function is provided, with information about esophageal function during eating, sleeping, and other daily activities. Information is recorded in response to >1,000 swallowing episodes. Ambulatory manometry can be combined with 24-hour pH monitoring to provide information regarding reflux.

15. How is information provided by esophageal manometry processed and used?

The information recorded is gathered by a data storage device and downloaded onto a computer. Analysis is carried out by computer algorithm that recognizes wave-form patterns. Events that occur during the monitoring session can be logged and compared with normal esophageal activity.

16. What is the normal esophageal activity over a circadian cycle?

- Esophageal activity is greatest during meals.
- Awake activity is greater than sleeping activity.
- Contractile forces are highest during meals to provide bolus propulsion down the esophagus.

BIBLIOGRAPHY

1. Bremner RM, Costantini M, et al: Normal esophageal body function: A study using ambulatory esophageal manometry. Am J Gastroenterol 93:183–187, 1998.
2. Dent J, Holloway RH: Esophageal motility and reflux testing. Gastroenterol Clin North Am 25:51–73, 1996.
3. Ergun GA, Kahrilas PJ: Clinical applications of esophageal manometry and pH monitoring. Am J Gastroenterol 91:1077–1089, 1996.

4. Fuller L, Huprich JE, et al: Abnormal esophageal body function: Radiographic-manometric correlation. Am Surgeon 65:911–914, 1999.
5. Marco PG, Lawrence WW: Evaluation and treatment of primary esophageal motility disorders. West J Med 166:263–269, 1997.
6. Orringer MB: Disorders of esophageal motility. In Sabiston (ed): Textbook of Surgery, 15th ed. Philadelphia, W.B. Saunders, 1997, pp 712–728.
7. Peters J, Demeester T: Esophagus and diaphragmatic hernia. In Schwartz (ed): Principles of Surgery, 7th ed. New York, McGraw Hill, 1999, pp 1081–1179.
8. Stein HJ: Clinical use of ambulatory 24-hour esophageal motility monitoring in patients with primary esophageal motor disorders. Dysphagia 8:105–111, 1993.

6. ESOPHAGEAL MOTILITY DISORDERS

Harry W. Donias, M.D., and Hratch L. Karamanoukian, M.D.

1. List the primary motor disorders of the esophagus.
- Achalasia
- Diffuse esophageal spasm
- Hyperperistalsis (nutcracker or supersqueeze esophagus)
- Hypertensive lower esophageal sphincter (LES)
- Nonspecific esophageal motility disorders

2. List systemic diseases that may result in secondary motility disorders of the esophagus.
- Collagen vascular disease
  - Scleroderma
  - Mixed connective tissue disease
  - Dermatomyositis
  - Polymyositis
- Chagas' disease
- Diabetes mellitus
- Idiopathic intestinal pseudo-obstruction
- Neuromuscular disorders
  - Cerebrovascular disease
  - Demyelinating disorders
  - Chorea-related disorders
  - Myasthenia gravis
  - Muscular dystrophies
- Alcoholism

3. Who should undergo esophageal motility studies?
Patients with a normal endoscopy who have consistent occurrence of dysphagia with ingestion of solids, especially if this has developed over the preceding few months, if there is associated weight loss, or if dysphagia is causing significant impairment of lifestyle. Another indication is in patients with noncardiac chest pain after coronary artery disease is ruled out by the appropriate tests. In such patients, achalasia and other esophageal motility disorders are major diagnostic possibilities.

4. Define the three types of contractions that are recorded in the esophagus by manometry.
1. **Primary peristalsis**—normal propulsive waves in response to the stimulation of normal voluntary deglutition.
2. **Secondary peristalsis**—normal waves occurring without voluntary deglutition. When distended or irritated, this type of wave appears at the point of distention in an attempt to empty the esophagus of its content.
3. **Tertiary peristalsis**—usually abnormal if they occur after deglutition. Waves may appear spontaneously between swallowing. Numerous stimulating factors are known to influence this spontaneous activity.

5. Discuss the classic symptoms of achalasia.
Dysphagia to solids and liquids is a major symptom of achalasia. The pattern of dysphagia, especially in patients with a dilated esophagus, is unique. Patients often augment food passage by drinking large amounts while eating or applying maneuvers such as straightening the back, raising the arms over the head, standing, or jumping. Weight loss can be seen in about half of these patients. The average duration of dysphagia before the patient seeks medical attention is 2 years. 60–90% experience regurgitation, and one third to one half complain of chest pain. Long-term esophageal food retention leads to a progressive esophageal dilation, in which setting regurgitation, especially nocturnal regurgitation, becomes a prominent symptom. Pulmonary symptoms may be prominent and may be the initial complaints, with wheezing, coughing, and choking frequently awakening the patient because of nocturnal aspiration of regurgitated liquid material from the dilated obstructed esophagus.

6. What are the characteristic radiologic findings of achalasia?

The diagnosis is often apparent on routine chest radiograph. Characteristic findings during a barium swallow show aperistalsis, esophageal dilation, and minimal LES opening. A bird's-beak deformity in the distal esophagus with more proximal esophageal dilation is characteristic and found in 90% of patients with achalasia. A fluid level in the upper part of the esophagus resulting from the retention of esophageal secretion and ingested material may be seen. Depending on the severity and duration of achalasia, the esophagus often shows marked dilation with a tortuous course (**sigmoid-shaped esophagus**).

7. What is pseudoachalasia?

Achalasia signs and symptoms caused by malignancy. It is most often due to adenocarcinoma of the gastric cardia but has been described in lymphoma as well as metastatic pancreatic, lung, liver, and prostate malignancies. Clinical clues, such as age > 55, duration of dysphagia < 1 year, and weight loss > 15 lb, may suggest a secondary cause. If clinical suspicion is high, CT scan and endoscopic ultrasound should be considered. Pseudoachalasia accounts for 5% of cases and can mimic completely the clinical and manometric presentation of achalasia. Malignant tumors produce an achalasia syndrome by infiltrating the gastroesophageal junction (GEJ) and creating a relative obstruction with secondary esophageal dilation. This potential risk mandates endoscopy as part of the diagnostic evaluation of achalasia.

8. Describe the manometric findings of achalasia.

The esophageal body reveals contraction abnormalities over its entire length, which are diagnostic. These include:

1. Absence of peristalsis in the body of the esophagus with all of the contractions seen in response to voluntary swallowing being nonpropulsive. They show the classic mirrorlike activity at all recording levels.

2. Elevated resting intraesophageal pressure that remains constantly elevated with regard to atmospheric and intragastric pressures.

3. Normal or hypertensive LES resting pressure.

4. Incomplete or absent relaxation of the LES with swallowing.

Cholinergic medications create an exaggerated motor response. Bethanechol chloride progressively increases resting pressure as well as strength and duration of contraction. This frequently results in chest pain and regurgitation, but these symptoms are abolished by the administration of atropine.

9. What is vigorous achalasia?

A variant of achalasia that has many features of achalasia but lacks the severe esophageal dilation typical of achalasia. These patients may have chest pain and dysphagia with radiographic changes of esophageal spasm. Manometry reveals high-amplitude and repetitive contractions.

10. What is the most effective nonsurgical treatment of achalasia?

Pneumatic dilation (PD) is reported to improve about 70% of patients who undergo this form of treatment. The dilator is placed fluoroscopically so that the balloon is centered on the GEJ. To achieve long-term benefit, dilation to a diameter of at least 3 cm must be performed. The main complication of dilation is perforation, which occurs in approximately 4% of patients. Presence of a hiatal hernia or epiphrenic diverticulum increases perforation risk and is considered a relative contraindication. Although some advocate medical management with bowel rest and broad-spectrum antibiotics for perforation, the element of functional obstruction that remains at the LES may lead to worsening mediastinitis. When these perforations are repaired immediately with the addition of a myotomy, long-term results are comparable to myotomy alone. Gastroesophageal reflux as a complication of dilation has been reported in 2–17% of patients.

11. Which patients tend to have a poor response to PD?

Patients who have not had success with dilation are unlikely to respond to a second attempt (<20%). Other predictors of a poor response are age <40 years and duration of symptoms < 5 years.

12. For which patients is surgical myotomy for achalasia appropriate?

1. **Patients in whom surgical therapy is recommended primarily because of their young age.** The results of PD are largely age-dependent. In patients <40 years old, PD is < 50% effective with the first treatment and < 70% effective ultimately. The incidence of esophageal perforation is 2–7%. Myotomy is approximately 90% successful and free of morbidity and mortality. In this setting, myotomy should be recommended as primary therapy. The same is true for childhood achalasia.

2. Patients **with recurrent symptoms after botulinum toxin (BoTx) injection or PD therapy.** Several studies comparing surgery and PD show a higher rate of recurrent dysphagia after PD. The long-term failure rate is not known, but in the short-term it appears that 15–35% of patients undergoing PD ultimately require a Heller myotomy.

3. **Patients in whom PD is thought to be excessively risky.** These include those with a tortuous distal esophagus, esophageal diverticula, or previous surgery of the GEJ (either a previous incomplete myotomy or an improperly constructed Nissen fundoplication). Although some of these patients may be temporarily treated with BoTx injections, the difficult endoscopic access to the GEJ may make precise injection of the LES with BoTx difficult.

4. **Patients who choose myotomy over PD.** Patients may choose myotomy because of its better long-term results with a single treatment or because of the lower perforation rate associated with controlled division of the LES than with forceful disruption with a pneumatic dilator.

13. How does BoTx serve as a treatment of achalasia?

BoTx has been proposed as an alternative nonsurgical treatment for patients with achalasia. BoTx, a potent inhibitor of acetylcholine release from nerve endings, counterbalances the selective loss of inhibitor neurons in the myenteric plexus, resulting in unopposed excitation of the esophageal smooth muscle by acetylcholine. It is injected directly into the LES by a sclerotreatment needle during upper endoscopy. In the short-term, results have been as good as that with PD. The effect of BoTx is eventually reversed by sprouting terminal axons that form new synapses, and its efficacy at 12 months drops to 18–36%. BoTx needs to be repeated annually, and at each visit there is a one third failure rate. Although the immediate complications of BoTx are few, the disruption with sacrifice of the submucosal plane makes myotomy difficult. For these reasons, BoTx should be reserved for patients in whom PD and surgical myotomy are contraindicated.

14. How does PD compare with surgery for achalasia?

A prospective, randomized control study of 39 patients treated with PD and 42 patients treated with myotomy found similar responses initially, but good-to-excellent responses 5 years after therapy were sustained in 95% of surgical patients versus 65% of patients managed with PD.

15. Describe the surgical treatment of achalasia.

The **esophageal myotomy** has been the gold standard for treatment of achalasia since it was first described by Heller in 1914. A short 5–7-cm myotomy is completed on the distal esophagus. It extends on the gastric wall for a distance of 1 cm. After the longitudinal and circular muscle layers are divided, the difference in the vascular supply of the mucosa is observed at the junction between the esophageal and gastric linings. The mucosa is dissected free from the muscularis over 50% of the esophageal circumference, allowing its protrusion between the cut muscle margins.

16. List the different approaches used for esophageal myotomy.

- Left thoracotomy
- Laparotomy
- Laparoscopic technique
- Thoracoscopic technique
- Video-assisted technique*

*Video assisted techniques have been shown to be as safe and as effective as conventional myotomy by laparotomy or thoracoscopy with little morbidity, shorter hospital stay, and quicker return to daily activities.

17. Currently, what is the preferred approach to esophageal myotomy for achalasia?

Laparoscopic myotomy with the addition of a partial fundoplication. Although the thoracoscopic and laparoscopic without antireflux procedures have shown good long-term symptomatic improvement, a high proportion of these patients have myotomy-induced reflux on postoperative pH testing. Although these patients are largely asymptomatic, the addition of an antireflux procedure to the myotomy simultaneously eliminates the symptoms of achalasia and avoids reflux. It is believed that better exposure of the GEJ with the ability to carry the myotomy to the stomach is afforded with the laparoscopic technique, decreasing the incidence of inadequate myotomy.

18. Which patient populations are best served by a thoracoscopic myotomy?

- Patients with insurmountable abdominal adhesions precluding a laparoscopic approach.
- Patients with diffuse esophageal spasm who do not need complete division of the LES but who require further exposure of the intrathoracic esophagus.

19. What type of fundoplication should accompany a myotomy for achalasia?

The two most popular fundoplications performed in conjunction with myotomy are the **Dor anterior 180° fundoplication** and the **Toupet posterior 180° fundoplication.** For the very dilated esophagus, a posterior fundoplication may increase outflow obstruction by excessively angling the esophagus anteriorly. An anterior (Dor) fundoplication that does not alter the geometry of the GEJ is recommended. A posterior (Toupet) fundoplication is performed on patients with mild-to-moderate esophageal dilation, especially young patients. This fundoplication has the advantages of holding the cut edges to the muscularis open and is probably a better antireflux procedure for long-term control of GER after sphincter division. A fundoplication that is excessively competent and may not allow the GEJ to open freely, such as the Nissen fundoplication, should not be performed after myotomy. Such a valve may increase outflow obstruction of the esophagus to the point that dysphagia is inadequately relieved.

20. Describe the early complications seen after esophageal myotomy.

Subphrenic and mediastinal abscesses may represent leaks that sealed before they could be detected. Mucosal perforation occurring during the procedure is well described; however, simple mucosal repair with fine interrupted sutures has proved extremely successful in preventing postoperative leakage. The most common early complication is pneumonia, which occurs in 2–3% of patients, and may be a complication of thoracotomy, laparotomy, general anesthesia, or perioperative aspiration of esophageal contents.

21. What are the late complications associated with esophageal myotomy?

Persistence of dysphagia and gastroesophageal reflux symptoms. Persistence or relapse of dysphagia is generally due to an incomplete myotomy area or to the inefficiency of myotomy in a decompensated sigmoid esophagus. Reflux disease is the most feared long-term complication, with the potential to evolve from reflux esophagitis to Barrett's esophagitis with dysplasia and adenocarcinoma. Many antireflux repairs have been suggested at the time of myotomy to prevent this complication. Adding an antireflux operation at the end of an atonic esophagus may lead to emptying problems as seen with total fundoplication. A partial fundoplication offers satisfactory control of reflux symptoms without causing undue emptying problems. It has been shown that 25% of patients treated with PD or esophageal myotomy have abnormal pH profiles after sphincter disruption, but after myotomy and partial fundoplication, the frequency of abnormal 24-hour pH probes is <5–10%.

22. What is the most severe complication seen with achalasia?

Squamous cell carcinoma, which occurs in 1–10% at an average of 20 years after diagnosis of achalasia. These tumors are diagnosed late because they have a longer evolution without causing obstruction in the dilated esophagus and they carry a poorer prognosis. Therapy does not eliminate the cancer risk, however, the absolute risk of cancer remains small, and surveillance endo-scopies are not advocated by national gastroenterology societies.

23. What triad of clinical features is seen in diffuse esophageal spasm (DES)?
1. Symptoms of dysphagia and chest pain
2. Abnormal esophageal contractions on barium esophagram
3. Characteristic esophageal manometric findings

The **pain** of DES may be variable, ranging from dull to colicky, mild to severe, and extremely brief to persistent. It is usually substernal but may radiate into the jaws and neck, down the arms, or through to the back. Because of the character of the pain and the fact that it may be relieved with sublingual nitroglycerin, these patients commonly are admitted to coronary care units and may even have angiograms before the origin of the pain is determined. The **dysphagia** is typi-cally intermittent in occurrence and rarely progressive in DES.

On barium swallow, the most suggestive presentation is the simultaneous segmental **con-tractions** observed in the smooth muscle section of the esophagus. Immediately below the upper esophageal sphincter, contractions appear normal. From the aortic arch level down to the GEJ, tertiary activity may be seen. These contractions are usually repetitive and simultaneous and may obliterate the esophageal lumen, causing the typical corkscrew or rosary bead appearance.

The major **manometric criteria** of DES are simultaneous repetitive tertiary contractions (triphasic or more) for at least 30% of wet swallows, with normal peristalsis between the abnormal contractions. Occasionally a sustained **tetanic** contraction may be seen during manometric stud-ies, with reproduction of the patient's chest pain. Amplitudes of 140 mm Hg are commonly seen.

24. Discuss the common presentation of hyperperistalsis (nutcracker esophagus)?
Hyperperistalsis or nutcracker esophagus is usually discovered in patients seen for chest pain. It is the most common esophageal motility abnormality reported in patients with noncardiac chest pain. Coronary artery disease is ruled out by the appropriate investigations. Heartburn, regurgi-tation, and dysphagia are generally absent. The diagnosis is suggested when motility studies show the presence of normal peristalsis but with distal peristaltic contraction amplitudes >2 standard deviations of normal (mean values >180 mm Hg) and prolonged duration of peristaltic contrac-tions (>6 seconds). Nutcracker esophagus is a manometric, not a radiologic, diagnosis. Radio-logic examination is usually normal or shows only nonspecific findings, such as tertiary contrac-tions. Esophageal transit time is also normal.

25. How is hypertensive LES characterized?
This is a manometric finding that presents with dysphagia or chest pain. It is characterized by the following findings on esophageal manometry:
- LES pressure >45 mm Hg
- LES relaxation >75%
- Normal esophageal peristalsis

Hypertensive LES has a distinct clinical and pathophysiologic significance because most patients respond to symptom-directed medical therapy, with only a few carefully selected patients requir-ing surgery. It is important to separate it from other clinical entities that may show a hypertensive LES but require different therapeutic modalities, such as:

- Achalasia
- DES
- Nutcracker esophagus
- Previous Nissen fundoplication
- Gastroesophageal reflux disease
- Carcinoma of the gastric cardia

26. What is nonspecific esophageal motility disorder?
A catchall category used for patients with motility disturbances that defy specific classifica-tion. These patients often have dysphagia or chest pain, but their motility studies, although out-side the normal manometric range, are not part of a fixed pattern. These include intermittent ab-sence of peristalsis on ≥20% of swallows, low-amplitude peristalsis, repetitive or triple-peaked

contractions, or spontaneous tertiary activity. When these recordings are not part of a fixed pattern, their recording must not produce a wrong diagnosis, leading to the wrong management.

27. What is the role of surgical therapy in patients with DES, nutcracker esophagus, hypertensive LES, and nonspecific esophageal motility disorder?

For **DES,** surgical treatment is considered only after full psychologic assessment and a prolonged trial at medical control of symptoms with sublingual nitroglycerin or calcium channel blockers. Significant incapacitation with chest pain and dysphagia with adverse effects on normal life must be present. In these selected patients, a long esophagomyotomy by a thoracotomy or thoracoscopic approach may be indicated. The length of the myotomy depends on the extent of the disease as determined by esophageal manometry. Most require myotomy only to the level of the aortic arch, but myotomies of the entire thoracic esophagus have been described. The results are not as good as that of achalasia; however, long esophagomyotomy provides good to excellent results in 67–70% of operated patients.

Long esophagomyotomy has also been conducted for nutcracker esophagus, hypertensive LES, and nonspecific esophageal motility disorders with varying success. The mainstay of treatment remains smooth muscle relaxants, anxiety medications with psychologic assessment, and support.

28. Discuss medications used for esophageal motility disorders.

Pharmacotherapy has traditionally used agents that act to decrease smooth muscle tone. Despite the multitude of drugs that have been used to treat primary esophageal motility disorders, no single agent has emerged as the drug of choice. The greatest experience has been with the use of **nitrates, anticholinergics,** and **calcium channel blockers.** Overall, responsiveness to these agents has been inconsistent and disappointing, with improvement of manometric parameters not reliably translating into symptom relief. For disorders such as achalasia, in which excellent results may be obtained with PD or surgical myotomy, drug therapy should be reserved for patients with minimal symptoms, as an adjunct to PD or myotomy for patients with continued difficulty, and for nonsurgical candidates. Many of the hypermotility disorders, such as DES and nutcracker esophagus, show an association with a high prevalence of psychiatric disorders, and symptom reduction may be achieved with the use of mild sedatives or antidepressants.

29. What is presbyesophagus?

Originally defined as abnormal esophageal motility associated with aging. The manometric findings included decreased incidence of normal peristalsis or absent peristalsis after swallowing, increased frequency of nonperistalsis, repetitive contractions, and occasional incomplete LES relaxation. These findings were thought to be a normal response to aging. In the original patients studied, however, many had diabetes mellitus, senile dementia, peripheral neuropathy, or all three. More recent manometric studies of healthy elderly individuals have shown relatively minor changes in esophageal motility with age. Many of the manometric criteria of presbyesophagus are similar to those used for **nonspecific esophageal motility disorder,** which has become the preferred term to describe the esophageal dysfunction seen in these patients.

BIBLIOGRAPHY

1. Achem SR, Kolts BE, Burton L: Segmental versus diffuse nutcracker esophagus: An intermittent motility pattern. Am J Gastroenterol 88:847–851, 1993.
2. Castell DO: Achalasia and diffuse esophageal spasm. Arch Intern Med 136:571–579, 1976.
3. Dent J, Holloway RH: Esophageal motility and reflux testing state-of-the-art and clinical role in the twenty-first century. Gastroenterol Clin North Am 25:51–73, 1996.
4. DiSimone MP, Felice V, Mattioli S, et al: Onset timing of delayed complications and criteria of follow-up after operation for esophageal achalasia. Ann Thorac Surg 61:1106–1111, 1996.
5. Duranceau A: Disorders of the esophagus in the adult. In Sabiston DC, Spencer FC (eds): Surgery of the Chest, 6th ed. Philadelphia, W.B. Saunders, 1995.

6. Ellis FH Jr: Esophagomyotomy for noncardiac chest pain resulting from diffuse esophageal spasm and related disorders. Am J Med 92:129S–131S, 1992.

7. Eypasch EP, DeMeester TR, Klingman RR, Stein HJ: Physiologic assessment and surgical management of diffuse esophageal spasm. J Thorac Cardiovasc Surg 104:859–869, 1992.

8. Graham AJ, Finley RJ, Worsley DF, et al: Laparoscopic esophageal myotomy and anterior partial fundoplication for the treatment of achalasia. Ann Thorac Surg 64:785–789, 1997.

9. Hunter JG, Richardson WS: Surgical management of achalasia. Surg Clin North Am 77: 993–1015, 1997.

10. Katada N, Hinder RA, Hinder PR, et al: The hypertensive lower esophageal sphincter. Am J Surg 172:439–443, 1996.

11. Koshy SS, Nostrant TT: Pathophysiology and endoscopic/balloon treatment of esophageal motility disorders. Surg Clin North Am 77:971–992, 1997.

12. Ott DJ: Motility disorders of the esophagus. Radiol Clin North Am 32:1117–1134, 1994.

13. Patti MG, Pellegrini CA, Horgan S, et al: Minimally invasive surgery for achalasia an 8-year experience with 168 patients. Ann Surg 230:587–594, 1999.

14. Spiess AF, Kahrila PJ: Treating achalasia from whalebone to laparoscope. JAMA 280:638–642, 1998.

15. Vaezi MF, Richter JE, Wilcox CM, et al: Botulinum toxin versus pneumatic dilatation in the treatment of achalasia: A randomised trial. Gut 44:231–239, 1999.

7. ACHALASIA

Marco Ricci, M.D., Ph.D., and Raffy L. Karamanoukian, M.D.

1. What is achalasia?

An esophageal motility disorder primarily characterized by abnormal or absent relaxation of the lower esophageal sphincter (LES). This condition, regardless of its cause, ultimately results in abnormal transit of esophageal contents from the distal esophagus into the stomach and in progressive esophageal dilation.

2. What is Chagas' disease?

A parasitic infestation, endemic in some areas of South America, that has been identified as one of the causes of achalasia. This disease is caused by *Trypanosoma cruzi,* which enters and selectively destroys ganglion cells of Auerbach's plexus, which represents the autonomic nervous system of the esophageal wall located between the longitudinal and circular muscle layers. Such destruction of ganglion cells of the myenteric plexus invariably alters esophageal motility, primarily affecting the LES, causing progressive esophageal dilation.

3. What is the cause of achalasia?

Although pathologic studies have shown that patients affected with achalasia unrelated to Chagas' disease invariably display a significant loss of ganglion cells of the myenteric plexus in the distal esophagus, the cause of such a severe derangement of the autonomic nervous system of the esophageal wall remains largely **unknown.**

4. Describe the clinical manifestations of achalasia.

Clinical manifestations of achalasia progressively worsen with failure of LES relaxation and the consequent esophageal dilation and impaired transit of ingested food from the esophagus into the stomach. As for other esophageal pathologies and motility disorders of the esophagus, symptoms characteristically include **dysphagia,** which is often more pronounced for liquids than solids. This is in contrast to esophageal carcinoma, in which symptoms of dysphagia appear, at least initially, with the ingestion of solid food. Patients with achalasia commonly experience **retrosternal discomfort during swallowing, regurgitation of undigested food,** and **halitosis.** As regurgitation of undigested food becomes more frequent and severe, particularly at night, symptoms related to recurrent bronchopneumonia, bronchiectasis, and lung abscess formation may become manifest.

5. How is the diagnosis usually made?

In the presence of symptoms suggestive of esophageal motor disorder, **barium esophagogram** should be performed initially, followed by **esophagoscopy** and **manometric studies.** These diagnostic studies may allow for the identification of achalasia as the cause of dysphagia, excluding other motility disorders of the esophagus (e.g., diffuse esophageal spasm) and esophageal carcinoma.

6. What findings are suggestive of achalasia on barium esophagogram?

Various degrees of esophageal dilation, in combination with narrowing of the distal esophagus and esophagogastric junction; this pattern of tapering of the distal esophagus is commonly referred to as **bird-beak appearance. Massive esophageal dilation** and **absence of peristalsis** on fluoroscopy are highly suggestive of long-standing history of achalasia. Undigested food may be shown within the distended distal esophagus.

7. Discuss the role of esophagoscopy.

Esophagoscopy is frequently performed not only to confirm the diagnosis of achalasia, but also to exclude other causes of dysphagia, such as carcinoma of the esophagus, adenocarcinoma involving the esophagogastric junction, and esophageal strictures resulting from severe gastroesophageal reflux disease. This technique permits accurate definition of the presence, severity, and extent of esophagitis. During esophagoscopy, esophageal biopsies may be performed to diagnose or exclude esophageal dysplasia and to define its severity (mild, moderate, or severe). The presence of esophageal carcinoma can be investigated and excluded.

8. Discuss the role of esophageal manometry.

Esophageal motility studies can confirm the diagnosis of achalasia, excluding other motility disorders, such as diffuse esophageal spasm. Typical findings suggestive of achalasia include lack of relaxation of the high pressure zone, which corresponds to the LES, after swallowing. Although esophageal contractions after swallowing may be relatively well preserved during the initial stages of the disease, these are markedly reduced, or absent, during the advanced stages of achalasia, in which a massively dilated esophagus may be observed (**megaesophagus**).

9. List the therapeutic alternatives when dealing with achalasia.
- Medical management
- Esophageal dilation
- Botulinum toxin (BoTox) therapy
- Surgical esophagomyotomy

10. What is the medical management of achalasia?

Calcium channel blockers and **nitroglycerin** may, only transiently, alleviate symptoms in the setting of milder forms of achalasia. Their use is limited largely to the treatment of initial stages of the disease or to patients who are not considered surgical candidates as a consequence of various coexistent medical conditions.

11. Discuss BoTox therapy for achalasia.

The injection of BoTox into the LES reduces the tone of the LES, ameliorating the transit of ingested food into the stomach. Despite initial favorable short-term results, the role that BoTox may have in accomplishing long-lasting relief of symptoms remains largely unknown. As such, it may be useful in combination with, or as an alternative to, mechanical dilation, particularly in elderly patients, as well as in those who are poor surgical candidates because of coexistent medical conditions.

12. Describe mechanical endoscopic dilation.

Mechanical endoscopic dilation, pneumatic or hydrostatic, has been employed frequently with success in the treatment of achalasia. This technique allows for forceful dilatation of the distal esophagus and LES, relieving symptoms and facilitating transit of ingested food into the stomach. Concerns have been raised regarding the development of gastroesophageal reflux disease after forceful dilation. Its occurrence seems to be low, however. Endoscopic dilation may be repeated in patients presenting with recurrent symptoms.

13. Which technique is preferred: mechanical dilation or esophageal myotomy?

Although the superiority of one technique over the other has not been shown conclusively by prospective, randomized trials, large retrospective series have shown that **esophageal myotomy** is associated with a lower risk of esophageal perforation and more frequently leads to long-lasting relief of symptoms. In a landmark study from the Mayo Clinic, esophageal myotomy was accompanied by a lower mortality rate (0.2% vs. 0.5%) and a lower rate of esophageal perforation (1% vs. 4%), than mechanical dilation. Surgical intervention was required in 50% of the patients who developed esophageal perforation after forceful dilation, and the operative mortality in this subgroup of patients was substantial (20%). In regard to long-term results, esophageal myotomy provided long-lasting relief of symptoms with good-to-excellent results in 85% of the patients versus 65% of patients treated by dilation.

14. What are the indications for surgical intervention?

Severe, symptomatic achalasia, as the primary treatment modality or after unsuccessful mechanical dialation.

15. How is esophageal myotomy (Heller myotomy) performed?

Through a transthoracic or transabdominal approach. It is accomplished by dividing the longitudinal and circular muscular fibers along the distal 7–10 cm of esophagus, prolonging the myotomy through the esophagogastric junction onto the proximal portion of the anterior wall of the stomach for 1–2 cm.

16. Is a concomitant antireflux procedure necessary?

Controversy exists as to whether esophageal myotomy should be combined with an antireflux procedure. Arguments against a concomitant antireflux procedure are mainly based on the fact that gastroesophageal reflux is uncommon if the gastric extension of the myotomy incision remains limited to the first centimeter of proximal stomach. This approach may result in incomplete division of the muscular fibers with consequent unsatisfactory relief of symptoms in 20% of patients. Extending the distal aspect of the myotomy to the proximal 2 cm of stomach may decrease the risk of treatment failure or recurrence, although it invariably risks development of gastroesophageal reflux disease because it creates incompetence of the cardia. Based on these considerations, these patients would be served best by **combining the esophageal myotomy with an antireflux procedure.** Most surgeons believe that some sort of antireflux procedure should be performed in combination with esophageal myotomy.

17. Describe the types of gastric fundoplication.

Although a complete, **floppy Nissen fundoplication** (360°) has been advocated by some in combination with the Heller myotomy in the treatment of achalasia, several studies have shown that a circumferential fundoplication in the setting of severely compromised esophageal motility may lead to long-term failure and distal obstruction. Partial fundoplication techniques are more commonly employed, including the **Belsey fundoplication** (270°), which is performed through a left thoracotomy approach, and Toupet (180° posterior) and Dor (180° anterior) fundoplications, using the transabdominal route. None of these techniques has been shown conclusively to be superior to the others.

As a result of advances in laparoscopic and thoracoscopic surgery, new endoscopic approaches have been developed. Data from the literature have shown that esophageal myotomy can be performed effectively thoracoscopically or laparoscopically. When using the transthoracic approach, an antireflux procedure may be avoided because the limited distal extension of esophageal myotomy and the minimal dissection of the esophageal hiatus theoretically reduce the risk of developing reflux disease. When a laparoscopic approach is used, esophageal myotomy frequently is combined with a partial anterior fundoplication (Toupet).

BIBLIOGRAPHY

1. Little AG, Soriano A, Ferguson MK: Surgical treatment of achalasia: Results of esophagomyotomy and Belsey repair. Ann Thorac Surg 45:489, 1988.
2. Malthaner RA, Todd TR, Miller L, Pearson FG: Long-term results in surgically managed esophageal achalasia. Ann Thorac Surg 54:1343, 1994.
3. Okike N, Payne WS, Neufeld DM, et al: Esophagomyotomy versus forceful dilatation for achalasia of the esophagus: Results in 899 patients. Ann Thorac Surg 28:119–126, 1979.
4. Pasricha PJ, Rai R, Ravich WJ, et al: Botulinum toxin for achalasia: Long-term outcome and predictors of response. Gastroenterology 110:1410–1415, 1996.
5. Pellegrini C, Wetter A, Patti M, et al: Thoracoscopic esophagomyotomy: Initial experience with a new approach for treatment of achalasia. Ann Surg 54:1046–1052, 1992.
6. Rosati R, Fumagalli U, Bonavino L, et al: Laparoscopic approach to esophageal achalasia. Am J Surg 169:424–429, 1995.

8. ESOPHAGEAL DIVERTICULA

Colin J. Powers, M.D., and Hratch L. Karamanoukian, M.D.

1. What are esophageal diverticula?

Outpouchings of the esophagus that emanate from the lumen and involve the esophageal wall. These structures may be considered **true** diverticula if they comprise a mucosal, submucosal, and muscular layer. Certain examples are considered **false** diverticula secondary to the involvement of only the mucosal and submucosal layers proceeding through the muscular component as a hernia defect. Other categories of classification consider the cause of the diverticula or whether it is congenital in origin versus acquired. The most common classification of esophageal diverticula is based on anatomic location.

2. List the three classic esophageal diverticula based on anatomic location.

1. Pharyngoesophageal
2. Midesophageal
3. Epiphrenic

3. What is Zenker's diverticulum?

The eponym for the pharyngoesophageal type of esophageal diverticula. These are the most common of the esophageal diverticula, with an incidence of 1.8–2.3% in patients with a complaint of dysphagia and a prevalence of 0.01–0.11% in the general population. Zenker's diverticula are found as a herniation of the hypopharyngeal mucosa and submucosa between the oblique fibers of the inferior pharyngeal constrictor and the transverse fibers of the cricopharyngeus muscle. Although the exact mechanism remains unknown, the most current theory holds that a failure of the cricopharyngeus muscle to relax completely during swallowing leads to a high pressure zone and subsequent diverticula formation.

4. How does Zenker's diverticulum present?

Many patients with small pharyngoesophageal diverticula may remain asymptomatic; however, the natural course of this process is for the diverticula to enlarge with time and generate symptoms secondary to retention of the food bolus or introduction of particulate matter into the respiratory tract. Specific complaints include:

- Dysphagia
- Halitosis
- Retrosternal pain
- Alterations in voice tone or character
- Coughing or wheezing after episodes of aspiration

5. List possible complications of Zenker's diverticulum.

- Fistula formation from the esophagus into the respiratory tract
- Weight loss and poor nutrition secondary to dysphagia
- Sequelae of aspiration, such as pneumonitis or lung abscess
- Squamous cell carcinoma arising within the chronically inflamed pouch

6. How is the diagnosis of Zenker's diverticulum made?

- Most patients present with symptoms of dysphagia. Contrast radiographic studies are the key element in making the diagnosis, with a barium swallow having a high degree of sensitivity and specificity.
- The role of endoscopy is not yet strictly defined. Many experienced surgeons believe that it does little to add to the overall workup and presents a definite risk of perforation. Others

state that endoscopy can be useful in cases in which a high degree of suspicion exists for malignancy or when impacted food materials inhibit an appropriate radiographic examination or surgical procedure.

- Esophageal manometry, although a key element in investigating the cause of this disorder, is of little use in the patient with an established and symptomatic diverticulum. A low threshold should exist, however, for employing esophageal manometry if the patient's history and complaint complex are suggestive of an esophageal dysmotility syndrome.

7. When should operative intervention be considered?

Small, asymptomatic diverticula may be followed with the physician advising the patient to masticate all foods thoroughly and follow meals with water. There is no effective medical therapy for this entity. Once a pharyngoesophageal diverticulum becomes symptomatic, surgical intervention is justified because the natural progression of the diverticulum will dictate further complaints and complications.

8. How are these diverticula surgically repaired?

- Diverticulectomy
- Diverticulopexy
- Cricopharyngeal myotomy
- Endoscopic or transluminal resection of the esophagodiverticular wall

The most commonly used procedure involves a left cervical incision to access the esophagus, excision of the diverticulum at its base using a linear stapling device, and performance of a cricopharyngeal myotomy extending several centimeters distal to the cricopharyngeus proper. This procedure is thought not only to remove the diverticulum, but also to eliminate the pathologic state responsible for the original herniation.

9. Are midesophageal diverticula pulsion diverticula or traction diverticula?

Midesophageal diverticula are historically believed to be caused by the adherence of the esophagus to adjacent lymph nodes and lesions involved in inflammatory reactions, such as histoplasmosis or tuberculosis (**traction diverticula**). These diverticula are found most frequently at the interbronchial level and are composed of mucosal, submucosal, and muscular components (making them **true** diverticula). This is in contrast to the mucosal and submucosal histology of the **pulsion** or **false** diverticula.

10. Can midesophageal diverticula be managed nonoperatively?

Yes. These diverticula are usually quite broad at their base and are directed in a cephalad direction (this is due to their creation as traction diverticula). This results in scant retention of swallowed materials and a generally asymptomatic existence. Most are discovered incidentally on barium esophagram during evaluation for other clinical conditions or esophageal dysmotility syndromes.

11. How should midesophageal diverticula be evaluated?

- Endoscopic examination to assess for the presence of malignancy or esophagitis
- Esophageal manometry to rule out associated or underlying dysmotility syndromes
- CT scan to evaluate the lymph nodes, pleura, and lung fields

12. When is surgical intervention necessary for midesophageal diverticula?

Although typically benign and asymptomatic, infrequent complications secondary to the inflammatory reaction of the initiating granulomatous or infectious disease can lead to acute surgical emergency. Fistulization of a diverticulum to the tracheobronchial tree or a thoracic great vessel can lead to rapid cardiopulmonary instability. Such a situation demands **thoracotomy** and **correction of the fistula** with interpositioning of a pleural or muscular flap to enhance the repair.

13. Where are epiphrenic diverticula located?

Typically within the last 10 cm of the thoracic esophagus. These pulsion diverticula usually arise from the right posterior wall and may exist as an isolated diverticulum or an area of multiple herniations.

14. How are these diverticula formed?

As pulsion diverticula, the epiphrenic variety are believed to arise from esophageal motor dysfunction or more distal luminal obstruction (i.e., stricture or neoplasm). Whether the essential esophageal abnormality is achalasia, diffuse esophageal spasm, or hypertension of the lower esophageal sphincter, a zone of increased intraluminal pressure results with subsequent herniation of the mucosal and submucosal layers through an area of muscular weakness. Many studies have shown what would then be expected, that a high proportion (approximately two thirds) of individuals with epiphrenic diverticula also have definable esophageal dysmotility disorders.

15. List the symptoms associated with epiphrenic diverticulum.

- Dysphagia
- Chest pain
- Regurgitation
- Complaints arising from episodes of aspiration

Because these diverticula are often found to co-exist with esophageal dysmotility states, whether the symptoms are secondary to the diverticulum or a result of the dysmotility syndrome is questioned.

16. How should epiphrenic diverticulum be evaluated?

- Barium esophagography
- Endoscopic examination
- Esophageal manometry
- Esophageal pH testing in patients with complaints consistent with gastroesophageal reflux disease

17. List complications that can arise from the presence of epiphrenic diverticula.

- Esophagitis
- Squamous cell carcinoma
- Bezoar formation
- Possible perforation

18. Is early surgery an appropriate means to address this entity?

No. Many authors have shown that most epiphrenic diverticula are asymptomatic. Many individuals benefit from a thorough evaluation for esophageal dysmotility and subsequent management where warranted. No clear correlation between diverticula size and clinical complaints or clinical progression has been proved. Current recommendations are surgical repair or revision only in patients with severe and intractable symptoms.

19. How is the surgical repair of epiphrenic diverticula performed?

A left posterolateral thoracotomy, diverticulectomy, and long esophagomyotomy performed from the stomach through the length of the esophagus shown to have dysmotility.

20. Is an antireflux procedure a necessary component of the operation?

Although remaining a point of contention, the most recent literature holds that an antireflux procedure is not a necessary addition to the diverticulectomy and long esophagomyotomy. It should be considered when a preexisting hiatal hernia exists or there is evidence of preoperative gastroesophageal reflux disease. In these cases, a less obstructing procedure, such as Belsey Mark IV, would be advised rather than the more typical Nissen fundoplication.

21. What are the risks associated with surgical repair of epiphrenic diverticula?

Data from the Mayo Clinic report perioperative mortality of 9% and complications in one of every three patients postoperatively, including a postoperative esophageal leak rate of approximately 20%.

22. What is esophageal intramural pseudodiverticulosis?

An extremely rare condition that manifests with patients complaining of dysphagia and radiographic contrast studies showing diffuse 1–5 mm diverticula throughout the esophagus. The exact mechanism of formation is unknown, yet current thought holds that these diverticula represent dilated mucous glands from chronic irritation. Further evidence on behalf of this theory consists of the roughly one third to one half of patients with esophageal intramural pseudodiverticulosis who also have *Candida albicans* infections. Present management consists of conservative treatment with medical therapy of gastroesophageal reflux and *Candida* infection where appropriate and dilation of associated strictures as necessary.

BIBLIOGRAPHY

1. Benacci J, Deschamps C, Trastek V, et al: Epiphrenic diverticulum: Results of surgical treatment. Ann Thorac Surg 55:1109–1114, 1993.
2. Ellis F: Pharyngoesophageal (Zenker's) diverticulum. Adv Surg 28:171–189, 1995.
3. Just R, Fulp S: Esophageal diverticula. In Castell O (ed): The Esophagus, 2nd ed. Boston, Little, Brown, 1995, pp 345–359.
4. Orringer M: Diverticula and miscellaneous conditions of the esophagus. In Sabiston D (ed): Textbook of Surgery, 15th ed. Philadelphia, W.B. Saunders, 1997, pp 729–735.
5. Tirnaksiz M, Deschamps C: Diverticula of the esophagus. In Cameron J (ed): Current Surgical Therapy, 6th ed. St. Louis, Mosby, 1998, pp 29–33.
6. Tobin R: Esophageal rings, webs, and diverticula. J Clin Gastroenterol 27:285–295, 1998.

9. GASTROESOPHAGEAL REFLUX DISEASE

Harry W. Donias, M.D., and Hratch L. Karamanoukian, M.D.

1. What is gastroesophageal reflux disease (GERD)?

Any symptomatic condition or histopathologic alteration resulting from gastroesophageal reflux (GER). Normal individuals have daily physiologic reflux, which causes neither symptoms nor histologic abnormalities. When reflux episodes cause symptoms, by an increase in amount, change in composition, or increase in frequency, the pathologic entity of GERD is present.

2. Discuss the prevalence of GERD.
- It is the most common GI condition in the United States.
- At least $10 billion is spent annually on prescription drugs for heartburn or dyspepsia.
- Approximately 40–45% of American adults experience heartburn, the cardinal symptom of GERD, at least once a month; 14% describe weekly heartburn; and 7% report having the symptom on a daily basis.
- The exact prevalence of the disease is difficult to determine because only 50–65% of patients with symptoms of GER have esophagitis or other complications of GERD at endoscopy, compared with a 3–4% prevalence of esophagitis in the general population.
- Only 65% of patients with esophageal inflammation complain of frequent heartburn, and 25% of patients with Barrett's esophagus have no GER symptoms.

3. How does age affect the prevalence of GERD?
- The prevalence of GERD-related symptoms, extent of mucosal injury, and incidence of Barrett's esophagus **increase** with age.
- In elderly patients, women are affected more frequently by reflux symptoms, and men are affected more frequently by esophagitis.

4. List the symptoms of GERD.

Typical
- Heartburn (pyrosis)
- Regurgitation—common after large meals or after stooping
- Dysphagia/odynophagia
- Water brash (excess salivation)
- Chest pain

Atypical
- Pulmonary aspiration
- Severe chest pain
- Asthma (adult onset)
- Chronic hoarseness
- Choking, difficulty initiating swallows
- Chronic cough
- Dental erosions

5. What percentage of patients with esophagitis develop complications?
Approximately 20%.

6. What esophageal complications are associated with reflux esophagitis?

COMPLICATION	%
Stricture	4–20
Barrett's esophagus	10–15
Esophageal ulcer	2–7
Hemorrhage	2

7. Describe the principal mechanism of GER and GERD.

Reflux occurs in normal subjects and in patients with GERD primarily as a result of transient relaxations of the **lower esophageal sphincter (LES)** and **crural diaphragm.** Transient relaxation of the LES is a neural reflux that is mediated through the brain stem. The efferent pathway for such relaxation is in the vagus nerve, and nitric oxide is the postganglionic neurotransmitter. The mechanism of relaxation of the crural diaphragm is not known. In contrast to healthy subjects, patients with GERD have more frequent transient LES relaxations, which permit a reflux of gastric contents into the esophagus. Once reflux has occurred, whether damage results depends on several factors. The duration of contact depends on the number of reflux episodes per unit time, the efficiency of esophageal peristalsis to clear the refluxed material, and the efficiency of salivary neutralization, which neutralizes the remaining gastric acid. Acid and pepsin together are more damaging to the esophageal epithelium than either one alone, and the addition of bile salts increases the damage.

8. Is a hiatal hernia an essential component of GERD?

No. Type I hiatal hernia can be seen radiographically in about half of individuals > 50 years old and is observed at the same frequency when endoscopists estimate the position of the gastroesophageal junction. Because <50% of the general population has **pathologic GER,** it is hard to implicate a hiatal hernia as more than a cofactor in GER. About 50% of patients with GER and GERD have a hiatal hernia, and the patients with the worst complications of GERD usually have a large or complicated hiatal hernia. The precise relationship between hiatal hernia and GER is still unclear, but it is believed that a hiatal hernia displaces the LES from its normal anatomic position, altering the anatomic barrier to reflux in some patients. Early retrograde flow of gastric contents into the esophagus is possible because the hernia acts as a reservoir, and, because of its altered positioning, the active contractions of the diaphragm, which normally enhance LES pressure during inspiration, may not be as effective.

9. What is the MUSE classification?

Used for staging the severity of endoscopic findings of GERD:
>   **M—metaplasia**
>   **U—ulcers**
>   **S—strictures**
>   **E—erosions**

10. How is mucosal damage scored in the MUSE classification?
Metaplasia
>   0—absent
>   1—on one esophageal fold
>   2—on two or more folds
>   3—circumferential

Ulcer
>   0—absent
>   1—junctional ulcer (Wolf or Savary)
>   2—Barrett's ulcer in esophagus
>   3—combined (Wolf + Barrett's)

Stricture
>   0—absent
>   1—<9 mm
>   2—≥9 mm
>   3—stricture and short esophagus

Erosions
>   0—absent
>   1—on one fold
>   2—on two or more folds
>   3—circumferential

11. What is unequivocal evidence of GERD by 24-hour ambulatory pH monitoring?

The **gold standard** test to confirm the presence of GER is a 24-hour esophageal pH assessment that quantifies the number and duration of episodes of acid reflux into the esophagus. This test correlates subjective symptoms with reflux events and differentiates between upright and supine GER. Normal individuals have acid pH levels (pH <4.0) in the distal esophagus 4% of the time. An acid exposure 4–7% of total recording time is by itself only equivocal evidence of reflux disease. Exposure to acid of 7–12% is unequivocal evidence of reflux disease and suggests the probability of mucosal damage, whereas acid reflux >12% of recording time usually is found in the more severe form of reflux disease. The sensitivity of prolonged pH monitoring in identifying pathologic GER is 50–100% (mean 85%), and the specificity is somewhat higher.

12. What is the Bernstein test?

A test to confirm that symptoms are due to esophageal sensitivity to acid. It is performed during esophageal manometry by alternatively infusing sterile water and dilute 0.1 N hydrochloric acid into the lower esophagus; an assessment for reproduction of the patient's symptoms after acid instillation is made. The sensitivity of the Bernstein test for GERD is 30–100% (mean 75%), and its specificity in 40–100% (mean 80%).

13. Name the goals of medical treatment of GERD.

- Heal the injured esophageal mucosa
- Eliminate symptoms
- Prevent or treat complications of GERD

14. How are the symptoms of GERD managed?

- Patients with mild symptoms of GERD usually can be managed empirically with lifestyle modifications along with antacids and histamine₂-receptor antagonists (H₂RAs).
- Patients who do not respond to this first level of therapy or who have unusual symptoms or significant manifestations that may indicate complications (dysphagia, odynophagia, and GI hemorrhage) require, at the minimum, endoscopy for diagnosis and to exclude other causes.
- By identifying esophageal inflammation, hiatal hernia, Barrett's esophagus, or stricture, endoscopy helps to determine patients who likely would require more intensive or prolonged pharmacologic therapy or antireflux surgery.

15. List some lifestyle modifications recommended to GERD patients.

- Elevating the head of the bed 6–10 inches using blocks or a foam wedge
- Weight reduction
- Smoking cessation
- Reduced alcohol consumption
- Limiting potentially precipitating activities, such as bending over or strenuous exercise
- Avoiding meals 2–3 hours before bedtime
- Dietary modifications with smaller meals and reduced fat content
- Avoiding chocolate, spearmint, peppermint, raw onions, caffeine, and acidic foodstuffs
- Discontinuation or substitution of reflux-promoting medications, such as calcium channel blockers, anticholinergic agents, narcotics, theophylline, estrogens, and nitrates

16. Describe the effects of H₂RAs.

The H₂RAs, cimetidine, ranitidine, famotidine, and nizatidine, decrease gastric acid secretion by reversible competitive inhibition of histamine-stimulated acid secretion and are considered equivalent in acid suppression when given in equipotent doses. Short-term standard doses are successful in symptomatic relief for 60–70% of patients. Nighttime dosing, which is effective in peptic ulcer disease, does not work as well with GER. The best time to take these medications is after breakfast and after the evening meal. Short-term therapy with standard doses is successful in healing esophagitis in approximately two thirds of patients. Tolerance often develops to these drugs, resulting in an approximate 50% decrease in efficacy that is usually not overcome by increasing the dose. Only 25–45% of patients with esophagitis remain free of mucosal injury after 1 year. Except for patients with mild GER, standard doses of H_2RAs probably have a limited role in modern medical therapy of GERD.

17. How do proton-pump inhibitors (PPIs) work?

The PPIs, **omeprazole, lansoprazole, pantoprazole,** and the newly approved **rabeprazole,** reduce gastric acid secretion by inhibiting activity of the gastric hydrogen/potassium adenosine triphosphate (H^+/K^+-ATPase) pump. These agents are protonated in the acidic gastric environment to active forms, which bind irreversibly to sulfhydryl groups on the H^+/K^+-ATPase molecule, rendering it inactive. PPIs are effective in 85–96% of patients with severe esophagitis, including those who initially failed other therapies. The best time to take PPIs seems to be early in the morning, and their effectiveness is dose-dependent. The activity of PPIs results in a profound, long-lasting acid suppression, which recovers only when therapy is discontinued and the newly synthesized H^+/K^+-ATPase from parietal cells is not blocked. Today, PPIs are the primary treatment for patients with GERD in the United States. Nearly half of patients on maintenance PPIs require increasing doses to maintain esophageal healing.

18. Discuss complications of long-term usage of PPIs.

Omeprazole has been shown to increase gastrin levels two to four times in patients during its use. Hypergastrinemia during PPI treatment has been shown to be of little if any recognized clinical significance. One study showed that >30% of patients on omeprazole for 5 years developed atrophic gastritis. Although the risk of atrophic gastritis remains unclear, it could lead to an increased risk of gastric cancer. In the study, only omeprazole-treated patients with *Helicobacter pylori* infections developed atrophic gastritis, suggesting that *H. pylori* is the most significant risk factor. There are no reports of GI tumors in humans taking omeprazole for 6 years, and PPIs still represent the best long-term medical treatment option for most patients with frequent, severe, or complicated GER.

19. Describe the role of prokinetic drugs in the treatment of GERD.

Theoretically, prokinetic drugs (**cisapride, bethanechol,** and **metoclopramide**) increase LES pressure, enhance gastric emptying, and increase the force of esophageal contractions. Bethanechol and metoclopramide are only minimally effective as solitary agents and provide only a moderate benefit when combined with H_2RAs. Bethanechol has the cholinergic potential for increasing gastric acid secretion, bronchoconstriction, and bladder contraction, and metoclopramide has a 20–50% incidence of fatigue, restlessness, tremor, parkinsonism, or tardive dyskinesia. Cisapride acts by releasing acetylcholine only within the myenteric plexus, minimizing its extraintestinal actions. Cisapride is superior to placebo for healing mild esophagitis, improving symptoms, and preventing relapse when used as a single agent, and it works synergistically with H_2RAs. The main disadvantage of cisapride is its frequent dosing regimen (four times a day). Cisapride alone or in combination with H_2RAs does not show more benefit than PPIs.

20. When can medical treatment of GERD be stopped?

For most patients, the answer is **never.** GERD is a chronic disease that when medically treated requires lifelong pharmacologic therapy in most patients. Despite effective initial treatment, recurrence of reflux esophagitis is rapid once treatment with acid-suppressing drugs is withdrawn. Of patients, 80% experience symptomatic recurrence within 6 months if not given adequate maintenance therapy. The recurrence appears to be progressive in some patients, in that they may suffer a relapse to a more severe grade of esophagitis or develop a complication. Controlled clinical trials have shown that patients suffering from reflux esophagitis can remain in clinical and endoscopic remission for as long as adequate acid-suppressing therapy is continued.

21. What is Barrett's esophagus?

An acquired condition in which the normal squamous epithelium of the distal esophagus is replaced by a metaplastic columnar epithelium characterized by the presence of goblet cells and villous architecture. It represents a peculiar form of healing that can occur at any time in patients with reflux esophagitis. Barrett's esophagus is a premalignant lesion because it is the initiating factor of a metaplasia-to-dysplasia-to-carcinoma sequence. The incidence of Barrett's adenocarcinoma is rising faster than that of any other tumor, with an incidence of about 3 per 100,000 white men in developed countries. Esophageal adenocarcinoma now accounts for most esophageal cancers in this population.

22. What types of columnar epithelium are seen in Barrett's esophagus?

The histologic hallmark of Barrett's esophagus is the finding of **intestinal metaplasia.** Mucin-containing goblet cells are in the epithelium. Goblet cell intestinal metaplasia constitutes most of the area of Barrett's esophagus. This histologic type is found in >95% of cases in which the endoscopist has seen a long segment (>3 cm) of Barrett's esophagus. This type of epithelium is associated with an increased risk of esophageal adenocarcinoma and requires endoscopic and biopsy surveillance. If the columnar epithelium shows metaplasia resembling gastric cardia or junctional mucosa with no intestinal metaplasia, there is no increased risk of adenocarcinoma, and this may suggest that the biopsy specimens were obtained from columnar epithelium within a diaphragmatic hernia and not from the esophagus.

23. How is Barrett's esophagus managed?

For the control of symptoms and esophagitis, PPIs or antireflux surgery is effective; however, Barrett's epithelium and the risk of cancer remain. If high-grade dysplasia is suspected, confirmation by a second expert GI pathologist is recommended. Different grades of dysplasia often occur in different areas of the same patient's esophagus; the endoscopist should obtain systematic biopsy specimens from the entire columnar-lined esophagus to find the highest grade of dysplasia present. Any patient with **high-grade dysplasia** should be considered for an esophagectomy. If resection is a prohibitive risk, endoscopic mucosal ablation is an option; however, accelerated surveillance with biopsies every 6 months should be undertaken because whether mucosal ablation reduces the risk of cancer is yet to be proved. For patients with **low-grade dysplasia,** the findings need to be verified by repeat biopsies after 12 weeks of PPI therapy. If low-grade dysplastic changes persist, biopsies should be repeated annually. If the dysplastic changes are no longer present, the initial finding can be attributed to inflammation from reflux. For patients with visible Barrett's esophagus and **intestinal metaplasia** but no dysplasia, examination at 1 year, then every 2–3 years is recommended.

24. Is Barrett's esophagus curable?

No. Antireflux surgery does not produce shortening of the Barrett's segments. Long-term treatment with PPIs has not been shown conclusively to reduce the length of Barrett's segments, but it has been associated with the formation of **islands** of squamous mucosa within the area of columnar epithelium. The risk of cancer is not eliminated, and the need for continued surveillance is unchanged with anything short of surgical resection of the distal esophagus.

25. List some extraintestinal manifestations of GERD.

- Chronic hoarseness
- Posterior laryngitis
- Pharyngitis
- Laryngospasm
- Subglottic stenosis
- Laryngeal nodules and ulcers
- Laryngeal cancer
- Asthma
- Recurrent pneumonitis
- Lung abscesses
- Pulmonary fibrosis
- Nocturnal choking
- Dental disease

26. How does GERD contribute to asthma?

Several reports have indicated that 50% of patients with asthma have endoscopic evidence of esophagitis or increased esophageal acid exposure on 24-hour ambulatory pH monitoring. Two mechanisms have been proposed as the pathogenesis of reflux-induced asthmatic symptoms:

1. The **reflux theory** maintains that respiratory symptoms are the result of the aspiration of gastric contents.

2. The **reflex theory** maintains that vagally mediated bronchoconstriction follows acidification of the lower esophagus.

The latter can be explained by the common embryologic origin of the tracheoesophageal tract and a shared vagal innervation. Medical therapy with PPIs and antireflux surgery have resulted in decreased asthma symptoms and asthma medication use before and after therapy as well as increased pulmonary function test performance in patients with reflux-induced asthma. To date, antireflux surgery has been shown to ameliorate respiratory symptoms consistently in patients with reflux-induced asthma more effectively than the published trials of antisecretory therapy. **Antireflux surgery** improves respiratory symptoms in nearly 90% of children and 70% of adults with asthma and GERD.

BIBLIOGRAPHY

1. Bowrey DJ, Peters JH, DeMeester TR: Gastroesophageal reflux disease in asthma: Effects of medical and surgical antireflux therapy on asthma control. Ann Surg 231:161–172, 2000.
2. Cameron AJ: Management of Barrett's esophagus. Mayo Clin Proc 73:457–461, 1998.
3. Donahue PE: Basic considerations in gastroesophageal reflux disease. Surg Clin North Am 77:1017–1040, 1997.
4. Duranceau A, Jamieson GG: Hiatal hernia and gastroesophageal reflux. In Sabiston DC (ed): Textbook of surgery: The Biological Basis of Modern Surgical Practice, 15th ed. Philadelphia, W.B. Saunders, 1997.
5. Howden CW, Castell DO, Cohen S, et al: The rationale for continuous maintenance treatment of reflux esophagitis. Arch Intern Med 155:1465–1471, 1995.
6. Hunt RH: Importance of pH control in the management of GERD. Arch Intern Med 159:649–657, 1999.
7. Hunter JG, Trus TL, Branum GD, et al: A physiologic approach to laparoscopic fundoplication for gastroesophageal reflux disease. Ann Surg 223:673–687, 1996.
8. Ireland AP, Clark GWB, DeMeester TR: Barrett's esophagus: The significance of p53 in clinical practice. Ann Surg 225:17–30, 1997.
9. Kahrilas PJ: Gastroesophageal reflux disease. JAMA 276:983–988, 1996.
10. McKernan JB, Champion JK: Minimally invasive antireflux surgery. Am J Surg 223:673–687, 1996.
11. Mittal RK, Balaban DH: Mechanisms of disease of the esophagogastric junction. N Engl J Med 336:924–932, 1997.
12. Pope CE: Current concepts in acid-reflux disorders. N Engl J Med 331:656–660, 1994.
13. Richardson WS, Trus TL, Hunter JG: Laparoscopic antireflux surgery. Surg Clin North Am 76:437–450, 1996.
14. Soper NJ: Laparoscopic management of hiatal hernia and gastroesophageal reflux. Curr Probl Surg 36:767–838, 1999.
15. Wo JM, Waring JP: Medical therapy of gastroesophageal reflux and management of esophageal strictures. Surg Clin North Am 77:1041–1062, 1997.

10. PARAESOPHAGEAL AND HIATAL HERNIA

Vivian Lindfield, M.D.

1. What is the phrenoesophageal membrane? What is its importance?

The phrenoesophageal membrane is a continuation of the diaphragmatic peritoneum. It inserts onto the esophagus at the level of the hiatus. This membrane marks the proximal margin of the intra-abdominal esophagus. This ligament helps provide a strong, but flexible airtight seal. One leaf of the fascia moves up through the hiatus to insert in the adventitia of the esophagus 1–2 cm above the gastroesophageal (GE) junction. The second leaf inserts into the adventitia of the abdominal fascia. The presence of this ligament varies with age. It is present in newborns, but in adults it becomes attenuated with fat accumulation. This ligament is usually not present in people with hernias.

2. What structures constitute the esophageal hiatus?

The esophageal hiatus is typically an elliptical opening present in the muscular portion of the diaphragm. It usually lies at the level of T10, just to the left of the midline. The diaphragmatic crura form the anterior and lateral margins of the hiatus. The median arcuate ligament usually forms the posterior margin. In 62% of people both crura formed the margins, with the right crus making up most of the border and the left crus making up the posterior. In 10%, the margins were made up of right and left crus equally. In another 10% the right crus exclusively formed the hiatus.

3. What structures pass through the esophageal hiatus?

Several other structures pass through the hiatus besides the esophagus. The anterior and posterior vagal trunks along with the esophageal arteries and veins, which arise from the left gastric vessels, also pass through this opening.

4. Describe the anatomy of the GE junction.

The distal esophagus is composed of two muscle layers, an inner circular layer and an outer longitudinal layer. These outer fibers continue through the hiatus and join the longitudinal gastric musculature. The circular muscle fibers at this region are asymmetrically thickened and therefore contribute to the high-pressure zone. All of these muscle fibers are composed of smooth muscle.

The submucosa joins the muscle layers and mucosa. This layer is quite strong due to the elastic and collagenous fibers that predominate. The mucosa is mainly squamous epithelium. Approximately 2 cm above the anatomic junction, the squamous epithelium changes to columnar. This area of change is known as the Z-line.

The vagal plexus, which surrounds the lower aspect of the esophagus, provides the major innervation. These nerves then form the anterior and posterior vagal trunks. The left gastric artery gives off several branches to supply the lower esophagus and the proximal stomach. Some of the posterior vascular supply comes from the splenic artery.

5. What is a hiatal hernia?

The basic definition of a hiatal hernia is ascent of the stomach through the esophageal hiatus into the thorax.

6. Is there more than one type of hiatal hernia?

Yes. There are four types of hiatal hernia:

1. **Type I or sliding hiatal hernia** is usually caused by a laxity in the phrenoesophageal ligament. Since this ligament no longer anchors the gastroesophageal in its normal intra-abdominal location, there is a cephalad migration of the junction and the stomach through the hiatus into the posterior mediastinum. Since the GE junction is no longer exposed to intra-abdominal pressure,

there is a common association of gastroesophageal reflux disease (GERD) with these hernias. There is usually no true hernia sac present. The stomach tends to make up the posterior wall of the sac with peritoneum anteriorly and laterally. The hiatus is also usually widened.

2. **Type II or primary paraesophageal hernia** is most commonly associated with normal abdominal positioning of the phrenoesophageal ligament and the GE junction. A hernia sac is almost always present and contains part of the gastric cardia. The opening of the hiatus tends to be anterior to the GE junction. These hernias are not usually associated with GERD.

3. **Type III hernia** is a combination of both types I and II. There is usually movement of the GE junction into the thorax plus a hernia sac containing gastric fundus. There may be mesoaxial or organoaxial rotation of the stomach associated with this hernia type. Both reflux and obstructive symptoms may be present.

4. **Type IV hernia** is usually associated with herniation of other organs such as colon, spleen or small intestine into the thorax.

7. What is the incidence of paraesophageal hernias?

The type II hernias are relatively uncommon, accounting for about 10% of all hiatal hernias. They tend to occur in older patients and are more common in females. The type I hernia is more common in younger or middle adult years.

8. What symptoms may be associated with hiatal hernias?

Type I hernias are usually associated with symptoms related to GERD. Type II hernias are different. These hernias tend to be asymptomatic. The paraesophageal hernias are more likely to be associated with symptoms related to obstruction, like chest pain, regurgitation, dyspnea, dysphagia, and vomiting. Symptoms may develop acutely due to obstruction or strangulation. The size of the hernia is usually not related to the presence of symptoms. If these hernias do obstruct and strangulate, there is a risk of perforation of the contents. This is similar to strangulation of any other hernia found elsewhere in the body.

9. What complications can occur with these hernias?

Paraesophageal hernia can result in gastric incarceration along with vascular compromise, which can then lead to gastric perforation. This complication is associated with a 50% mortality rate. Therefore, surgery is indicated for paraesophageal hernias to avoid this situation.

Erosion of the gastric mucosa can also occur and lead to occult or chronic blood loss. This erosion is thought to be due to "acid stasis" along with chronic venous engorgement.

10. What techniques are available to help diagnose paraesophageal hernias?

When a patient describes symptoms such as chest pain, early satiety, and regurgitation, a paraesophageal hernia should be part of the differential diagnosis. Chest x-rays may show an air-fluid level in the thorax. This is typically present posterior to the heart shadow. It is sometimes helpful to place a nasogastric tube prior to the chest x-ray. The tube may show up coiled in the thoracic stomach. The primary diagnostic test for paraesophageal hernia is the barium esophagogram and upper GI study.

11. What is the role of endoscopic exam in diagnosing paraesophageal hernia?

Endoscopic exam is important as a preoperative test. However, the insufflation of air during the exam can precipitate gastric incarceration, requiring emergent surgery. Therefore, this test is reserved until just prior to surgery. If esophagitis or evidence of reflux is noted, an antireflux procedure should be considered.

12. Is manometric pH monitoring necessary?

Sometimes passing the catheters can be very difficult. If there is no sign of reflux, these studies are usually not required. The lower esophageal sphincter pressure is relatively normal in patients with paraesophageal hernias compared to those with sliding hernias. Manometry is useful in determining how effective esophageal peristalsis is and if a fundoplication procedure is necessary.

13. What is the management of paraesophageal hernias?

Paraesophageal hernias have a high risk for serious complications, like obstruction and strangulation. Twenty to thirty percent of patients who are treated nonoperatively have complications associated with catastrophic results; therefore, medically stable patients should undergo elective repair of these hernias. If there are any symptoms of obstruction, anemia or strangulation, surgery should be considered.

14. How does the treatment of a sliding hernia differ from that for paraesophageal hernia?

Up to half of the siding hernias are asymptomatic and do not require therapy. If esophagitis is present, medical management should be attempted first. Simple lifestyle modifications such as keeping the head of the bed elevated, not lying down after eating, and a diet low in fat are all helpful in managing symptoms. Prokinetic agents like metaclopramide or cisapride can sometimes increase healing of esophagitis by increasing sphincter tone and peristalsis. An 8–12-week course of H2-blockers can be useful in treating mild to moderate disease. For more serious disease, proton pump inhibitors, like omeprazole, are more useful. Once these drugs are stopped, however, recurrence rates are high. Surgery is considered once medical management has been attempted and failed. Usually some form of an antireflux procedure, such as fundoplication, is performed.

15. What surgical therapies are currently being used to treat hiatal hernias?

The principle of surgical treatment for these hernias is the same as that for all hernia repairs. The contents of the hernia should be returned to their anatomic position, the hernia sac should be resected, and the defect repaired. In these hernias, the stomach is reduced by traction. Adhesions that may be present are lysed. The hernia sac is dissected from the diaphragm and the visceral pleura and resected. The diaphragm is repaired with nonabsorbable sutures in a tension-free repair. There may be a need to anchor the stomach in an intra-abdominal position by gastropexy to the anterior abdominal wall or arcuate ligament. The type of repair will depend on what type of hernia is present.

16. What approach is used to repair a paraesophageal hernia?

Usually an abdominal approach is indicated for a proper repair of these hernias. Thoracotomy is sometimes used, especially if there is shortening of the esophagus. A thoracotomy is also useful to manage those patients who are experiencing reflux symptoms after a fundoplication procedure. More recently, laparoscopic techniques have been used to repair paraesophageal hernias. The surgeon must be familiar with both the open and laparoscopic techniques if this approach is to be attempted, since any complication needs to be addressed via the open technique.

17. Is an antireflux procedure always necessary in the repair of paraesophageal hernias?

The use of fundoplication is still controversial. Paraesophageal hernias do not usually present with symptoms of reflux disease. Antireflux procedures are more commonly used in the repair of type I hernias associated with GERD. The fundoplication procedure is added to the repair based on preoperative symptoms and diagnostic tests that demonstrate reflux. It has been reported that the recurrence rates are much lower when a fundoplication procedure is performed with all repairs regardless of the type of hernia. This issue is still a matter of debate.

18. A patient presents with a paraesophageal hernia documented on chest x-ray. She has a short esophagus due to complications of GERD. What procedure should be used to repair this hernia?

If it is expected that there will not be enough esophageal length to restore the GE junction to an intra-abdominal position despite extensive dissection in the thorax, an esophageal lengthening procedure such as a Collis gastroplasty should be performed. In this procedure, a gastrointestinal anastomosis (GIA) stapler is positioned along the lesser curvature of the stomach to create a tubular extension of the esophagus. The new fundus that is created by the stapling is then wrapped around the new esophagus as a partial or total fundoplication to re-establish antireflux function. The repair is reduced without tension under the diaphragm. Sometimes a gastropexy procedure is also performed to help maintain the stomach in the abdomen. Usually, however, the fundoplication and reduction is all that is required.

19. What results can be achieved with repair of paraesophageal hernias?

Risk of mortality with open abdominal and transthoracic repairs of these hernias is about 1% in the short term. The risk of major complications associated with surgery is about 20%. Regardless of the approach, approximately 90% of patients have a good long-term result. The postoperative results with laparoscopic repair are very similar to those of the open procedures. However, shorter hospital stays, fewer nonfatal complications, and less pain are the advantages of the laparoscopic approach.

BIBLIOGRAPHY

1. Ferguson M: Paraesophageal hiatal hernia. In Cameron JL (ed): Current Surgical Therapy, 6th ed. St. Louis, Mosby, 1998.
2. Duranceau A, Jamieson G: Hiatal hernia and gastroesophageal reflux. In Sabiston DC Jr (ed): Textbook of Surgery: The Biological Basis of Modern Surgical Practice, 15th ed. Philadelphia, W.B. Saunders, 1997.
3. Landreneau R: Surgical management of paraesophageal herniation. In Nyhus LM, Baker RJ, Fischer JE (eds): Mastery of Surgery, 3rd ed. Boston, Little, Brown, 1997.
4. Pellegrini C, Way L: Esophagus and diaphragm. In Way L (ed): Current Surgical Diagnosis and Treatment. Norwalk, CT, Appleton & Lange, 1994.
5. Mason RJ, et al: The digestive system. In O'Leary JP (ed): The Physiologic Basis of Surgery, 2nd ed. Baltimore, Williams & Wilkins, 1996.

11. BARRETT'S ESOPHAGUS

Colin J. Powers, M.D., and Hratch L. Karamanoukian, M.D.

1. What type of epithelium is present in the normal esophagus?

The normal, healthy esophagus is lined with a stratified squamous epithelium.

2. What type of epithelium is present in Barrett's esophagus?

In Barrett's esophagus the stratified squamous epithelium is replaced by a circumferential columnar cell lining.

3. What cell type is crucial in identifying Barrett's esophagus?

The columnar epithelium of Barrett's esophagus can manifest in three varieties. The hallmark of the "specialized columnar epithelium" are the mucin-containing and -secreting **Goblet cells.** This histologic type comprises 80–95% of Barrett's esophagus and identifies the tissue as a focus of true intestinal metaplasia.

4. What can be done to enhance the staining of Goblet cells and subsequently improve their recognition?

Although Goblet cells respond to standard hematoxylin-eosin preparations, the use of alcian blue accents their presence significantly. Methylene blue is a vital stain that is occasionally used when obtaining the histologic specimen. This stain is selectively absorbed by the metaplastic epithelium when applied to living tissue. Hence, it aids in selecting sites for tissue sampling.

Various antibodies are also under investigation at the present time. 7E12H12 (also known as Mab DAS-1) is a monoclonal antibody directed against the Barrett's epithelium. This work is in a preliminary stages and has limited diagnostic use at present.

5. What stimulates this transition from the stratified squamous to immature columnar epithelium?

Reflux appears to be the main factor. The actual causative content is still a matter of argument. Some camps hold that the gastric acid is the key agent, while others state that bile acids or pancreatic enzymes contribute more substantially to the alteration of normal histology. The uniform opinion remains that Barrett's esophagus is an acquired condition that results from gastroesophageal reflux.

6. Why is the presence of Barrett's esophagus important?

Barrett's esophagus is by definition an area of metaplasia and as such has a definite association with the development of dysplasia and subsequent esophageal adenocarcinoma.

7. In whom does Barrett's esophagus most commonly occur?

The typical patient is a Caucasian male around 50–60 years of age at the time of diagnosis. The disease process is found infrequently in the African populations and male to female ratio is 3:1. Furthermore, patients with Barrett's esophagus have up to a 15% risk of eventually developing an esophageal adenocarcinoma. This represents at least a 40-fold increase over the incidence in the general population.

8. How do patients with Barrett's esophagus present?

Patients with Barrett's esophagus usually present with complaints arising from the primary pathologic process of reflux. Heartburn, dysphagia, and regurgitation are frequent at presentation.

9. Can patients with Barrett's esophagus be asymptomatic?

Yes. Long-standing exposure to gastroesophageal reflux can diminish the sensitivity of the esophageal mucosa. However, the absence of symptoms does not decrease the rate of dysplastic complications.

10. Besides esophageal adenocarcinoma, what other complications are associated with Barrett's esophagus?

Bleeding, esophageal stricture, ulceration, and mediastinitis are all possible complications from mucosal inflammation, dysplasia, or frank esophageal perforation.

11. How should these patients be evaluated?

While Barrett's esophagus may occur in asymptomatic patients, the possibility should be given substantial consideration in all patients with a history of long-standing gastroesophageal reflux disease (GERD) or symptoms suggestive of the associated complications. Swallow studies and contrast-enhanced radiographic techniques may demonstrate esophageal stricture and mucosal ulceration, but overall remain ineffective in detecting the fine tissue changes of this disease process. Similarly, nuclear medicine studies, potential difference testing, manometry, and pH studies are all described in the literature. Unfortunately, they too remain unreliable and nonspecific. The gold standard for detection and evaluation of Barrett's esophagus is endoscopy with biopsy.

12. How should the endoscopy and biopsy be performed?

The endoscopist needs to differentiate between the pink, sheen stratified squamous epithelium and the red, beefy areas of the columnar epithelium. Metaplastic regions may occur dispersely, but Barrett's esophagus typically arises in the area of the gastroesophageal junction and extends proximally. All grossly abnormal areas should be biopsied. Furthermore, in order to increase the test sensitivity to severe dysplasia and adenocarcinoma, circumferential regions of Barrett's esophagus should be sampled in each of the four quadrants every 2–3 cm in length. The normal-appearing tissue immediately adjacent to endoscopically abnormal esophageal mucosa should also be biopsied, as it tends to be an area of particular dysplasia and frequently missed malignancy.

13. Outline a reasonable medical treatment plan for the patient with Barrett's esophagus.

The medical treatment of Barrett's esophagus is the treatment of the underlying GERD. Patients should be advised to lose weight, refrain from eating before bedtime, elevate the head of their bed, and avoid large, fatty meals or known reflux-stimulating substances such as caffeine, alcohol, and nicotine.

Pharmacologic treatment includes the use of promotility agents, such as cisapride, and medications that decrease the secretion of gastric acid. H2-receptor blockers such as cimetidine and famotidine have proven efficacy, but fail to match the overall results of the proton pump inhibitors. Omeprazole and lansoprazole are the gold standard, but are expensive to use on a daily basis for an extended period of time.

The above steps can help reduce symptoms, but they do not reverse the histologic changes already in existence. Long-term follow-up of patients with effective medical management has shown very limited regrowth of islands of stratified squamous epithelium, yet the risk of progressive dysplasia and adenocarcinoma is unchanged.

14. At what point is surgical intervention warranted?

Surgical intervention should be considered in any patient who has no prohibitive operative risk following a reasonable trial of medical management. The excellent results obtained with laparoscopic Nissen fundoplication combined with the short recovery period make this procedure an extremely attractive option.

15. When do patients with known Barrett's esophagus need to be seen in follow-up?

There are no universally accepted protocols in the literature. However, a simple plan as set forth by the World Congress of the International Society of Diseases of the Esophagus in 1996 recommends follow-up endoscopy and biopsy every 2 years in patients who demonstrate no dysplasia on initial assessment. Individuals with low-grade dysplasia should be subject to annual exam and biopsy. Esophagectomy is recommended once high-grade dysplasia is detected and confirmed on repeat biopsy.

16. What options are available for the patient with epithelial dysplasia but prohibitive operative risk?

Esophagectomy is recommended for the patients with high-grade dysplasia detected on endoscopic biopsy. This recommendation is strengthened by studies showing that in up to 50% of these patients retrospective analyses of surgical specimens demonstrate carcinoma in situ.

Regardless of the specific operative technique used, esophagectomy is an inherently invasive procedure with substantial morbidity and mortality. Local endoscopic mucosal resection, Argon beam or YAG laser ablation, and photodynamic therapy are additional tools for patients with prohibitive operative risk. These less invasive techniques offer reduced rates of death and complication and hold considerable promise for the future, but have technical limitations and remain unable to detect or treat invasive adenocarcinoma.

BIBLIOGRAPHY

1. Brenner C, Brenner R: Barrett's esophagus. Surg Clin North Am 77:1115–1137, 1997.
2. Cameron A: Management of Barrett's esophagus. Mayo Clin Proc 73:457–461, 1998.
3. Fergusen M: Barrett's esophagus. In Baue AE, Geha AS (eds): Glenn's Thoracic and Cardiovascular Surgery, 6th ed. Stamford, CT, Appleton & Lange, 1996, pp 779–788.
4. Nandurkar S, Talley N: Barrett's esophagus: The long and short of it. Am J Gastroenterol 94:30–40, 1998.
5. Navaratnam R, Winsler M: Barrett's esophagus. Postgrad Med J 74:653–657, 1998.
6. Orringer M: Tumors of the esophagus. In Sabiston D (ed): Textbook of Surgery, 15th ed. Philadelphia, W.B. Saunders, 1997, pp 744–758.
7. Wolfe W, Sebastian M: Disorders of the esophagus in the adult: Benign and malignant tumors of the esophagus. In Sabiston D, Spencer F (eds): Surgery of the Chest, 6th ed. Philadelphia, W.B. Saunders, 1995, pp 919–934.

12. CAUSTIC ESOPHAGEAL INJURY

Jennifer I. Lin, M.D., Michael G. Caty, M.D., and Kathryn D. Anderson, M.D.

1. What is the most important first step in the evaluation of the child with a caustic ingestion?
To establish the patency of the airway. Alkaline substances can cause injury to the pharynx, larynx, or both. Ongoing swelling can obstruct the airway. Endotracheal intubation or tracheostomy may be necessary in these cases.

2. What substances do children ingest that may cause caustic injuries?
Both **acids** and **alkalis** are ingested. Strong alkalis in **household cleaners** are the most commonly ingested substances. Formerly battery acid was frequently ingested by toddlers. Bleach and ammonia do not usually injure children because they usually take only one swallow and stop their ingestion because of the taste.

3. What is the difference in injuries resulting from acid versus alkali?

Alkali	Acid
More viscous	Less viscous
Injury to proximal pharynx and esophagus	More distal injury
Deeper injury with liquefactive necrosis	Dramatic injury to stomach
	Coagulation necrosis

4. Describe the complications of caustic injuries.
The severity of complications relates to the depth of the injury. Superficial mucosal injury is painful but resolves without long-term sequelae. Deeper caustic injuries to the esophagus result in healing by fibrosis and subsequent stricture formation. Short-length esophageal strictures may require resection. Greater involvement of the esophagus may mandate esophageal replacement. Full-thickness injury to the esophagus may result in perforation and potential fistula formation to the trachea or, in extreme cases, the aorta.

5. Does it help to induce vomiting when a child has ingested a caustic substance?
No; vomiting is **contraindicated.** Regurgitation of a caustic substance can reinjure the esophagus, pharynx, or larynx. Regurgitation also places the child at risk for aspiration pneumonitis.

6. What age groups ingest caustic agents?
- Ingestion of corrosive substances: **< 5 years old** (boys more commonly than girls)
- Caustic ingestion as suicide attempts: **adolescent** (girls more commonly than boys)

7. When is esophagoscopy indicated to assess the potential injury to the esophagus?
Whenever a caustic injury is suspected. Esophagoscopy is best done within 24–48 hours after ingestion. The examination should be limited to the first level of injury to avoid perforation.

8. When is esophagoscopy contraindicated?
In any patient who lacks a secure airway. For example, in a patient presenting with stridor or evidence of pharyngeal burns, esophagoscopy without first controlling the airway may lead to a complete airway obstruction.

9. When is a contrast study indicated?
A contrast esophagogram with water-soluble contrast should be performed at the initial presentation if perforation is suspected and to assess the length of mucosal injury. An esophagogram is usually done 2–3 weeks after the ingestion to determine the presence of strictures.

10. How is an esophageal injury graded endoscopically?

0	Normal
I	Mucosal edema and hyperemia
IIa	Superficial injury
IIb	Superficial injury with limited areas of deeper or circumferential injury
IIIa	Small scattered necrotic areas
IIIb	Extensive necrosis

11. How does the endoscopic grade of the lesion affect patient management?
- For grade I injuries, no specific treatment is indicated. A contrast study may be performed after 2–3 weeks if symptoms of dysphagia are present.
- For more severe injuries, there is an increased risk of stricture formation. These patients require close follow-up with endoscopy and esophageal dilation.

12. List the indications for immediate surgical exploration.
- Free air in the peritoneum or mediastinum
- Evidence of contrast material extravasating from the esophagus or stomach
- Evidence of peritonitis

13. What is the role of antibiotics in managing caustic esophageal injury?
There are no data supporting the routine use of antibiotics as prophylaxis. Antibiotic therapy may be appropriate if there is evidence of systemic infection or transmural necrosis.

14. How is an esophageal stricture that results from a caustic ingestion managed?
Esophageal dilation should be performed, at least once a week, with a catheter that is 1–2F sizes smaller than the stricture. A lumen that remains inadequate after 9–12 months of frequent dilation suggests the presence of irreversible fibrosis, and resection of the stricture or replacement of the esophagus becomes necessary.

15. Is there an association between caustic injury to the esophagus and development of esophageal carcinoma?
Yes. There is a correlation between corrosive esophageal injuries and the development of esophageal carcinoma 15–20 years after the ingestion.

CONTROVERSY

16. Discuss the considerations of using steroid therapy in the management of corrosive injuries to the esophagus.
Theoretically, steroids would inhibit the inflammatory response and decrease the formation of strictures after a caustic ingestion. Although this has been shown in animal studies, no statistical benefits were demonstrated in trials conducted in human subjects. The use of high-dose dexamethasone in the management of caustic esophageal injuries also requires further study.

BIBLIOGRAPHY

1. Anderson KD, Rouse TM, Randolph JG: A controlled trial of corticosteroids in children with corrosive injury of the esophagus. N Engl J Med 323:637, 1990.
2. Millar AJW, Cywes S: Caustic strictures of the esophagus. In O'Neill JA, Rowe MI, Grosfeld JL Coran AG (eds): Pediatric Surgery, 5th ed. St. Louis, Mosby, 1998, pp 969–979.

13. ESOPHAGEAL PERFORATIONS

Mark R. Jajkowski, M.D., and Eddie L. Hoover, M.D.

1. What is the most common cause of esophageal perforation?

Most esophageal perforations (50–60%) are **iatrogenic,** resulting from endoscopy (leading cause), stricture dilation, operative injury, or nasogastric or endotracheal tube placement.

2. List other causes of esophageal perforation.
- Traumatic (20–25%)
- Barogenic (15%)
- Foreign bodies (7%)
- Carcinoma (7%)

3. What about the risk of esophageal perforation during endoscopy?

Risk of perforation may become less common as the use of rigid esophagoscopy decreases.

4. What is the distribution of perforations by location in the esophagus?
- Cervical, 25%
- Thoracic, 60%
- Abdominal, 15%

5. Discuss the mortality rate associated with esophageal perforation.

Esophageal perforation has a mortality rate of approximately 20%. This is due to the severe chemical mediastinitis or peritonitis and necrotizing infection that results from the leakage of GI secretions and oral flora. The mediastinitis is worse if the mediastinal pleura is not penetrated. Without perforation of the mediastinal pleura, a closed space infection results.

6. List mortality rates by site and by cause.

Site	Cause
Cervical, 6%	Instrumentation, 19%
Thoracic, 34%	Barogenic, 39%
Abdominal, 29%	Trauma, 5%

7. Where do perforations of the cervical esophagus usually occur?

Posteriorly, because the esophageal wall is thinnest in this area. **Iatrogenic** perforations are most common posteriorly and to the left side as a result of most endoscopists being right-handed.

8. Define Lannier's triangle.

The area of esophageal mucosa uncovered by muscularis and at high risk of perforation during instrumentation. Lannier's triangle is bordered by the pharyngeal inferior constrictor and the cricopharyngeus muscles.

9. List early signs of esophageal perforation in the cervical region.
- Neck stiffness or ache
- Hematemesis
- Odynophagia
- Subcutaneous emphysema in the neck
- Tachycardia
- Tachypnea
- A general sense of discomfort*

*The patient may describe a feeling of not being able to "get comfortable" or "not feeling right."

10. How is an esophageal perforation best diagnosed?

Contrast radiography is the standard method of diagnosis of a cervical esophageal perforation. We recommend using water-soluble contrast material because extravasation of this material may cause less of an inflammatory reaction and be less problematic at the time of surgery. Some authors prefer dilute barium sulfate, and others use a barium study if an initial water-soluble contrast study is negative. Regardless of the method, there is approximately a 10% false-negative rate associated with this modality. Endoscopy should not be relied on to visualize an esophageal perforation.

11. How is a cervical esophageal perforation treated?

Exploration of the esophagus is carried out through a left neck incision anterior to the sternocleidomastoid muscle and carotid sheath but lateral to the thyroid and trachea. Once the perforation is identified and débrided, it may be closed with a single-layer monofilament, nonabsorbable suture, although almost any reasonable suture closure gives a satisfactory result. The key to success is obtaining viable tissue. If the tissues are viable and have sufficient strength, reinforcement is probably not necessary. The neck and superior mediastinum are drained with a closed-suction catheter. Preoperatively, antibiotic coverage of oral flora is given. If the perforation is unable to be identified, drainage catheters are placed, and the operation is terminated.

12. In the presence of a perforation of the thoracic esophagus, on which side will a pleural effusion most likely develop?

Left.

13. Define Boerhaave's syndrome.

First described by Boerhaave in 1724, after autopsy of the High Admiral of the Dutch Navy, the Baron van Wessenaer. This refers to a barogenic rupture of the esophagus. The tear usually occurs longitudinally and lies on the left posterolateral wall of the esophagus 2–6 cm above the diaphragm. This rupture usually follows an intense episode of retching and vomiting and usually drains into the left pleural space or peritoneum.

14. Define Mackler's triad.

History of (1) vomiting, (2) sudden lower thoracic pain, and (3) subcutaneous emphysema at the base of the neck associated with a barogenic perforation.

15. List absolute indications for the operative treatment of an esophageal perforation.
- Pneumothorax
- Pneumoperitoneum
- Sepsis
- Shock
- Failure of nonoperative management (e.g., abscess, empyema)

16. Discuss the surgical treatment of a perforation of the thoracic esophagus.

The esophagus is approached through a right thoracotomy in the fifth to sixth intercostal space for lesions in the upper two thirds of the esophagus. The lower one third of the esophagus is reached through a left thoracotomy in the sixth to seventh intercostal space. If treated within 24 hours, the perforation may be closed in two layers (inner absorbable layer and outer nonabsorbable layer) after débridement of necrotic tissue. All of the tissue in the area may have a green discoloration and appear slimy and necrotic because of staining from gastric contents. All of this tissue cannot be débrided, and it is important to look at the mucosal edges for evidence of viability. It is advisable to buttress the repair with a mediastinal pleural pedicle flap, intercostal muscle, gastric wall (Thal patch), or a strip of diaphragm. If the last-mentioned is used, the strip should not be taken in a radial fashion so as not to denervate the diaphragm. Two large chest tubes are left in place for drainage of the mediastinum and pleural spaces.

17. What principles are adhered to when primarily repairing an esophageal perforation?
- Débridement of necrotic tissue
- Myotomy so as to expose the full extent of the mucosal injury
- Mucosal closure with reinforcement and drainage of the area

For drainage purposes, a right-angled chest tube sutured into the sulcus with 2–0 chromic catgut is recommended.

18. Is reinforcement of the primary repair always necessary?
The literature historically shows that without reinforcement primary repair carries a mortality rate of 25% and a fistula rate of 39%, in contrast to 6% and 13% rates for reinforced repairs. The key to success of primary repair probably lies in the viability of the tissues. If the tissues are healthy, reinforcement is an option but is probably not necessary.

19. List the options for repair reinforcement.
- Cervical — strap muscles
- Thoracic — intercostal muscles, diaphragm, pleura, gastric wall
- Abdominal — omentum, gastric wall

20. What are the criteria for nonoperative management of an esophageal perforation?
- Confinement of the perforation to the mediastinum
- Perforation is well drained back into the esophagus
- Patient has few to no symptoms
- No signs of sepsis

21. How is an esophageal perforation managed nonoperatively?
- NPO
- Broad-spectrum antibiotics for 1–2 weeks
- Drainage of any pleural effusions
- Total parenteral nutrition
- Nasogastric tube placed proximal to the perforation for drainage of oral secretions

22. What is the difference between early and late diagnosis of an esophageal perforation?
Early diagnosis is made within 24 hours of the perforation, and beyond this is considered late diagnosis. This is an important distinction because perforations >24 hours old are less likely to heal spontaneously or with primary closure. Early diagnosis carries a mortality rate of 15%, whereas late diagnosis has an associated 33–55% mortality. The golden period for closure of an esophageal perforation is within the first 12 hours. After 24 hours, at least half of primary repairs leak.

23. How is a late esophageal perforation treated?
Several methods have been devised and employed. We prefer operative débridement of the area and placement of a T tube or Malecot tube for larger defects into the esophagus for drainage. This creates a controlled esophagocutaneous fistula. The mediastinum is drained with multiple chest tubes, including a right-angled tube sutured into the sulcus with chromic catgut. Some authors also describe success with primary repair, reinforcement, and drainage if there is evidence of tissue viability. Resection is reserved for massive necrosis or the presence of a malignant obstruction. Alternatively an intraluminal stent may be placed in a patient with terminal, malignant disease. We prefer the expandable Wallstent, which is commonly used for prevention of bronchial stenosis in lung transplant patients.

BIBLIOGRAPHY

1. Abbott OA, Mansour KA, et al: Atraumatic so-called "spontaneous" rupture of the esophagus: A review of 47 personal cases with comments on a new method of surgical therapy. J Thorac Cardiovasc Surg 59:67–83, 1970.
2. Balkan ME, Ozdulger A, Tastepe L: One-stage operation for treatment after delayed diagnosis of thoracic esophageal perforation. Scand Cardiovasc J 31:111–115, 1997.
3. Bufkin BL, Miller JI Jr, Mansour KA: Esophageal perforation: Emphasis on management. Ann Thorac Surg 61:1447–1452, 1996.
4. Fell S: Esophageal perforation. In Pearson FG, et al (eds): Esophageal Surgery. New York, Churchill Livingstone, 1995, pp 495–515.
5. Handy JR, Reed CE: Esophageal injury. In Baue AE, et al (eds): Glenn's Thoracic and Cardiovascular Surgery. Stamford, CT, Appleton & Lange, 1996, pp 747–759.
6. McFadden DW, Zinner MJ: Benign disorders of the esophagus. In Zinner MJ, Schwartz SI, Ellis H (eds): Maingot's Abdominal Operations. Stamford, CT, Appleton & Lange, 1997, pp 843–858.
7. Scott-Mackie PL, Morgan RA, Mason R, Adam A: Treatment of a malignant esophageal perforation with a prototype conical Wallstent. Cardiovasc Interven Radiol 21:501–502, 1998.
8. Subhash P, Donahue PE: Esophageal perforation. In Wastell C, Nyhus LM, Donahue PE (eds): Surgery of the Esophagus, Stomach, and Small Intestine. Boston, Little, Brown, 1995, pp 344–350.
9. Symbas PN, Hatcher CR Jr, Harlaftis N: Spontaneous rupture of the esophagus. Ann Surg 187:634–640, 1978.
10. Symbas PN, Logan WD, Hatcher CR Jr, Abbott OA: Factors in the successful recognition and management of esophageal perforation. South Med J 59:1090–1096, 1966.
11. Wang N, Razzouk AJ, et al: Delayed primary repair of intrathoracic esophageal perforation: Is it safe? J Thorac Cardiovasc Surg 111:114–122, 1996.

14. BENIGN ESOPHAGEAL NEOPLASMS

Reginald Abraham, M.D.

1. What is the incidence of all benign esophageal neoplasms?
<1%

2. What is the most common presentation of a benign mass in the esophagus?
Dysphagia or substernal chest discomfort (or both). The esophagus can accommodate the gradual growth of a benign tumor mass.

3. What is the typical growth pattern?
Slow and balloonlike, compressing surrounding tissue.

4. Why do benign tumors present after many years and remain clinically silent?
There is often spontaneous cessation of growth, and the tumor may not change in size for many years.

5. At what size does obstruction of the esophageal lumen start to occur?
5 cm

6. Which benign tumors behave as if they were peptic strictures or cancer?
Annular constricting tumors, such as leiomyoma.

7. Describe the four layers of the esophagus.
   1. Inner mucosa
        Nonkeratinized stratified squamous epithelium
        Lamina propria—loose connective tissue with esophageal cardiac glands
        Muscularis mucosa—smooth muscle
   2. Submucosa—loose coonective tissue with few, widely spaced glands
   3. Muscularis propria (striated upper third, mixed mid third, smooth lower third)
        Inner circular
        Outer longitudinal
   4. Tunica adventitia—outer loose areolar tissue, which is replaced by serosa at gastro-esophageal junction

8. What lies between the circular and longitudinal muscles?
Autonomic myenteric plexus.

9. List the tumor types occurring in each of the four esophageal layers.

Mucosal layer	Submucosal layer
• Squamous papilloma	• Hemangioma
• Inflammatory pseudotumor	• Granular cell tumors
• Mucous retention cyst	• Neurilemoma
• Fibrovascular polyp	
• Adenomas	

Muscularis propria	Adventitial layer*
• Leiomyoma	• Schwannoma
• Rhabdomyoma	• Fibroma
• Neurofibroma	• Choristoma
• Granular cell tumor	

*Benign tumors occur rarely.

10. What is the most common benign intramural tumor?
Leiomyoma (67%).

11. How are most benign esophageal lesions found?
Serendipitously.

12. What has the highest yield for diagnosis?
Esophagoscopy, after careful history and physical examination.

13. List other diagnostic modalities that are helpful.
- Barium swallow
- Cine esophagogram
- Double-contrast radiographs
- CT-MRI
- Endoluminal ultrasound

14. Which are the echo-poor areas by endoluminal ultrasound?
The second and fourth layers (i.e., the muscularis propria). Leiomyomata arise from here.

15. What is the endoscopic appearance of a hemangioma?
Blue-gray, easily compressible submucosal polypoid mass.

16. Should biopsy be attempted if the mucosa is intact?
No, because they bleed.

17. What misdiagnosis can be applied to larger benign tumors?
Achalasia, especially if there is progressive esophageal dilation with pedunculated fibrovascular polyps.

18. What is the most common site of squamous cell papilloma?
Lower third of the esophagus.

19. Name a common malignant differential diagnosis for squamous cell papilloma.
Verrucous squamous cell carcinoma.

20. When is excision indicated?
- Obstructing symptoms
- Inability to rule out malignancy

21. What is the common location for fibrovascular polyps?
The upper esophagus, below the cricopharyngeus muscle sphincter.

22. What are the limitations for endoscopic excision?
- Size < 2 cm
- A thin pedicle

23. List five points that must be kept in mind regarding excision.
1. Pedunculated polyps are mobile inside the gullet and range over a distance of several inches.
2. Proper contrast examination is necessary for correct diagnosis.
3. Site of origin, size of the polyp, and thickness of pedicle must be determined at esophagoscopy, endoluminal ultrasound is helpful.
4. Aspiration is a dangerous complication if esophagoscopy is performed under local anesthesia.

5. Resection is indicated to prevent fatal asphyxiation from acute laryngeal obstruction.

24. What is the histologic origin of granular cell tumors?
Perineural (Schwann's cell).

25. What endoscopic appearance suggests the diagnosis of granular cell tumors?
Molar on the gingiva (as in a tooth).

26. Is endoscopic removal of a granular cell tumor advised?
No. The tumor is submucosal, and the tendency to recur with incomplete removal is high. Although these tumors remain stable over long durations, benign and malignant forms are similar, and surgical excision (enucleation by thoracotomy) for lesions > 2 cm is advised.

27. Where are inflammatory pseudotumors found?
Usually in the lower third of the esophagus (may be related to the mucosal ulceration).

28. What feature is most important with an inflammatory pseudotumor?
Distinguishing it from carcinoma.

29. What is the treatment for a reflux gastroesophageal polyp?
Treat the underlying problem (the reflux).

30. Who first described the esophageal leiomyoma?
Virchow, in 1863.

31. Where are leiomyomata located?
At all levels of the esophagus, more often in the lower third. They are usually discovered incidentally.

32. Describe the typical clinical characteristics of leiomyomata?
Sessile, firm to touch, round, eccentric, and lobulated. They are gray-white on section and consist of whorls of smooth muscle surrounded by a fibrous tissue capsule.

33. What is the epidemiology of esophageal leiomyoma?
Women in their 20s and 30s. They are associated with vulvar leiomyomata (Alport's syndrome).

34. What is the treatment for leiomyomata?
Lesions ≤2 cm or smaller can be watched. Rapidly growing (rare), symptomatic, or larger lesions must be enucleated. Diffuse symptomatic leiomyomatosis may have to be treated by esophagectomy.

35. What is thought to be the origin of esophageal cysts?
They are classified as developmental cysts arising from persistent vacuoles in the wall of the foregut during the development of the trachea and esophagus. They are the second most common tumorlike condition of the esophagus.

36. How can these cysts be distinguished by CT scan?
- Low density
- Fluid-filled
- Cyst content

37. How should symptomatic cysts or cysts increasing in size be managed?
Extramucosal resection.

38. To keep the problem of benign esophageal neoplasms in perspective, what percentage of benign esophageal tumors are symptomatic?
  <1%.

BIBLIOGRAPHY

1. Baue AE, Geha AS, Hammond GL, et al: Glenn's Thoracic and Cardiovascular Surgery, 6th ed. Stamford, CT, Appleton & Lange, 1996.
2. Coutinho DS, Soga J, Yoshikawa T, et al: Granular cell tumors of the esophagus: A report of two cases and review of the literature. Am J Gastroenterol 80:758, 1985.
3. Franco KL, Putnam JB: Advanced Therapy in Thoracic Surgery. Hamilton, Ontario, B.C. Decker, 1998.
4. Pearson FG, Deslauriers J, Ginsberg RJ, et al: Esophageal Surgery. New York, Churchill Livingstone, 1995.
5. Pearson FG, Deslauriers J, Ginsberg RJ, et al: Thoracic Surgery. New York, Churchill Livingstone, 1995.
6. Seremetis MG, Lyons WS, DeGuzman VC, et al: Leiomyomata of the esophagus: An analysis of 838 cases. Cancer 41:717, 1961.
7. Shields TW (ed): General Thoracic Surgery, 4th ed. Baltimore, Williams & Wilkins, 1994.
8. Van Lanschott JJ, Poublon RM, Zonderland HM, et al: Benign pedunculated tumors of the esophagus. Neth J Surg 39:83, 1987.

15. CANCER OF THE ESOPHAGUS

Carmine M. Volpe, M.D.

1. What is the annual incidence of esophageal cancer in the United States?

In 1998, 12,000 new cases of esophageal cancer were diagnosed, and an estimated 11,000 people died of their disease. The male-to-female ratio is 3:1. In most part of the world, including the United States, the incidence rates are 2–5 per 100,000 population. In endemic regions, this rate often exceeds 100 per 100,000 population.

2. Identify areas of the world considered endemic for esophageal cancer.

Northern provinces of China, the Transkei region of South Africa, the Normandy and Brittany provinces of France, the Gonbad region of Northern Iran, and the region of Asia northeast of the Caspian Sea. An **esophageal cancer belt** runs from northern China to the Middle East.

3. What are the most common histologic cell types?

Squamous cell and **adenocarcinoma**. Previously, squamous cell carcinoma (SCC) accounted for > 95% of esophageal malignancies. Since 1980, the incidence of adenocarcinoma dramatically increased, now accounting for a third of all esophageal cancers.

4. Describe the distribution of esophageal SCC.

In the United States, approximately 20% of SCC involves the upper third of the esophagus, from the cricopharyngeus to the aortic arch, a distance of 25 cm from the incisors endoscopically. About 50% of SCC occur in the middle third from the aortic arch to the inferior pulmonary vein, 25–32 cm from the incisors. The remaining 30% occur in the distal third of the esophagus, corresponding to a distance of 33–42 cm from the incisors.

5. Describe the distribution of adenocarcinoma.

Nearly 90% of adenocarcinomas occur in the distal third of the esophagus. Most of the remaining adenocarcinomas develop in the middle third, whereas only 1–2% arise in the upper third.

6. List the major risk factors for esophageal SCC.

In **endemic areas**:
- Ingestion of nitrosamines
- Consumption of food contaminated with fungi, most often *Geotrichum candidum*
- Hot beverages
- Betel leaf chewing
- Tobacco chewing

In **low-risk populations as well as in the high-risk European populations**
- Cigarette smoking
- Alcohol consumption (beer and liquor)
- Low socioeconomic status
- Diets deficient in fruits and vegetables

7. List the risk factors associated with esophageal adenocarcinoma.

- Cigarette smoking
- Low socioeconomic status
- Obesity
- Gastroesophageal reflux

8. Name and describe the lesions and conditions that are considered to be premalignant and predispose to the development of esophageal carcinoma.

- Achalasia
- Caustic strictures (lye)
- Barrett's esophagus (adenocarcinoma)
- Plummer-Vinson syndrome (sideropenic dysphagia)
- Tylosis
- History of head and neck SCC
- Esophageal diverticulum

Caustic strictures pose a risk for esophageal SCC 1000-fold greater than the general population. The latency period from the time of ingestion to the development of cancer is about 40 years. The incidence of Plummer-Vinson syndrome is highest in Scandinavia and Great Britain, typically seen in elderly women with iron deficiency anemia, atrophic oral mucosa, and cervical esophageal webs, in which cancers usually arise.

9. Describe the genetic alterations most often observed in esophageal cancers.

Esophageal cancer is a disorder of the tumor-suppressor gene system. *p53* gene mutations located on the short arm (p) of chromosome 17 are seen in at least half of all esophageal cancers. Other altered genes include the *APC* (adenosis polyposis coli) gene located on chromosome 5q, *CDKN2* (cyclin-dependent kinase 4 inhibitor) gene on chromosome 9p and *Rb* (retinoblastoma) gene on chromosome 13q. Loss of heterozygosity, homozygous deletion, and hypermethylation are mechanisms of inactivation (mutations) that commonly occur in these growth-suppressive genes.

10. Is esophageal cancer an inherited disease?

Yes. **Tylosis** (hereditary hyperkeratosis palmaris et plantaris) is an autosomal dominant disorder characterized by thickening of the skin on the palms and soles and is associated with a high risk of esophageal SCC. It usually presents with oral hyperkeratosis and follicular hyperkeratosis at 7–8 years of age. Nearly 50% of affected individuals develop esophageal cancer by age 45 and 95% by age 70. Tylosis is one of the palmoplantar keratodermas, a complex group of hereditary syndromes classified according to the presence or absence of epidermolysis and pattern of disease, focal or diffuse. Tylosis is a focal, nonepidermolytic form of palmoplantar keratoderma. The **tylosis oesophageal gene locus (TOC)** has been mapped to a 1-cM region on the long arm (q) of chromosome 17 by linkage analysis.

11. Is there any role for mass screening and surveillance of asymptomatic individuals?

The overall incidence of esophageal cancer is too low to justify mass screening in the United States. Low-risk countries should offer individuals with Barrett's esophagus, achalasia, caustic strictures, history of head and neck cancers, and with tylosis some form of surveillance.

BIBLIOGRAPHY

1. Chow WH, Blot WJ, Vaughan TL, et al: Body mass index and risk of adenocarcinomas of the esophagus and gastric cardia. J Natl Cancer Inst 90:150–155, 1988.
2. Dolan K, Garde J, Gosney J, et al. Allelotype analysis of oesophageal adenocarcinoma: Loss of heterozygosity occurs at multiple sites. Br J Cancer 78:950–957, 1998.
3. Endoscopic survellance of Barrett's esophagus: A cost-effectiveness comparison with mammographic surveillance for breast cancer. Am J Gastroenterol 93:911–915, 1998.
4. Gammon MD, Schoenberg JB, Ahsan H, et al: Tobacco, alcohol, and socioeconomic status and adenocarcinomas of the esophagus and gastric cardia. J Natl Cancer Inst 89:1277–1284, 1997.
5. Gore RM: Esophageal cancer: Clinical and pathologic features. Radiol Clin North Am 35:243–263, 1997.
6. Kelsell DP, Risk JM, Leigh IM, et al: Close mapping of the focal non-epidermolytic palmoplantar keratoderma (PPK) locus associated with oesophageal cancer (TOC). Hum Mol Genet 5:857–860, 1996.
7. Lagergren J, Bergstrom R, Lindgren A, et al: Symptomatic gastroesophageal reflux as a risk factor for esophageal adenocarcinoma. N Engl J Med 340:825–832, 1999.

8. Landis SH, Murray T, Bolden S, et al: Cancer 1998 statistics. CA Cancer J Clin 48:6–31, 1998.

9. Orringer MB: Tumors, injuries, and miscellaneous conditions of the esophagus. In Greenfield LJ, Mulholland MW, Oldham KT, et al (eds): Surgery Scientific Principles and Practice, 2nd ed. Philadelphia, Lippincott-Raven, 1997, pp 735–745.

10. Orringer MB: Tumors of the esophagus. In Sabiston DC (ed): Textbook of Surgery: The Biological Basis of Modern Surgical Practice, 15th ed. Philadelphia, W.B. Saunders, 1997, pp 744–759.

11. Shi ST, Yang GY, Wang LD, et al: Role of p53 gene mutations in human esophageal carcinogenesis: Results from immunohistochemical and mutation analyses of carcinomas and nearby non-cancerous lesions. Carcinogenesis 20:591–597, 1999.

12. Von Brevern M, Hollstein MC, Risk JM, et al: Loss of heterozygosity in sporadic oesophageal tumors in the tylosis oesophageal cancer (TOC) gene region of chromosome 17q. Oncogene 17:2101–2105, 1998.

13. Xing EP, Nie Y, Song Y, et al: Mechanisms of inactivation of p14[ARF], p15[INK4b], and p16[INK4a] genes in human esophageal squamous cell carcinoma. Clin Cancer Res 5:2704–2714, 1999.

14. Zhou X, Suzuki H, Shimada Y, et al: Genomic DNA and messenger RNA expression alterations of the CDKN2B and CDKN2 genes in esophageal squamous carcinoma cell lines. Genes Chromosomes Cancer 13:285–290, 1995.

16. STAGING OF ESOPHAGEAL CARCINOMA

Vivian Lindfield M.D., and Carmine M. Volpe, M.D.

1. What is clinical staging of esophageal cancer based on?
Clinical staging evaluates on the **anatomic extent** of the primary tumor. This can be determined before treatment with the following:
- Thorough history and physical examination
- Biopsy
- Laboratory studies
- Imaging and endoscopic examination

2. Is there a difference between clinical and pathologic staging?
Yes. Pathologic staging is based on surgical exploration and examination of the resected esophagus. It also is based on associated lymph nodes that may have been resected with the tumor.

3. Describe the staging of the primary tumor (T) in esophageal carcinoma.

Tx	Primary tumor cannot be assessed
T0	No evidence of primary tumor
Tis	Carcinoma *in situ*
T1	Tumor invades lamina propria or submucosa
T2	Tumor invades muscularis propria
T3	Tumor invades adventitia
T4	Tumor invades adjacent structures

4. Describe the staging for regional lymph nodes (N) in esophageal carcinoma.

Nx	Regional lymph nodes cannot be assessed
N0	No nodes present
N1	Regional lymph node metastasis

5. Describe the staging for distant metastasis (M) in esophageal carcinoma.

Mx	Distant metastasis cannot be assessed
M0	No distant metastasis
M1	Distant metastasis

6. What are the regional lymph nodes associated with the cervical esophagus and the intrathoracic esophagus?

Cervical Esophagus	Intrathoracic Esophagus
Scalene	Tracheobronchial
Internal jugular	Superior mediastinal
Upper cervical	Peritracheal
Periesophageal	Carinal
Supraclavicular	Hilar
Cervical	Periesophageal
	Perigastric
	Paracardial

7. What is a distant metastasis in esophageal carcinoma?
Involvement of more distant lymph nodes (i.e., **celiac nodes** or **cervical nodes**).

8. Describe the metastasis (M) classification for tumors of the thoracic esophagus.

Tumors of upper thoracic esophagus:

M1a	Metastasis in cervical nodes
M1b	Other distant metastasis

Tumors of midthoracic esophagus:

M1a	Not applicable
M1b	Nonregional nodes or other distant metastasis

Tumors of lower thoracic esophagus:

M1a	Metastasis in celiac lymph nodes
M1b	Other distant metastasis

9. Why is the M1a category not applicable for midthoracic esophageal tumors?

Tumors in this area with metastasis in distant lymph nodes have an equally poor prognosis as tumors with metastasis in distant sites.

10. Describe the stages of esophageal carcinoma based on the TMN system.

STAGE	TUMOR	NODES	METASTASIS
0	Tis	N0	M0
1	T1	N0	M0
2a	T2	N0	M0
	T3	N0	M0
2b	T1	N1	M0
	T2	N1	M0
3	T3	N1	M0
	T4	any N	M0
4	any T	any N	M1
4a	any T	any N	M1a
4b	any T	any N	M1b

11. List prognostic factors for esophageal carcinoma.
- Anatomic location
- Depth of invasion of the tumor (T)
- T, N, and M categories (independently)

12. What are the different histologic types of esophageal carcinoma?
- Squamous cell carcinoma (more common)
- Adenocarcinoma

13. Is the histologic type of cell found in the carcinoma important for prognosis?

No. An exception to this is found in **T1 lesions,** in which adenocarcinoma tends to be more favorable compared with squamous cell lesions.

14. List the methods for staging of esophageal carcinoma.
- Complete history and physical examination
- Chest radiograph
- Pulmonary function tests
- Laboratory tests
- CT scans of the chest and abdomen
- Bronchoscopy
- Endoscopic ultrasound (EUS)
- Video-assisted thoracoscopic surgery
- Positron emission tomography (PET)

15. How can EUS improve clinical staging?

- It provides imaging of the malignant esophageal mass and its relationship to the esophageal wall.
- It can provide evidence of depth of invasion through the layers of the wall.
- It provides a better way of assessing the T stage of the tumor with relative ease.
- It can assess whether the tumor is intraesophageal or extraesophageal.
- It is useful in the assessment of lymph nodes.

16. Compare the accuracy of EUS versus CT scan.

	EUS	CT SCAN
Determining tumor stage	80–90%	60%
Staging regional lymph nodes	80%	50%
Assessing early esophageal tumors	Good	Ineffective*
Assessing distant metastasis	Poor	Good

*CT scan is ineffective at differentiating early-stage tumors from more advanced tumors.

17. Discuss the surgical methods or invasive techniques available for staging.

- **Mediastinoscopy** is the classic approach to sampling of mediastinal lymph nodes. There are limitations, however: aortopulmonary window nodes, subcarinal nodes, and left paraaortic nodes are difficult to assess using this method
- **Thoracoscopic procedures** provide easier access to these difficult node locations. Thoracoscopy is as useful for lymph node staging in esophageal carcinoma as mediastinoscopy is for lung carcinoma. This method is minimally invasive and well tolerated by patients.

18. What is the goal of preoperative staging?

To identify patients who would benefit from further therapies: radiation, chemotherapy, or both in the neoadjuvant or adjuvant setting.

19. What is the role of PET scanning in esophageal tumors?

PET can be used to assess areas of increased metabolism that may be associated with malignancies. PET scans improve the ability to identify distant metastasis that may be missed by more conventional methods. PET scans, however, are not as accurate at identifying small regional lymph nodes compared with other methods, such as CT scans. PET scans can be used to identify those that could be considered for resection by identifying early metastases that may otherwise be missed.

BIBLIOGRAPHY

1. American Joint Committee on Cancer: Manual for Staging of Cancer, 5th ed. Philadelphia, Lippincott-Raven, 1998, pp 65–69.
2. Block MI, et al: Improvement in staging of esophageal cancer with the addition of positron emission tomography. Ann Thorac Surg 64:770–777, 1997.
3. Botet JF: Preoperative staging of esophageal cancer: Comparison of endoscopic ultrasound and dynamic CT. Radiology 181:419–425, 1991.
4. Brugge WR, et al: Endoscopic ultrasound staging criteria for esophageal cancer. Gastrointest Endosc 45:147–152, 1997.
5. Krasna MJ: Advances in staging of esophageal carcinoma. Chest 113:107S–111S, 1998.
6. Lightdale CJ, Botet JF: Esophageal carcinoma: Pre-operative staging and evaluation of anastomotic recurrence. Gastrointest Endosc 36(suppl):S11–S16, 1990.
7. Luketich JD, et al: Role of positron emission tomography in staging esophageal cancer. Ann Thorac Surg 64:765–769, 1997.
8. Tio TL, et al: Endosonography in the clinical staging of esophagogastric carcinoma. Gastrointest Endosc 36(suppl):S2–S10, 1990.

17. SURGICAL APPROACHES FOR ESOPHAGEAL CANCER

John D. Urschel, M.D.

1. What are the goals of esophagectomy for esophageal cancer?
- Palliate dysphagia
- Perform a **curative** cancer resection
- Minimize morbidity

2. What is the difference between a palliative and a curative esophagectomy for cancer?

If there is residual microscopic disease, the resection is termed an **R1 resection.** If there is residual macroscopic disease, the resection is termed an **R2 resection.** R1 and R2 resections are considered palliative, or incomplete, resections. A curative, or **R0 esophagectomy,** is defined by complete removal of the cancer (negative resection margins) and any involved lymph nodes (adequate lymphadenectomy). Although a curative (R0) resection does not guarantee cure, a palliative resection almost always results in cancer recurrence.

3. What is a lymph node ratio?

The lymphatic equivalent of tumor resection margins (**ratio of invaded to removed nodes**). It is important prognostically, and it is an indicator of completeness of resection. A ratio of <0.2 (20% of examined nodes positive for metastatic cancer) suggests a complete (R0) resection and a more favorable prognosis than higher ratios.

4. List the most important shortcomings of surgical therapy of esophageal cancer.
- >70% of patients eventually die of their malignancy.
- Approximately 10% of patients (less in high-volume centers) die postoperatively.
- Respiratory failure and anastomotic leaks are common causes of postoperative mortality.

5. Do cervical esophagogastric anastomoses have a greater propensity to leak than intrathoracic esophagogastric anastomoses?

Yes. The exact reasons are not completely understood. Experienced surgeons report leakage of the cervical esophagogastric anastomosis in >10% of patients. The incidence of intrathoracic anastomotic leakage is often <5%.

6. Does the location (neck or chest) of the anastomosis affect the severity of an anastomotic leak?

Yes. Intrathoracic leaks are less frequent than cervical anastomotic leaks, but they are generally more life-threatening. It is easier to drain a cervical leak; the neck incision is opened at the bedside and packed. It is a mistake to underestimate the lethal potential of cervical esophagogastric anastomotic leaks. Constructing an anastomosis in the neck does not guarantee that a leak will not contaminate the mediastinum.

7. What are the consequences of postoperative recurrent laryngeal nerve palsy?
- Hoarse voice
- Difficulty coughing
- Increased risk for pulmonary aspiration

8. Discuss the advantages and disadvantages of the transhiatal (laparotomy and cervico-tomy) esophagectomy.

Advantages	Disadvantages
• Near-total esophagectomy (generous proximal margin)	• Imprecision in esophageal and lymph node dissection
• Anastomosis in the neck (less severe leaks)	• Anastomosis in the neck (more frequent leaks)
• Reduced pain (no thoracotomy)	• Risk of recurrent laryngeal nerve injury

Transhiatal esophagectomy is best suited for tumors of the distal esophagus, but some enthusiasts use it for midthoracic tumors as well. Although the transhiatal esophagectomy has been criticized from an oncologic point of view, cancer survival appears equivalent to transthoracic esophagectomy approaches. Proponents of transhiatal esophagectomy often claim that this approach reduces pulmonary morbidity. There is no evidence to support this claim. Postesophagectomy pulmonary morbidity is multifactorial; the presence or absence of a thoracotomy incision is not the key issue.

9. List the advantages and disadvantages of the Lewis-Tanner (laparotomy and right thoracotomy) esophagectomy.

Advantages	Disadvantages
• Precise esophageal and lymph node dissection under direct vision	• Anastomosis in the chest (leaks often highly morbid)
• Anastomosis in the chest (low incidence of leaks)	• Pain from the thoracotomy (epidural catheter helpful)
• Infrequent recurrent laryngeal nerve injury	• Less than total esophagectomy

This approach is broadly applicable in esophageal cancer surgery.

10. Discuss the advantages and disadvantages of the McKeown (laparotomy, right thoracotomy, and cervicotomy) esophagectomy.

This approach is particularly useful for tumors of the proximal and midthoracic esophagus. It permits dissection under direct vision and a near-total esophagectomy. It combines the other advantages and disadvantages of the two previously discussed approaches (thoracotomy needed, anastomosis in the neck). This approach is time-consuming (three different positions), but it can be modified to reduce operating time. All three incisions can be made with a single patient positioning (French position) if the surgeon is willing to sacrifice exposure in both the chest and the abdomen. Alternatively the thoracotomy can be done first, then the laparotomy and cervicotomy done together (only one position change).

11. Discuss the advantages and disadvantages of the left thoracoabdominal esophagogastrectomy.

This approach gives excellent exposure to the stomach and distal esophagus, but the aortic arch and great vessels hamper exposure of the proximal esophagus. It is best suited to tumors of the gastric cardia. Disadvantages include:

• Painful incision
• Intrathoracic anastomosis
• Propensity for postoperative reflux
• Temptation to accept a close proximal resection margin

The operation has a bad reputation because too many surgeons accept inadequate proximal resection margins; anastomotic recurrences are common. One can obtain a better proximal margin and construct the anastomosis above the aortic arch if a second intercostal incision (same skin incision) is made to facilitate proper exposure. Alternatively, this approach can be combined with a left cervicotomy for the anastomosis.

12. Do laparoscopic and thoracoscopic approaches for esophagectomy reduce perioperative morbidity?

These approaches probably do not reduce morbidity. **Thoracoscopic esophagectomy** appears to cause more pulmonary morbidity than conventional operations. Prolonged intraoperative single-lung ventilation may be responsible. **Laparoscopic esophagectomy** (modification of the transhiatal operation) is more appealing, but it is technically demanding. Its role is not yet defined.

13. What are the common causes of esophagogastric anastomotic leaks?

Leaks are multifactorial in origin, but **technical errors** and **inadequate perfusion of the gastric conduit** are the common causes. The fundus of the stomach or the proximal tip of the gastroplasty tube often has marginal tissue perfusion.

14. Are anastomotic leaks less common with stapled esophagogastric anastomoses?

No. Equivalent leak rates are shown for stapled and hand-sewn anastomoses; either technique is acceptable.

15. What is the best method for performing a hand-sewn esophagogastric anastomosis?

Single-layer, two-layer, interrupted, and running suture methods are all acceptable. The skill with which a surgeon applies an anastomotic technique is more important than the choice of anastomotic technique itself.

16. What are the keys to good outcomes in esophageal cancer surgery?

Well-trained and experienced surgeons working in high-volume centers.

CONTROVERSIES

17. Discuss the three major areas of controversy in the surgical treatment of esophageal cancer.

Controversies in (1) operative approach, (2) extent of resection, and (3) multimodality treatment are interrelated. For example, certain operative approaches (transhiatal esophagectomy) are suitable for conservative esophageal resections, whereas other approaches (transthoracic) are needed to accomplish a radical esophagectomy. Similarly, clinicians favoring radical surgery for esophageal cancer often question the need for additional chemotherapy and radiotherapy, whereas surgeons performing conservative esophageal resections emphasize the need for effective systemic therapy.

18. A surgeon's goal is to achieve a complete (R0) resection. In practical terms, how extensive should the esophageal resection (and lymphadenectomy) be?

The definition of a complete, or R0, resection, is not as straightforward as it initially may appear. Achieving negative proximal and distal resection margins is usually not difficult, but vital structures in the mediastinum pose a problem at the radial margin of dissection. Some surgeons recommend radical en bloc resection of the esophagus to achieve an adequate radial margin. This operative strategy has conceptual inconsistencies; it entails radical removal of nonessential radial tissues (pleura, mediastinal fat, pericardium, thoracic duct), while preserving vital structures situated in close proximity to the tumor (aorta, heart, spine, trachea, main bronchi). The issue of lymphadenectomy is also controversial (see next question).

19. Removing lymph nodes helps with postoperative cancer staging, but is it therapeutic?

As for many solid tumors, there is some evidence to suggest a small survival benefit for lymphadenectomy, but the evidence is not compelling. Lymphadenectomy does not address the issue of systemic disease, and its survival benefit, if any, is modest. It is desirable to remove diseased lymph nodes and to obtain a **margin** of normal lymph nodes as well. Extensive lymphadenectomies, such as the three-field (abdominal, thoracic, cervical) lymphadenectomy, increase morbidity without obviously improving survival.

20. Should a pyloromyotomy be done to ensure adequate gastric emptying?

Probably. At least one randomized trial supports this contention. It is simplistic to think that the state of the pylorus is solely responsible for gastric emptying after esophagectomy, however. Other factors, such as the size of the gastric conduit and partial intrathoracic gastric volvulus, are also important.

BIBLIOGRAPHY

1. Bartels H, Stein HJ, Siewert JR: Preoperative risk analysis and postoperative mortality of oesophagectomy for resectable oesophageal cancer. Br J Surg 85:840–844, 1998.
2. Beitler AL, Urschel JD: Comparison of stapled and hand-sewn esophagogastric anastomoses. Am J Surg 175:337–340, 1998.
3. Goldminc M, Maddern G, Le Prise E, et al: Oesophagectomy by a transhiatal approach or thoracotomy: A prospective randomized trial. Br J Surg 80:367–370, 1993.
4. Iannettoni MD, Whyte RI, Orringer MB: Catastrophic complications of the cervical esophagogastric anastomosis. J Thorac Cardiovasc Surg 110:1493–1501, 1995.
5. Miller JD, Jain MK, de Gara CJ, et al: The effect of surgical experience on results of esophagectomy for esophageal carcinoma. J Surg Oncol 65:20–21, 1997.
6. Nigro JJ, DeMeester SR, Hagen JA, et al: Node status in transmural esophageal adenocarcinoma and outcome after en bloc esophagectomy. J Thorac Cardiovasc Surg 117:960–968, 1999.
7. Nishimaki T, Suzuki T, Suzuki S, et al: Outcomes of extended radical esophagectomy for thoracic esophageal cancer. J Am Coll Surg 186:306–312, 1998.
8. Orringer MB, Marshall B, Iannettoni MD: Transhiatal esophagectomy: Clinical experience and refinements. Ann Surg 230:392–403, 1999.
9. Peracchia A, Rosati R, Fumagalli U, et al: Thoracoscopic esophagectomy: Are there benefits? Semin Surg Oncol 13:259–262, 1997.
10. Roder JD, Busch R, Stein HJ, Siewert JR: Ratio of invaded to removed lymph nodes as a predictor of survival in squamous cell carcinoma of the esophagus. Br J Surg 81:410–413, 1994.
11. Swanstrom LL, Hansen P: Laparoscopic total esophagectomy. Arch Surg 132:943–949, 1997.
12. Tilanus HW, Hop WC, Langenhorst BL, van Lanschot JJ: Esophagectomy with or without thoracotomy: Is there any difference? J Thorac Cardiovasc Surg 105:898–903, 1993.
13. Urschel JD: Esophagogastrostomy anastomotic leaks complicating esophagectomy—a review. Am J Surg 169:634–640, 1995.

18. ADJUVANT, NEOADJUVANT, AND COMBINED-MODALITY THERAPY FOR ESOPHAGEAL CARCINOMA

Monica Spaulding, M.D.

1. Discuss the differences between neoadjuvant, adjuvant, and combined-modality therapy in esophageal carcinoma.

Neoadjuvant therapy refers to therapy that is used to shrink a tumor before definitive therapy. It is used for tumors that are not known to have metastases but are thought to be potentially curable with some form of locally directed therapy. Definitive therapy comprises a surgical resection of the esophagus, surrounding tissues, and regional nodes or full course of radiation therapy to the tumor and draining lymph nodes (6,000 cGy). The neoadjuvant approaches used for esophageal cancer include chemotherapy before surgery or radiation therapy, radiation therapy before surgical resection, or the administration of concurrent chemotherapy and radiation therapy before surgical resection.

Adjuvant therapy generally refers to chemotherapy or radiotherapy used postoperatively to improve the likelihood of long-term cure. Adjuvant therapy is recommended in situations in which the tumor has been completely resected, but based on the disease removed, there is believed to be a high likelihood of recurrence. Recurrence rates are high in patients with tumor invading through the wall of the esophagus and when there is tumor involvement of regional nodes.

Combined-modality treatment is a more general phrase that can be used to describe any situation in which more than one modality is used to treat cancer. It is used to describe the use of systemic chemotherapy in combination with radiotherapy, as a primary treatment or as a preoperative treatment: radiation therapy alone plus surgery or chemotherapy alone plus surgery.

2. What is the justification for use of more than single-modality treatments for esophageal carcinoma?

Five-year Survival of Patients with Esophageal Carcinoma According to Pathologic Stage

STAGE	TNM	5-YEAR SURVIVAL (%)
I	TIN0M0	50
IIA	T2,T3N0M0	40
IIB	T1,T2NIM0	20
III	T3N1,T4Nany	15
IV	anyTanyN M	0

Even patients with no involved nodes at the time of surgery have a low 5-year survival. Such statistics encourage the study of more than single-modality treatments.

3. Discuss the reasons for great interest in using more than one modality for the standard management of localized esophageal carcinoma.

Surgery has been the standard option for patients with localized esophageal carcinoma, although radiation therapy has a role for patients who are too debilitated for a resection or who have other life-limiting diseases. With either modality, there is a high rate of treatment failure. Various autopsy studies have shown residual local or metastatic disease is 75% of patients undergoing an esophagectomy for cure. The high failure rate reflects difficulties with selection of patients for resection of esophageal cancer. Only patients with T1 and T2 disease treated by surgery alone have a cure rate >50%. Those with tumor extending through the esophageal wall or with lymph

71

node involvement usually die of local and distant metastases. Early esophageal cancer has few symptoms, suggesting that patients have had their cancer for a long time before the diagnosis is made. During that asymptomatic period, tumor cells have spread longitudinally along lymphatics in the esophagus. Through lymphatics, cancer cells can spread to nodal stations ranging from the supraclavicular to celiac area. Hematogenous spread may also occur. Tumor is found in the lungs and liver in most patients dying of esophageal cancer.

4. Describe some of the newer modalities or techniques that have been studied for better staging of esophageal carcinoma.

Overall accuracy of staging has been improved by the addition of several modalities. **Endoscopic ultrasound** is an excellent tool for evaluating the depth of tumor invasion into the esophageal wall. It is also good at detecting involvement of contiguous and nearby lymph nodes. Rosch reported the accuracy of endoscopic ultrasound as 84% for the T (tumor) stage and 77% for the N (nodal) stage. He had performed endoscopy in >1,000 patients before surgical resection so that there was pathologic confirmation of his findings. Endoscopic ultrasound is limited in detecting celiac node and tracheobronchial involvement. It is also limited in its use by stenotic tumors; however, stepwise dilation can sometimes allow its use.

The ability to detect distant metastatic lesions has been improved by the use of **CT scanning.** Celiac nodal involvement; liver metastases; and local invasion of tumor into the trachea, bronchi, or pericardium may be suggested by this technique. Its sensitivity and specificity for detecting adjacent organ involvement range from 85–95%.

The **thoracoscopy** and **limited laparotomy** have also improved the staging of esophageal carcinoma. Krasna has done a multi-institutional study in which patients scheduled for an esophageal resection underwent staging thoracoscopy before the more definitive surgery. This procedure allowed visualization of periesophageal nodes as well as occult pleural or pulmonary metastases. A minilaparotomy may be done to characterize celiac nodes before a more extensive esophageal resection.

Positron emission tomography, a procedure in which ^{18}F-labeled glucose-6-phosphatase is administered before a whole-body positron scan, has been shown to be an accurate, noninvasive way to detect mediastinal and celiac node involvement with a high degree of accuracy.

5. How could the new staging procedures be used in the development of clinical trials?

Staging procedures should help select patients with limited disease who are better candidates for single-modality therapy, primarily surgery. Staging should also help select patients who have more advanced disease and might benefit from participation in a trial of multimodality therapy.

6. List potential advantages and disadvantages of the preoperative (adjuvant) use of radiation therapy.

Advantages	Disadvantage
• May make tumor more resectable	• May increase rate of postoperative complications
• May decrease likelihood of tumor spread at surgery	

7. Discuss the results of trials of preoperative radiotherapy in patients with resectable carcinoma of the esophagus.

Mei et al. have reported the results of a randomized trial in which patients received radiotherapy followed by surgery or surgery alone. Patients eligible to be randomized had tumors <8 cm in length, were younger than age 65, and were able to take a semiliquid diet. Patients treated with preoperative radiotherapy received 4,000 cGy to the mediastinum and draining gastroepiploic nodes before they went to surgery. More patients underwent a curative resection in the group receiving preoperative radiation, and they had fewer lymph node metastases. Local recurrence rate was less in the irradiated group. None of these differences were significant, and survival was not changed. The rate of postoperative complications was no higher in patients receiving radiotherapy before surgery. There have been at least four other randomized trials comparing surgery alone with radiotherapy followed by surgery. In none of them has there been an advantage to the use of preoperative radiotherapy.

8. Discuss the role of postoperative (adjuvant) radiotherapy in esophageal carcinoma.

The major advantage of postoperative radiotherapy is more accurate selection of patients based on pathologic findings. The physician has direct knowledge of the tumor extent and can plan radiotherapy to treat areas at high risk. The potential disadvantage is that there could be a higher incidence of strictures at anastomotic sites or delay in postoperative recovery. Fijuka et al. reported a series of patients who received postoperative radiotherapy (5,000 cGy) to the mediastinum and supraclavicular area. The patients were compared with a group of similar patients receiving radiotherapy before surgery. Patients with postoperative treatment survived longer; however, there is a selection bias in the study because only patients who could be resected or did not have postoperative complications received postoperative radiotherapy. There was no mention of delayed radiotherapy-related complications. Teniere reported the results of 221 patients with squamous cell tumors randomized to surgery alone versus postoperative radiotherapy. Postoperative radiotherapy had no impact on survival, although there was a decrease in local recurrence in patients receiving radiotherapy who had no lymph node involvement at the time of surgery. Fok et al. reported that similar trials with similar results showed an increased incidence of gastric complications and fibrosis after therapy.

9. What is the role of neoadjuvant chemotherapy in locally advanced carcinoma of the esophagus?

Many drugs have shown activity against metastatic esophageal carcinoma. Several investigators have developed randomized protocols in which patients received chemotherapy before standard surgery or standard surgery alone. The pretherapy staging procedure was the same for patients in each arm. Roth reported a study in which the neoadjuvant therapy included two courses of cisplatin, vindesine, and bleomycin. Schlag developed a similar study in which half the patients received preoperative chemotherapy with cisplatin and 5-fluorouracil. There was no difference between the two treatments in either study. Although Roth reported that the responders to chemotherapy had a longer survival, the numbers are small. The Schlag study was stopped early because of increased postoperative morbidity in the neoadjuvant arm. Kelson et al. reported an interesting study done at Memorial Sloan-Kettering in which patients were randomized to preoperative chemotherapy or preoperative radiotherapy. There were no differences in resectability, operative mortality, or survival between the two groups. At present, preoperative (neoadjuvant chemotherapy) alone should not be considered a standard of care.

10. List some drugs that are active against metastatic esophageal carcinoma and are also known to have activity as radiosensitizers.
- Cisplatin
- 5-Fluorouracil
- Bleomycin
- Mitomycin C
- Carboplatin
- Taxol

11. What are the potential benefits and risks of administering chemotherapy and radiotherapy together?

The concurrent administration of chemotherapy and radiotherapy is done to obtain more tumor shrinkage than can be expected from the radiotherapy alone; it also means that there may be enhanced radiation effect on normal tissues. As applied to the esophagus, there may be more mucositis and esophagitis than would be expected with radiotherapy alone. There may be a life-threatening acute effect from administering the two modalities together. Physicians need to be aware of this side effect because even patients who are swallowing at the beginning of their therapy will be unable to swallow when severe esophagitis occurs. Nutritional supplements may be needed by gastrostomy or jejunostomy tube or venous hyperalimentation.

12. Have there been any studies to suggest that concurrent chemotherapy and radiation might be better than radiotherapy alone?

The Radiation Therapy Oncology Group performed a multi-institutional trial in which patients with locally advanced disease received either radiation therapy alone (64 Gy) or radiotherapy given with two courses of concurrent chemotherapy. The chemotherapy was cisplatin and infusion 5-fluorouracil. Two additional courses of the same chemotherapy were given at the completion of the radiotherapy. The study was stopped early because there was a significant difference in median survival (12.5 vs. 8.5 months) and 2-year survival (30% vs. 10%) favoring the combined therapy arm. Overall survival statistics are not satisfactory, and newer approaches are needed.

13. Discuss the results of trials of combined-modality therapy using chemotherapy plus radiotherapy before surgical resection in selected patients with esophageal carcinoma.

Walsh et al. reported a randomized trial in which patients with locally invasive adenocarcinoma of the esophagus were randomized to receive surgery alone or two courses of cisplatin and 5-fluorouracil with 40 Gy of radiotherapy followed by surgery. The results showed a striking improvement in survival for patients receiving the combined-modality therapy. Median survival was 16 months for the combined-modality group versus 11 months for those receiving surgery alone. After 3 years of follow-up, only 6% of those receiving surgery alone were alive, whereas 32% percent of those treated by the combination therapy were alive. The study is impressive for the differences between the two arms; however, it has been criticized for the poor survival in the control arm. It is worse than historical data would have expected. Selection for therapy was also not based on endoscopic staging, and it is not clear as to whether the arms were balanced at randomization. Other investigators are looking at treatment regimens that include radiation therapy along with carboplatin and taxol, taxol alone, irinotecan, and gemcitabine. Each of these drugs is active against esophageal cancer and has radiosensitizing potential.

14. Is there presently any evidence that different combined-modality approaches need to be developed based on cell type of esophageal carcinoma (adenocarcinoma or squamous cell carcinoma)?

No. Studies suggest that adenocarcinoma and squamous cell carcinoma respond similarly to chemotherapy, radiotherapy, or combined-modality therapy.

BIBLIOGRAPHY

1. Fok M, Sham JST, Choy D, et al: Postoperative radiotherapy for carcinoma of the esophagus: A prospective randomized controlled trial. Surgery 113:138–147, 1993.
2. Forastiere AA, Urba S: Combined-modality therapy for cancer of the esophagus. Upd Princ Pract Oncol 11:1–15, 1996.
3. Herskovic A, Martz K, Al-Saraf M, et al: Combined chemotherapy and radiotherapy compared to radiotherapy alone in patients with cancer of the esophagus. N Engl J Med 326:1593–1598, 1992.
4. Iizuka T, Ide H, Kakegawa T, et al: Preoperative radioactive therapy for esophageal carcinoma. Chest 93:1054–1058, 1988.
5. Kelsen DP, Minsky BD, Smith M, et al: Preoperative therapy for esophageal carcinoma: A randomized comparison of chemotherapy versus radiotherapy. J Clin Oncol 8:1352–1361, 1990.
6. Krasna MJ, Reed CE, Jaklitsch MT, et al: Thoracoscopic staging of esophageal cancer: Cancer and Acute Leukemia Group B Thoracic Surgeons. Ann Thor Surg 60:1337–1340, 1995.
7. Luketich JD, Schauer PR, Meltzer CC, et al: Role of positron emission tomography in staging esophageal carcinoma. Ann Thor Surg 64:765–769, 1997.
8. Mei W, Xian-Zhi G, Weibo Y, et al: Randomized clinical trial on the combination of preoperative irradiation and surgery in the treatment of esophageal carcinoma: Report on 206 patients. Int J Radiat Oncol Biol Phys 16:325–327, 1988.

9. Noh HM, Fishman EK, Forastiere AA, et al: CT of the esophagus: Spectrum of disease with emphasis on esophageal carcinoma. Radiographics 15:113, 1995.
10. Rosch T: Endosonographic staging of esophageal carcinoma: A review of literature results. Gastrointestinal Endosc 5:537–547, 1995.
11. Roth JA, Putnam JB Jr: Surgery for carcinoma of the esophagus. Semin Oncol 21:453, 1994.
12. Roth JA, Pass HI, Flanagan MM, et al: Randomized trial of preoperative therapy and postoperative adjuvant therapy with cisplatin, vindesine and bleomycin for carcinoma of the esophagus. J Thor Cardiovasc Surg 96:242–248, 1988.
13. Schlag PM: Randomized trial of preoperative chemotherapy for squamous cell carcinoma of the esophagus. Arch Surg 127:1446–1450, 1988.
14. Teniers P, Hay JM, Fingerhut A, et al: Postoperative radiation therapy does not increase survival after resection for squamous cell carcinoma of the middle and lower esophagus as shown by a multicenter controlled trial. Surg Gynecol Obstet 173:123–130, 1991.
15. Tummula R, Williams SR: Esophageal cancer. In Djulbegovic B, Sullivan DM (eds): Decision Making in Oncology. New York, Churchill Livingstone, pp 169–178.
16. Walsh TN, Noonan N, Hollywood D, et al: A comparison of multimodality therapy and surgery for esophageal carcinoma. N Engl J Med 335:462–467, 1996.

III. The Lungs

19. EMBRYOLOGY AND SURGICAL ANATOMY OF THE LUNGS

Scott C. Boulanger, M.D., Ph.D., Vivian Lindfield, M.D., and Philip L. Glick, M.D.

1. When does the development of the respiratory system begin?

The primordium of the respiratory system begins development at about 4 weeks' gestation, with the appearance of an outgrowth from the ventral wall of the foregut, called the **respiratory diverticulum.** This eventually partitions along the dorsal/caudal axis to form two channels. The ventral channel gives rise to the trachea and lung buds, whereas the dorsal channel becomes the esophagus.

2. How do the origins of the epithelial lining of the respiratory system differ from the origins of the muscular and cartilaginous components?

The epithelium is derived from the foregut and is of endodermal origin. The muscle and cartilage derive from the splanchnic mesenchyme surrounding the foregut.

3. How do the bronchi arise?

During separation from the esophagus, the respiratory diverticulum gives rise to the trachea and lung buds. The lung buds are lateral outpouchings from the trachea. The right lung bud divides into three main bronchi, whereas the left lung bud bifurcates into two main bronchi; this eventually results in the development of three pulmonary lobes on the right and two on the left.

4. How are the pleural cavities formed?

The lung buds continue to branch in a dichotomous manner and grow in a caudal and lateral direction into a space called the **pericardioperitoneal canal.** These canals are eventually separated from the peritoneal and pericardial cavities to form the pleural cavities.

5. What is the origin of the pleura?

The **visceral pleura** arises from the mesoderm covering the outside of the lung. The **parietal pleura** comes from the somatic mesoderm covering the body wall from the inside.

6. Approximately how many times do the main bronchi divide?

The main bronchi divide dichotomously approximately 23 times; 17 of these divisions occur by 6 months' gestation, whereas the others occur postnatally.

7. How do the divisions of the main bronchi affect the size of the airways?

Even though the diameter of the peripheral airways becomes progressively smaller, the cross-sectional area increases markedly as a result of the asymmetric dichotomous branching pattern.

8. Discuss the four major stages of lung development.

1. The **pseudoglandular stage** begins at week 5 and lasts to week 17 of gestation. During this phase, the major airways develop and the lung has a glandular appearance.

2. The **cannilicular stage** lasts between weeks 17 and 26 of gestation. During this stage, the lung develops to the stage of the terminal bronchioles, and cartilage, muscle, and blood vessels develop from the mesenchyme.

3. The **saccular stage** lasts from week 24 until birth. It is called saccular because the terminal bronchioles begin to differentiate into immature alveoli, or saccules, which are capable of some inefficient gas exchange. The surfactant system also develops during this stage.

4. The **alveolar stage** takes place postnatally and is marked by development of alveoli and maturation of airways.

Some experts refer to the development of the pulmonary system during the first 4 weeks of gestation as the **embryonic stage.** During this period the lung develops to the level of the major bronchi.

9. What percentage of alveoli are formed postnatally?

Approximately 90%. Alveolar development continues until approximately age 8 years, although some workers have suggested that alveolar development is complete by 2 years of age.

10. Name the segments of the right and left lung.

The right lung has ten segments: apical, posterior, anterior, lateral, medial, superior, medial basal, anterior basal, lateral basal, and posterior basal. The only difference in the left lung is that there is no medial basal segment.

11. What percentages of the lung volume are provided by the right and left lung?

The right lung provides 55% and the left lung 45% of the total lung volume.

12. What is the anatomic explanation for the more frequent foreign body aspiration on the right side?

The angle of take-off of the right main stem bronchus is not as sharp as the left.

13. Which is shorter, the right or left main bronchus?

The right main stem bronchus; this is due to the take-off of the right upper lobe.

14. What is an azygos lobe?

During development, the precursor to the azygos vein along with the pleura penetrates the right upper lobe. This causes a part of the lobe to be trapped and separated from the rest of the lobe.

15. How often is an azygos lobe present?

In pproximately 0.7% of individuals.

16. Define Clara cells.

First-order bronchi contain ciliated columnar epithelium. As they continue to divide, this epithelium is replaced with nonciliated columnar cells that contain a rounded, protruding cytoplasm. These cells are thought to secrete the carbohydrate component of surfactant and an antiprotease. After further division, Clara cells give way to cuboidal epithelium.

17. How many types of cell are present in human alveolar epithelium?

There are two cell types: **squamous alveolar cells** (type I) and **great alveolar cells** (type II). Type I cells are 30% less numerous than type II cells, but they occupy about 95% of the alveolar surface area. Their function is to serve as a protective barrier between the air and the alveolar septum. Type II cells cover only 5% of the alveolar surface. They are cuboidal in shape compared with the thin, broad shape of type I cells. Type II cells secrete surfactant.

18. Describe the functions of the type II alveolar cell.

In addition to being the source of surfactant, these cells serve as the stem cell for the alveolar surface in case of injury. They can regenerate the alveolar surface 5 days. They secrete complement factors, arachidonic acid metabolites, and connective tissue components of the basement membrane (e.g., fibronectin).

19. State the relationship of the pulmonary arteries to the main bronchi.

The right pulmonary artery is located below the right main bronchus; whereas the left pulmonary artery lies above the left main stem bronchus.

20. What primarily determines the diameter of pulmonary veins?

Lung volume. This is due to the fact that pulmonary veins are connected directly to pulmonary tissue by connective tissue. This mechanism serves to promote venous return in a low-pressure system.

21. What are pores of Kohn?

Pores between alveoli that allow collateral ventilation in the event of bronchiole obstruction. Bronchoalveolar communications also exist and serve as another means of collateral ventilation.

22. What are N1 and N2 lymph nodes?

The two main groups of lymph nodes draining the lungs. N1 or **pulmonary lymph nodes** contain four groups of nodes: hilar, interlobar, lobar, and segmental. N2 or **mediastinal lymph nodes** also are classified into four groups: anterior mediastinal, posterior mediastinal, tracheo-bronchial, and paratracheal lymph nodes.

23. Describe the arterial blood supply to the lungs.

The lungs have a dual blood supply. The pulmonary arteries supply deoxygenated blood to the alveoli for gas exchange. The bronchial arteries arise directly or indirectly from the aorta and supply the lung parenchyma, bronchi, and inferior trachea. The right side is usually supplied by a branch of the third intercostal artery. The left usually has two branches that come directly from the aorta. The bronchial arteries supply the bronchial wall to the level of the respiratory bronchioles, then anastomose with branches of the pulmonary arteries. The pulmonary arteries are derived embryologically from the left sixth aortic arch. They are closely associated with the main stem bronchus and provide arterial branches to the bronchial ramifications.

24. What is the eparterial bronchus?

The right upper or right superior lobar bronchus (first branch off the right main bronchus). It is so named because it is the only bronchus that lies superiorly to the pulmonary artery.

25. Describe the venous system of the lungs.

The bronchial veins form two distinct systems:

1. The **deep bronchial veins** start at the intrapulmonary bronchiolar plexuses and communicate freely with the pulmonary veins. These eventually form a single trunk, which ends in a main pulmonary vein or in the left atrium.

2. The **superficial bronchial veins** drain extrapulmonary bronchi, visceral pleura, and hilar lymph nodes. These also communicate with pulmonary veins and end in the azygos vein on the right or the superior intercostal or accessory hemiazygos veins on the left.

There are two pulmonary veins for each lung that drain the pulmonary capillaries. These small veins coalesce at the capillary level to form larger branches that traverse the lung independently of the pulmonary arteries and bronchi. These eventually form larger vessels that ultimately accompany the arteries and bronchi to the hilum. The main pulmonary veins develop as outgrowths of the cardiac atria, whereas the intrapulmonary veins are derived from mesenchyme.

26. Is a bronchopulmonary segment a complete vascular unit with an individual bronchus, artery, and vein?

No. Veins do not travel with the bronchi and arteries. In a bronchopulmonary segment, usually a bronchus and its branches are central and accompanied by arteries. There are many tributaries of pulmonary veins running between segments and serving adjacent segments (which may drain into more than one vein). In resection of segments, it is noted that the planes between segments are not avascular but are crossed by veins and arterial branches. This pattern of bronchi, arteries, and veins is highly variable, with the veins being the most variable.

27. How many lymphatic systems does the lung contain?

Two—a superficial and a deep system. The **superficial system** lies in the pleura, whereas the **deep system** is associated with the bronchi and pulmonary arteries and veins. The two systems anastomose in the pleura and in the hilum. Lymphatics are not found in the alveoli.

BIBLIOGRAPHY

1. Banister L: Respiratory system. In Williams PL, Bannister LH, et al (eds): Gray's Anatomy, 38th ed. New York, Churchill-Livingstone, 1995.
2. King TC, Smith CR: Chest wall, pleura, lung and mediastinum. In Schwartz SI, Shires GT, Spencer FC, et al (eds): Principles of Surgery. New York, McGraw-Hill, 1994.
3. Sadler TW (ed): Langman's Medical Embryology, 6th ed. Baltimore, Williams & Wilkins, 1990.
4. Wagner HN: The lungs. In Zuidema GA (ed): The Johns Hopkins Atlas of Human Functional Anatomy. Baltimore, The Johns Hopkins University Press, 1992.
5. Wolfe WG, Lilly RE: Disorders of the lungs, pleura and chest wall. In Sabiston DC Jr (ed): Textbook of Surgery, 15th ed. W.B. Saunders, Philadelphia, 1991.

20. NONINVASIVE THORACIC IMAGING

Harry W. Donias, M.D., and Hratch L. Karamanoukian, M.D.

1. How frequently is chest radiography performed?
It is the principal imaging examination employed in the investigation of thoracic disease and is the most frequent examination performed in most radiology departments, constituting 30–50% of studies.

2. What is the cost of chest radiography?
About $11 billion per year in North America.

3. What is the patient radiation dose from a chest radiograph?
Approximately 20–30 mrem per view. This is comparable to the background radiation individuals receive on a monthly basis in the United States from radon and cosmic radiation.

4. What is the patient radiation dose from a chest CT scan?
Approximately 2000 mrem (100 times that of a single-view chest radiograph).

5. List the indications for a chest CT scan.
- The staging of bronchogenic carcinoma
- A solitary pulmonary nodule, mass, or opacity
- Diffuse infiltrative lung disease
- Widened mediastinum, a mediastinal mass, or other abnormality of the mediastinum
- An abnormal hilum
- Pleural abnormalities or the need to differentiate pleural from parenchymal abnormalities
- Chest wall lesions
- Detection of metastatic disease in tumors with a propensity for metastasis to the lungs
- Hemoptysis or suspected bronchiectasis
- Evaluation of the thymus in patients who have myasthenia gravis
- Evaluation of patients with endocrine abnormalities that are associated with a suspected lung tumor or with parathyroid adenoma
- Search for an unknown source of infection, especially in immunocompromised patients
- Evaluation of the pulmonary parenchyma in patients with normal chest films and suspected diffuse infiltrative lung disease or emphysema
- Suspicion of aortic dissection or aneurysm

6. How is conventional CT performed?
The x-ray tube and detectors rotate around the stationary patient in a full circle to acquire data in a single axial image. There is a brief pause as the tube is advanced incrementally, then the x-ray tube and detectors rotate in the opposite direction because the cables supplying the x-ray tube in the circular gantry need to be unwound after each image is obtained.

7. How is spiral (helical) CT performed?
The electric current is supplied to the x-ray tube through the contact of slip rings and brushes; the tube is free to rotate continuously in the same direction around the patient. During this continuous x-ray exposure, the patient moves through the scanner without stopping. This results in a helical volume of data over the length of the thorax. Because spiral scanning acquires continuous images of a patient's body, it provides imaging data between the actual slices displayed. This complete data set of the patient's body can be retrieved and reprocessed into additional images. Image reconstruction is used to search for anatomic structures that are smaller than the CT scan

slice, to delineate better an anatomic structure without obtaining additional images, and to create three-dimensional imaging.

8. Discuss the role of spiral CT in the diagnosis of pulmonary embolism.

Until the early 1990s, the standard diagnostic imaging procedures for evaluation of pulmonary embolism were ventilation-perfusion (V/Q) scintigraphy and pulmonary angiography. There has been a progressive replacement of pulmonary angiography with spiral CT angiography because this allows noninvasive identification of intravascular clots. The sensitivity of spiral CT is greater than that of V/Q scintigraphy (75–92% vs. 36–65% [mean values, 85% vs. 50%]). The main advantage of spiral CT is the lower percentage of nondiagnostic examinations because the lung parenchyma, mediastinum, and thoracic wall structures are also evaluated. Consequently, alternative causes of the clinical signs and symptoms may be identified, which have been shown to be present in 11–33% of cases. Several authors suggest that spiral CT should be the initial modality of choice, especially in patients known to be associated with a high rate of indeterminate V/Q scintigraphic studies, including all inpatients and patients with chronic obstructive pulmonary disease.

9. List alternative causes of clinical signs and symptoms of pulmonary embolism that have been identified by spiral CT.

- Pneumothorax
- Pneumonia
- Lung cancer
- Septic emboli
- Bronchiectasis
- Emphysema

10. When should pulmonary angigraphy be employed in the diagnosis of pulmonary embolism?

In patients in whom clinical suspicion for pulmonary embolism remains high despite normal results of spiral CT and duplex ultrasonography of the legs.

11. What is virtual bronchoscopy (VB)?

A noninvasive imaging technique that takes advantage of three-dimensional reconstruction of spiral CT images. Commercially available programs have been designed to create a three-dimensional tracheobronchial tree model automatically from spiral CT scan images of the thorax. To create the three-dimensional airway, the programs use the natural contrast between air in the tracheobronchial tree and the soft tissue of the airway wall and mediastinum to create an airway caste along the lumen of the tracheobronchial tree. The caste is generated into a three-dimensional airway. Once the virtual airway is created, the imager can travel within or navigate through the lumen as if using a simulated bronchoscope. In contrast to actual bronchoscopy, with VB, the imager is able to view the contents of the airway simultaneously as well as the extraluminal mediastinal and hilar structures. The mediastinum and hila may be viewed through the airway walls, which may be rendered semitransparent, or by superimposing multiplanar or three-dimensional volume–rendered mediastinal images. Another feature of VB is the ability to rotate images on the computer monitor.

12. Discuss some current uses of VB.

- VB is helpful in evaluating **obstructive airway lesions.** By displaying the airway three-dimensionally, VB can display the level of obstruction and the extent to which the obstruction narrows the airway, helping to determine the presence of airway patency beyond the obstruction.
- Measuring the width and length of airway stenosis and displaying the exact location of abnormal lymph nodes allows one to determine whether a bronchoscope can be passed through an area of narrowing or the best approach for transbronchial needle sampling. This information can be used in **preoperative planning** for resection of tracheobronchial tumors or palliative stent placement in airways constricted by tumor or scar.

- Because VB is noninvasive, it is useful for **follow-up** in determining the patency of airways in conditions such as stenosis, surgical reconstruction, lung transplantation, or stent placement.

13. Describe contraindications for iodinated CT contrast administration.

- The only **absolute contraindication** is significant contrast allergy, specifically **anaphylaxis.** Steroid premedication is advised before imaging in these patients.
- **Renal insufficiency** is a **relative contraindication** because iodine can exacerbate renal insufficiency. A serum creatinine level of $>1.8–2.0$ mg/dL is used as a cut-off value. This is particularly important in patients with underlying diabetes or dehydration, in whom the potential toxic effects of iodine are increased.

14. How frequently is chest MRI used?

MRI has not had extensive application in the thorax mainly because of problems resulting from motion artifacts secondary to cardiac and respiratory movements. The normal lung does not produce a magnetic resonance signal because of magnetic susceptibility effects. MRI does provide excellent images of the mediastinum and the chest wall, however, and does permit direct imaging in the coronal and sagittal as well as the axial planes.

15. List the indications for chest MRI.

- Evaluation of the mediastinum or vascular structures in patients in whom contrast media are contraindicated
- Diagnosis of aortic dissection and congenital abnormalities of the aorta
- Evaluation of superior sulcus tumors
- Imaging of chest wall lesions and brachial plexus abnormalities
- Staging of bronchogenic carcinoma with particular reference to direct chest wall and mediastinal invasion
- Evaluation of posterior mediastinal masses
- Follow-up of patients with lymphoma.

16. How does MRI produce an image?

MRI relies on the mobile hydrogen concentration of blood and tissues to generate an image. When placed in an external magnetic field, the individual magnetic moments of all hydrogen atoms in the body align themselves with the external field. Energy in the form of a radiofrequency pulse is used to energize the aligned nuclei to varying degrees. The relaxation of these hydrogen atoms produces a signal that is used to generate an image. The final MRI signal is a function of the following:

- Concentration of hydrogen atoms
- Relaxation time
- Motion
- Blood flow
- Scanning parameters
- Imaging protocol

17. List contraindications to MRI.

- Metallic foreign bodies in the orbit
- Ferrous intracranial aneurysm clips
- Cochlear implants
- Shrapnel in critical locations
- Implanted electronic devices, including cardiac pacemakers

An additional risk of MRI is the attraction of **ferromagnetic objects** by the magnetic field. Pens, scissors, and medical equipment such as stethoscopes all are potentially lethal objects in the scanning room, and meticulous attention to objects on, in, and around the patient is required.

18. How are thoracic aortic aneurysms diagnosed?

- Plain radiographs (diagnosis not definitive)
- Aortography
- CT scanning
- MRI

19. Compare aortography, MRI, and CT scanning in diagnosing thoracic aortic aneurysm.
- **Aortography** is considered the gold standard, but drawbacks include radiation exposure, invasiveness of the procedure, and contrast administration.
- **MRI** has the advantage of imaging in multiple planes without additional radiation exposure or contrast administration; however, scan times can be long, requiring hemodynamically stable patients.
- Common indications for **CT scanning** of the thoracic aorta include preoperative planning for aneurysm repair, suspected aortic dissection, and aortic injury after blunt trauma.

20. Discuss the advantages CT scanning has over other modalities in evaluating the aorta.
- CT scanners far outnumber MRI scanners available for imaging in the emergency setting, and scans can be performed by on-call technologists without the need for an in-house radiologist.
- Modern spiral CT scanners are capable of producing images of the entire aorta in a matter of seconds. Patients are usually on and off the table within a few minutes.
- CT scanning is minimally invasive, requiring only a peripheral venous injection of contrast material.
- CT scanning can diagnose other thoracic pathology that can mimic the clinical presentation of aortic dissections and aneurysms, including pulmonary embolism, pneumothorax, and pneumonia.

21. Define FDG-positron emission tomography (PET).
PET is a noninvasive means to evaluate primary and recurrent lung cancer and to differentiate malignant from benign solitary pulmonary nodules. It is a promising noninvasive technique in detecting regional lymph node metastases of non-small cell lung cancer and defining the systematic extent of lung cancer by whole-body imaging. Focal metabolic differences between tumor and surrounding tissue can be imaged effectively using PET. It has been shown that neoplasms, particularly lung cancers, use glucose to a greater degree than normal tissue. [^{18}F] Fluorodeoxyglucose (FDG) can be used as a glucose analog. FDG is taken up by the glucose transporter, is phosphorylated, and remains trapped intracellularly and accumulates within tumor tissue. The radioactive label ^{18}F is a positron-emitting isotope. After absorption of their kinetic energy, positrons undergo an annihilation reaction with an electron, and two resulting gamma rays are sensed by detectors surrounding the patient's body.

22. Discuss the diagnostic studies that are available for evaluating focal lung abnormalities.
- Imaging with **chest radiography, CT,** or **MRI** rarely characterizes focal lung abnormalities definitely as benign or malignant.
- **Bronchoscopy,** including bronchial washings and brushings, has a sensitivity of 65% for malignancy; the addition of transbronchial biopsy increases the sensitivity to 79%.
- Peripheral lesions can be biopsied with CT-guided **transthoracic needle aspiration** with a sensitivity of 94–98% and specificity of 91–96%. Negative results from transbronchial or transthoracic needle aspiration cannot always be accepted as true negatives. Transthoracic needle aspiration has an 18–26% risk of pneumothorax.
- **Thoracoscopic lung** biopsy, or biopsy with thoracotomy, provides a definitive diagnosis, but many of the radiologically indeterminate nodules resected are benign. Many patients undergo an invasive and potentially avoidable surgical procedure.
- **FDG-PET** is evolving as a noninvasive study that can be performed after the identification of a pulmonary abnormality by an anatomic study (chest radiography, CT, or MRI) to evaluate the metabolic activity of a lesion in an attempt to distinguish a benign from a malignant process.

23. What is the role of FDG-PET in evaluating focal lung abnormalities?
FDG-PET has shown an average sensitivity of 95% and specificity of 88% for the detection

of malignancy in focal lung abnormalities. The optimal algorithm incorporating PET for the evaluation of pulmonary abnormalities has not been identified. FDG-PET is used on an individual basis, mostly in patients unable or unwilling to undergo biopsy of a focal lung abnormality. FDG-PET evaluation of solitary pulmonary nodules can identify metabolically inactive lesions likely to be benign, and these patients can be followed by sequential imaging studies rather than undergoing invasive sampling procedures. The individual decision is still based on whether a missed cancer diagnosis or an unnecessary invasive procedure represents the greater risk for the patient.

24. What diagnostic studies are used in staging thoracic lymph nodes?

Current noninvasive methods for evaluating the mediastinum include CT, MRI, and FDG-PET.

CT and **MRI** depend primarily on anatomic imaging features, including lymph nodes >1 cm in short-axis diameter and the presence of centralized calcification. They have a reported sensitivity of 52–69% in staging mediastinal lymph nodes and are considered by many to be only complementary to mediastinoscopy with lymph node sampling. Staging of the mediastinum can be performed by **mediastinoscopy,** which has a sensitivity of 87–91%, but it is an invasive procedure.

FDG-PET is noninvasive and depends primarily on the metabolic characteristics of tissue for the diagnosis of disease. The average sensitivity and specificity of PET imaging for evaluating nodal disease is 88% and 91%. The average sensitivity of PET for nodal disease is near that reported for mediastinoscopy. FDG-PET as a complementary adjunct to CT scanning has the potential to evolve into a more accurate noninvasive means of staging lymph nodes in lung cancer, resulting in improved treatment planning and prognostic information, while decreasing the need for invasive diagnostic procedures such as mediastinoscopy.

BIBLIOGRAPHY

1. Aquino SL, Vining DJ: Virtual bronchoscopy. Clin Chest Med 20:725–730, 1999.
2. Chai J, Spritzer CE: Role of computed tomographic scans in cardiovascular diagnosis. In Baue AE (ed): Glenn's Thoracic and Cardiovascular Surgery, 6th ed. Stamford, CT, Appleton & Lange, 1996.
3. Guhlmann A, Strock M, Kotzerke J, et al: Lymph node staging in non-small cell lung cancer: Evaluation by [(18) F] FDG positron emission tomography (PET). Thorax 52:438–441, 1997.
4. Hansell DM: Thoracic imaging—then and now. Br J Radiol 70:S153–S161, 1997.
5. Lipchik RJ, Goodman LR: Spiral computed tomography in the evaluation of pulmonary embolism. Clin Chest Med 20:731–738, 1999.
6. Lowe VJ, Naunheim KS: Current role of positron emission tomography in thoracic oncology. Thorax 53:703–712, 1998.
7. McLoud TC: Thoracic radiology: Imaging methods, radiographic signs, and diagnosis of chest disease. In McLoud TC (ed): Thoracic Radiology: The Requisites. St. Louis, Mosby, 1998.
8. Prauer HW, Weber WA, Romer W, et al: Controlled prospective study of positron emission tomography using the glucose analogue [(18) F] fluorodeoxyglucose in the evaluation of pulmonary nodules. Br J Surg 85:1506–1511, 1998.
9. Remy-Jardin M, Remy J: Spiral CT angiography of the pulmonary circulation. Radiology 212:615–636, 1999.
10. Slone RM: Chest imaging and diagnostic testing. In Slone RM, Gutierrez FR, Fisher AJ (eds): Thoracic Imaging: A Practical Approach. New York, McGraw-Hill, 1999.
11. Spritzer CE: Role of magnetic resonance imaging in cardiovascular diagnosis. In Baue AE (ed): Glenn's Thoracic and Cardiovascular Surgery, 6th ed. Stanford, CT, Appleton & Lange, 1996.
12. Tai NRM, Atwal AS, Hamilton G: Modern management of pulmonary embolism. Br J Surgery 86:853–868, 1999.
13. Urban BA, Bluemke DA, Johnson KM, Fishman EK: Imaging of thoracic aortic disease. Cardiol Clin North Am 17:659–682, 1999.

21. BRONCHOSCOPY

Kurt VonFricken, M.D.

1. What are the types of indications for bronchoscopy?
Diagnostic and therapeutic.

2. List the diagnostic indications for bronchoscopy.
Symptoms
- Hemoptysis
- Unexplained, persistent cough

Clinical situations
- Recurrent or unresolved pneumonia
- Suspected airway stricture
- Suspected foreign body aspiration
- Positive sputum cytology

Radiologic findings
- Persistent local infiltrate or diffuse bilateral infiltrates
- Deviation of the trachea or bronchi
- Hilar mass
- Peripheral lesion
- Lung abscess
- Unexplained pleural effusion
- Positive sputum cytology

3. Describe the therapeutic indications for bronchoscopy.
- Pulmonary secretions causing atelectasis can be aspirated.
- Blood, foreign bodies, and vomitus can be removed.
- Many modalities used to treat malignant obstruction of the airway are administered via the bronchoscope.
- Stenting of the airway is performed with a bronchoscope.
- A bronchoscope can aid in a difficult intubation and is especially useful in the placement of a double-lumen endotracheal tube.

4. Can bronchoscopy cause infection by contaminating the lungs with oropharyngeal bacteria?
Probably not.

5. Is it possible to spread infection from one part of the lung to another?
It has been suggested but has not been proved.

6. Should prophylactic antibiotics be given?
Only in patients with a history of endocarditis, a prostatic valve, or a shunt.

7. List the advantages of a rigid bronchoscope.
- Better for removing foreign bodies
- Better for managing massive hemoptysis
- Better for treating airway obstruction
- Better for use in infants

8. List the disadvantages of a rigid bronchoscope.
- Less comfortable in the awake patient
- Smaller field of view

9. List the advantages of flexible bronchoscopy.
- More comfortable in the awake patient
- Greater field of view, allowing good segmental visualization

10. List the disadvantages of flexible bronchoscopy?
- A small lumen makes aspiration more difficult.
- A small lumen limits the size of instruments that can be placed through the scope.
- Foreign bodies generally are too large to pass through the lumen, so once the foreign body is grasped, the whole scope must be withdrawn.

11. What premedication should be given for the awake, conscious patient?
- Sedative
- Drying agent
- Antitussive

12. What type of monitoring is required?
All patients should be monitored with an electrocardiogram and pulse oximetry. Intravenous access is needed.

13. List the types of tissue sampling that can be obtained with bronchoscopy.
- Washings
- Brushings
- Biopsies

14. What technique generally is used for treatment of benign strictures causing airway obstruction?
Progressive dilation.

15. What technique generally is used for treatment of malignant strictures?
Core out the tissue causing the obstruction and extract it with forceps.

16. List other treatment modalities that are available.
- Lasers, used to release benign strictures and to excise malignant strictures
- Brachytherapy, often combined with laser excision for longer-lasting results
- Electrocautery
- Cryotherapy
- Photodynamic therapy

17. State the main purpose of airway stents.
To maintain patency of the airway after a stricture has been treated.

18. How are foreign bodies in the airway diagnosed?
- **History** of a foreign body ingestion.
- **Symptoms** such as wheezing or coughing.
- **Radiographic findings** such as an opaque foreign body or an infiltrate or atelectasis.

19. What are the two main types of foreign bodies?
Organic and inorganic.

20. Which type of foreign body has the potential to be worse?
Organic, because they tend to absorb water, swell, and produce obstruction or infection if not removed.

21. What type of anesthesia is best for foreign body removal?
General.

22. What type of bronchoscope usually is better for foreign body removal?
Rigid.

23. How is rigid bronchoscopy performed on someone under general anesthesia?

There is a ventilation port on the side of the bronchoscope, and the end of the scope can be capped off with an eyepiece.

24. Is coagulopathy, platelet dysfunction, or prolonged bleeding time a contraindication to a bronchoscopy?

Only if brushings, aspirations, or biopsies are to be performed.

BIBLIOGRAPHY

1. Cooper JD, Pearson FG, Patterson GA, et al: Use of silicone stents in the management of airway problems. Ann Thorac Surg 47:371–378, 1989.
2. Dumon JF: A dedicated transbronchial stent. Chest 97:328–332, 1990.
3. Edens ET, Sia RL: Flexible fiberoptic endoscopy in difficult intubations. Ann Otol 90:307–309, 1981.
4. Lan RS, Lee CH, Chiang YC, et al: Use of fiberoptic bronchoscopy to retrieve bronchial foreign bodies in adults. Am Rev Respir Dis 140:1734–1737, 1989.
5. Mantor PC, Tuggle DW, Tunell WP: An appropriate negative bronchoscopy rate in suspected foreign body aspirations. Am J Surg 158:622–624, 1989.
6. McElvin RB: Bronchoscopy: Transbronchial biopsy and bronchoalveolar lavage. In Baue AE, Geha AS, Hammond GL, et al (eds): Glenn's Thoracic and Cardiovascular Surgery, 6th ed. Stamford, CT, Appleton & Lange, 1996, pp 169–180.
7. Schray MF, McDougall JC, Martinez A, et al: Management of malignant airway compromise with laser and low dose rate brachytherapy: The Mayo Clinic experience. Chest 93:264–269, 1988.
8. Weissberg D, Schwartz I: Foreign bodies in the tracheobronchial tree. Chest 91:730–733, 1987.

22. PULMONARY INFECTIONS

Asif Muhammad, M.D.

1. List the clinical features of acute sinusitis.
- Purulent nasal discharge
- Postnasal drip
- Nasal congestion
- Headache
- Facial pain
- Fever

2. List the risk factors for acute sinusitis.
- Recent viral upper respiratory infection
- Allergic rhinitis
- Orofacial trauma
- Periapical dental disease
- Nasotracheal intubation
- Frequent use of topical decongestants
- Smoking
- Intranasal use of cocaine
- Human immunodeficiency virus (HIV) infection

3. What are the common pathogens involved in acute sinusitis?
Major causes are *Streptococcus pneumoniae,* nontypable *Haemophilus influenzae, Strepto-coccus pyogenes,* and, less often, *Staphylococcus aureus.*
- Oral anaerobes are the common pathogens in patients with odontogenic sinusitis.
- Nosocomial sinusitis involves bacteria such as methicillin-resistant *S. aureus,* gram-negative bacilli such as *Escherichia coli* and *Pseudomonas aeruginosa,* and yeasts such as *Candida albicans.*

4. How is acute sinusitis diagnosed?
Clinically. **Transillumination** is helpful in the diagnosis. Sinus **radiographs** and **CT scanning** may be necessary in complicated cases, especially those of ethmoid and sphenoid sinusitis.

5. Discuss treatment of acute sinusitis.
Empiric antibiotics with activity against *S. pneumoniae* and *H. influenzae,* such as ampicillin, amoxicillin, and trimethoprim-sulfamethoxazole, should be used initially for 3–7 days. Many bacteria are resistant to amoxicillin, including β-lactamase–producing *H. influenzae* and penicillin-resistant *Pneumococcus.* For such cases, amoxicillin-clavulanate, cefuroxime, cefpodoxime, or cefixime should be used for at least 7 days. Patients allergic to sulfonamides or β-lactams can be treated with clarithromycin. **Decongestants,** such as phenylephrine and oxymetazoline nasal spray, are useful but should not be used for > 1 week.

6. List the common complications of sinusitis of different anatomic sites.

Maxillary sinusitis
- Periorbital cellulitis
- Facial cellulitis
- Osteomyelitis
- Parapharyngeal abscess

Frontal and ethmoid sinusitis
- Orbital cellulitis
- Epidural abscess
- Subdural abscess
- Intracranial abscess
- Cavernous sinus thrombosis

Sphenoid sinusitis
- Meningitis
- Cavernous sinus thrombosis
- Cerebral infarction
- Retroorbital abscess

7. Which viruses are involved in infection of the respiratory tract?

VIRUS	RESPIRATORY TRACT INFECTION
Adenovirus	Common cold
	Bronchitis
	Pharynoconjunctival fever
	Pneumonia
Influenza virus	Influenza
	Common cold
	Pharyngitis
	Bronchitis
	Bronchiolitis
	Pneumonia
Parainfluenza and respiratory syncytial virus (RSV)	Common cold
	Bronchitis
	Bronchiolitis
	Pneumonia
Herpes simplex virus (HSV)	Acute and chronic pharyngitis
	Tracheitis
	Pneumonia in immunosuppressed
Cytomegalovirus (CMV)	Mononucleosis
	Acute and chronic pharyngitis
	Pneumonia in immunosuppressed
Varicella-zoster virus (VZV)	Pneumonia
Epstein-Barr virus	Mononucleosis
	Acute and chronic pharyngitis
Papillomavirus	Laryngeal and tracheobronchial papillomatosis
HIV	Pharyngitis
	Secondary infections

8. Who is at risk for developing viral pneumonia?

- Children attending day care centers or school
- Adult patients with chronic pulmonary or cardiac conditions
- Patients from nursing homes or correctional facilities
- Pregnant women
- Immunocompromised patients
  - HIV infection
  - Malignancy
  - Chemotherapy or radiation therapy
  - Extensive burns

9. What antiviral agents are available for the treatment of viral pneumonia?

DRUG	VIRUS
Acyclovir	HSV, VZV
Ganciclovir	CMV
Amantadine/rimantadine	Infuenza A
Ribavirin	RSV, influenza A and B, hantavirus
Interferon-alfa	CMV, HSV, VZV, rhinovirus

10. Describe the clinical features of influenza.

This is an acute respiratory illness caused by influenza virus A and B mainly in the winter season in the form of an epidemic. There is abrupt onset of fever, chills, headache, myalgias, malaise, cough, sore throat, conjunctival injection, and clear nasal discharge. The frequency and severity of symptoms are significantly greater in smokers than nonsmokers. Patients with uncomplicated influenza gradually improve over 2–5 days. In some, the recovery may be delayed for up to a week.

11. What are the complications of influenza?

In children
- Otitis media
- Sinusitis
- Reye's syndrome

In adults
- Pneumonia
- Myocarditis
- CNS syndromes (encephalitis, transverse myelitis) manifestations (mimicking acute appendicitis)
- Myositis
- Rhabdomyolysis
- Toxic shock syndrome

12. What are the risk factors for developing primary influenza pneumonia?

Primary influenza pneumonia occurs in 2–18% of adults **hospitalized with pneumonia** during an epidemic. Most patients are > **40 years** old. Other risk factors are:

- Underlying cardiac or pulmonary disease
- Diabetes mellitus
- Renal disease
- Malignancy
- Corticosteroid or cytotoxic therapy
- Hemoglobinopathy
- HIV infection

13. How is influenza diagnosed?

Influenza occurring in an epidemic can be diagnosed clinically. Individual or sporadic cases may be difficult to diagnose and may require special testing. The most widely used test is the isolation of virus in **tissue culture** (sputum, nose and throat swabs, and nasal washes), which usually can be accomplished within 72 hours of inoculation. Serologic diagnosis takes a longer time than virus isolation or antigen detection techniques. Commonly used methods are hemagglutination-inhibition test, complement-fixation test, and enzyme-linked immunosorbent assay (ELISA). A $\geq$ 4-fold rise in antibody titers shown between serum obtained during acute illness and convalescent serum specimen obtained 10–14 days later is considered diagnostic by **hemagglutination-inhibition test** in 80% of cases. **Complement-fixation testing** detects a rise in about 70% of infections but is not able to distinguish the subtype of influenza A virus causing a particular infection. Serologic responses determined using **ELISA** antibodies are more sensitive than other tests. Rapid viral diagnostic tests employing immunofluorescence, radioimmunoassay, and enzyme immunoassay are available for the detection of influenza virus antigens in respiratory secretions. These appear to be less sensitive than tissue culture techniques.

14. Discuss the treatment of influenza and its complications.

Amantadine and rimantadine are effective against influenza A when administered within 48 hours of the onset of illness. These agents reduce the duration of fever and other systemic symptoms by 1–2 days, reduce the duration and quantity of virus shedding in respiratory secretions, and result in more rapid return to daily activities. The recommended dose of amantadine or rimantadine for therapy of influenza is 200 mg/d for 3–7 days. The efficacy of these agents in preventing complications of influenza or for the treatment of established complications, such as influenza pneumonia, has not been studied adequately. **Ribavirin,** a nucleoside analogue, has been shown to provide some reduction in fever and systemtic symptoms when given by aerosol in influenza A and B infections. Orally administered ribavirin is ineffective against influenza, and the intravenous form of the drug is used to treat influenza myocarditis. **Zanamivir** inhibits influenza virus neuraminidase and shortens the duration of symptoms. It is available in powder form and is used with a Diskhaler delivery device. The adult dosage is 2 inhalations twice daily for 5 days beginning within 48 hours of onset of symptoms.

15. Discuss available preventive measures for influenza.

Immunoprophylaxis

The currently available inactivated influenza vaccine reduces the risk of influenza virus–related morbidity and mortality. Vaccine efficacy in preventing clinical influenza is 50–80%. In nursing home residents, vaccine efficacy against influenza is found to be at best 45%. Vaccine may cause local redness and induration for 1–2 days and less commonly fever and constitutional symptoms lasting 48 hours. Because the vaccine is prepared from the viruses grown in eggs, extreme caution should be exercised in using vaccine in patients who have documented allergies to eggs or egg products.

Chemoprophylaxis

Amantadine and rimantadine are effective only for prevention of influenza A infections. These agents are 70–100% effective when taken orally and have to be given for the duration of the epidemic (6–10 weeks). Another approach is to use amantadine for 2 weeks along with immunization of the patients to provide protection for the first 2 weeks until the response to immunization develops. Amantadine is associated with CNS side effects, such as insomnia, jitteriness, anxiety, lightheadedness, and difficulty concentrating. Rimantadine is equally effective as amantadine when given in the same dosage and is associated with less frequent CNS side effects.

16. Which are the target groups for influenza and immunization?
- Adults and children with chronic pulmonary and cardiovascular disease, including asthma
- Residents of chronic care facilities and nursing homes
- Adults and children with chronic metabolic diseases (renal insufficiency, anemia, diabetes mellitus, immunosuppression)
- Children and teenagers receiving long-term aspirin therapy (may be at risk for Reye's syndrome)
- Health care providers with high-risk patient contact
- Household contacts of high-risk patients
- Adults who provide essential community services (police, firefighters)
- Any person who wants to reduce risk of influenza infection

Based on recommendations of the Advisory Committee for Immunization Practices (ACIP).

17. How common is community-acquired pneumonia?

In the United States, pneumonia is the sixth leading cause of death, and the number one cause of death from infectious diseases. It is estimated that about 4 million cases of community-acquired pneumonia occur annually, and one fifth of these require hospitalization.

18. Which patient populations are affected by community-acquired pneumonia?
- Older patients
- Patients with coexisting medical illnesses
  - Chronic obstructive lung disease
  - Renal insufficiency
- Diabetes mellitus
- Congestive heart failure
- Chronic liver disease
- Alcoholic
- Smokers

19. What are the common pathogens involved in community-acquired pneumonia?
- *S. pneumoniae*
- *Mycoplasma pneumoniae*
- Respiratory viruses
- *Chlamydia pneumoniae*
- *H. influenzae*
- *Legionella pneumophila*

Aerobic gram-negative bacilli are more common in patients with comorbidities. *S. aureus* can complicate viral respiratory tract infection and cause pneumonia.

20. List the risk factors for mortality or a complicated course of pneumonia.
- Age > 65 years
- Coexisting medical conditions
- Chronic obstructive pulmonary disease, bronchiectasis, cystic fibrosis
- Chronic renal failure
- Congestive heart failure

- Diabetes mellitus
- Chronic liver disease
- Suspicion of aspiration
- Altered mental status
- Postsplenectomy state
- Chronic alcohol abuse or malnutrition
- Physical findings
    Respiratory rate > 30 breaths/min
    Systolic blood pressure < 90 mm Hg and diastolic blood pressure < 60 mm Hg
    Temperature > 38.3°C (101°F)
    Presence of extrapulmonary site of infection
- Laboratory findings
    White blood cell count < 4,000/μL or > 30,000/μL
    PaO_2 < 60 mm Hg or $PaCO_2$ > 50 mm Hg on room air
    Blood urea nitrogen > 20 mg/dL or serum creatinine > 1.2 mg/dL
    Hemoglobin < 9 g/dL or hematocrit < 30%
    Metabolic acidosis
    Increased prothrombin time or partial thromboplastin time
    Decreased platelets or fibrin split products > 1:40
- Need for mechanical ventilation
- Unfavorable chest radiographic findings
    More than one lobe involved
    Pleural effusion
    Cavitary lesion
    Rapid spreading of infiltrates to other regions of lungs

21. When is community-acquired pneumonia called severe?

If one or more of the following factors are present:
1. Respiratory rate > 30 breaths/min on admission
2. PaO_2:FiO_2 ratio < 250
3. Presence of shock (systolic blood pressure < 90 mm Hg, diastolic blood pressure < 60 mm Hg)
4. Requirement for vasopressors
5. Chest radiograph showing increase in infiltrates by $\geq$ 50% within 48 hours of admission
6. Need for mechanical ventilation
7. Urine output < 20 mL/h

22. Should all patients with severe community-acquired pneumonia be admitted to the intensive care unit (ICU)?

Yes.

23. Discuss diagnostic studies that are appropriate for community-acquired pneumonia.

A complete history and physical examination is important, as are posteroanterior and lateral chest radiographs. Chest radiographs reveal the extent and type (alveolar vs. interstitial) of pneumonic infiltrate, presence of pleural effusion, cavities, abscesses, or atelectasis. Although Gram's stain of expectorated sputum commonly is used to guide therapy, its role in diagnosis is controversial because of the low sensitivity and specificity. However, special sputum stains for *Legionella, Mycobacterium,* fungi, and *Pneumocystis carinii* may be diagnostic. Complete blood count and routine serum chemistries are helpful to assess the risk and severity of pneumonia and should be performed in all hospitalized patients. Two sets of blood cultures should be obtained from hospitalized patients. A diagnostic thoracentesis should be performed in patients with pleural effusion.

24. What is the outpatient and in-hospital treatment of community-acquired pneumonia?

• **Initial** treatment is with **empiric antibiotics** selected on the basis of severity of illness, patient's age, and comorbidities.

• In **outpatients,** the preferred antimicrobials are macrolides (azithromycin, clarithromycin, or erythromycin), fluoroquinolones (levofloxacin, sparfloxacin, or grepafloxacin) or doxycycline.

• Patients with **suspected aspiration** should be treated with amoxicillin/clavulanate.

• Patients admitted to the **general medical ward** should be treated with ceftriaxone or cefotaxime with or without a macrolide. Fluoroquinolones also can be used as a single agent in these patients.

• Patients admitted to the ICU should be treated with a combination of ceftriaxone or piperacillin/tazobactam **plus** erythromycin or azithromycin or a fluoroquinolone.

• Patients with **structural disease of the lung,** such as bronchiectasis, should receive piperacillin **plus** a macrolide or fluoroquinolone **plus** an aminoglycoside.

25. What is nosocomial pneumonia (NP)?

Infection of the lung acquired after being in the hospital for $\geq$ 48 hours. Among hospital-acquired infections, it is the second most common infection and the leading cause of death. For each 1,000 hospital admissions, there are 5–10 cases of NP. Although 10% of patients requiring ICU care after general surgery develop this infection, 20% of patients intubated and 70% of patients with adult respiratory distress syndrome develop NP. The mortality rate can exceed 50% in mechanically ventilated patients, especially if the infection is caused by resistant enteric gram-negative organisms, such as *P. aeruginosa* and *Acinetobacter* species.

26. What is ventilator-associated pneumonia?

A form of NP that refers to the pneumonia developing in a mechanically ventilated patient > 48 hours after intubation. It is an independent determinant of mortality in patients receiving mechanical ventilation. The incidence is related to the duration of ventilation, occurring at a rate of 1% per day during the first month of ventilation. This risk applies to medical and surgical ICU patients.

27. What are the risk factors for the development of NP?

Patient-related factors	**Therapy-related factors**
• Age	• Use of sedatives
• Malnutrition	• Corticosteroids
• Sepsis	• Antacids
• Shock	• Cytotoxic agents
• Respiratory failure	• Antibiotic therapy
• Extrapulmonary infection	• Enteral feeding
• Diabetes mellitus	• High gastric volume
• Azotemia	• Endotracheal intubation
• Chronic obstructive pulmonary disease	• Reintubation
• CNS dysfunction	• Nasal intubation
• Head trauma	• Circuit change in < 48 hours
• Lung trauma	• Supine position
• Prolonged or complicated surgery	**Infection-control factors**
	• Failure to wash hands routinely
	• Failure to isolate patients with resistant pathogens

28. What are the common pathogens involved in NP?

When a patient has no unusual risk factor or if the pneumonia develops within the first 4 days of hospitalization (i.e., early-onset NP), the **core** group of pathogens are common:

• *E. coli*	• *Serratia marcescens*
• *Klebsiella*	• *H. influenzae*

- *Proteus*
- *Enterobacter*

- *S. pneumoniae*
- Methicillin-sensitive *S. aureus*

When risk factors are present or if the pneumonia develops on or after day 5 (i.e., late-onset NP), in addition to being at risk for the "core" group of organisms, patients with coma, head injury, diabetes, or renal failure are at risk for *S. aureus* infection; those with witnessed aspiration are at risk of anaerobic infection; those receiving high-dose steroids are at risk of *Legionella* infection; those with prolonged ICU stay and prior antibiotic use are at risk for *P. aeruginosa, Acinetobacter,* and methicillin-resistant *S. aureus* infection.

29. How is NP diagnosed?

Clinical diagnosis requires the presence of a new or progressive lung infiltrate **plus** at least two of the following: fever, purulent sputum, or leukocytosis.

The role of **quantitative cultures of respiratory secretions** obtained bronchoscopically (by PSB or BAL) or with a blind catheter is controversial because it uses predetermined microbiologic threshold concentrations (PSB $> 10^3$ and BAL $> 10^4$ or 10^5 colony-forming units/mL), above which pneumonia is diagnosed. This approach can cause false-negative results in the early stages of pneumonia when the diagnostic threshold is not met or if the patient has received antibiotics before collecting the specimen. When such invasive methods are used, results are delayed until growth of the quantitative cultures has occurred, emphasizing the use of early and appropriate empiric antibiotics.

If patients who are mechanically ventilated, finding of $> 5\%$ BAL cells that contain intracellular bacteria is specific for the presence of ventilator-associated pneumonia. **Non-quantitative culture of endotracheal aspirate** is a sensitive but nonspecific method of evaluating the lower airway microflora because it often contains pathogens and colonizing organisms. Endotracheal cultures have a significant negative predictive value and can be used to exclude certain pathogens and modify initial empiric antibiotic therapy.

30. Discuss the treatment of NP.

- In patients with no risk factors and who develop NP in < 5 days of hospitalization, the core group of pathogens play an important role. These patients can be treated with a single agent, such as nonpseudomonal third-generation cephalosporin (ceftriaxone) or β-lactam/β-lactamase inhibitor (ampicillin/sulbactam).
- If the patient is allergic to penicillin, a fluoroquinolone or clindamycin plus aztreonam can be used.
- If the patient has risk factors or if the pneumonia develops ≥ 5 days after hospitalization, infection with *P. aeruginosa, Acinetobacter,* or methicillin-resistant *S. aureus* can occur. Such patients always should be started empirically on dual antipseudomonal therapy until the culture results become available. The following regimens can be used: aminoglycoside or ciprofloxacin **plus** antipseudomonal penicillin, ceftazidime, imipenem, or β-lactam/β-lactamase inhibitor with or without vancomycin (if methicillin-resistant *S. aureus* is a concern).
- If *P. aeruginosa* is present in cultures, combination therapy should be continued.
- If *P. aeruginosa* is not present in tracheal cultures, therapy can be changed from combination therapy to monotherapy with agents such as ciprofloxacin, imipenem, or ceftazidime.
- Clindamycin should be used in patients at risk of anaerobes (postsurgical, witnessed aspiration), vancomycin in patients at risk of *S. aureus* (coma, head trauma, diabetes), and erythromycin with or without rifampin in patients at risk of *Legionella* (high-dose steroids).
- The length of treatment in cases of NP caused by **core** group of organisms can be 7 to 10 days, whereas that in case of *Pseudomonas* or *Acinetobacter* infection should be 2 to 3 weeks.

31. What is the effect of antibiotic administration on survival of NP?

Survival of NP patients is improved when **adequate** antibiotic therapy is used as opposed to inadequate antibiotic therapy. The timing of adequate antibiotic therapy is important; if patients receive adequate therapy **immediately,** their survival may be much better than if the same therapy is administered 1, 2, or 3 days later.

32. List noninfectious conditions that can mimic NP.
- Inflammatory lung disease
- Alveolar hemorrhage
- Pulmonary edema
- Pulmonary embolism
- Chemical or radiation pneumonitis
- Persistent atelectasis
- Infiltrative tumor

33. List some preventive strategies for NP.
- Hand washing
- Isolation of patients with multi-resistant pathogens
- Adequate nutritional support (enteral rather than parenteral)
- Careful handling of ventilator tubing
- Continuous aspiration of subglottic secretions
- Avoidance of large gastric residuals
- Lateral rotational bed therapy
- Semierect positioning of patient

34. What is aspiration pneumonia?
The infectious process of lung that results from the abnormal entry of fluid into the lower respiratory tract. Aspirated material may consist of a combination of particulate exogenous substances and endogenous secretions contaminated by pathogenic organisms. The most common segments involved in aspiration are the posterior segments of the upper lobes and the superior segments of the lower lobes.

35. List factors that predispose to aspiration.
- Reduced consciousness
- Impaired cough reflex
- Impaired glottic closure
- Dysphagia
- Vomiting
- Seizures
- Nasogastric tubes
- Large-volume feedings
- Recumbent position
- Periodontal disease or gingivitis

36. What pathogens are involved in aspiration pneumonia?

Community-acquired
- *S. aureus*
- *S. pneumoniae*
- *Bacteroides*
- *Fusobacterium nucleatum*
- *Peptostreptococcus*
- *Prevotella*
- *Eikenella corrodens*

Nosocomial
- *S. aureus*
- *E. coli*
- *Klebsiella*
- *Proteus*
- *Enterobacter*
- *P. aeruginosa*

37. How is aspiration pneumonia treated?
Community-acquired

Clindamycin or alternatively penicillin G combined with metronidazole. Metronidazole should not be used as monotherapy because it is associated with a failure rate of 50% in the treatment of anaerobic pulmonary infections.

Nosocomial

Ceftriaxone, piperacillin/tazobactam, imipenem, or clindamycin combined with fluoroquinolones.

38. What is the preventive therapy for tuberculosis based on the tuberculin skin test?
Isoniazid in a single daily dose of 300 mg for adults and 5 to 10 mg/kg body weight for children. The therapy should be given for at least 6 months except in persons with HIV infection or patients with large areas of scarring on radiograph, in whom it should be given for 12 months.

39. How is the tuberculin skin test interpreted?

> 5 mm: All individuals receive prophylaxis without respect to age

Known/suspected HIV infection, contacts of the active tuberculosis cases, chest radiograph suggests prior active tuberculosis

> 10 mm: Patients < 35 years old receive prophylaxis

Diabetes mellitus, renal failure, hematologic malignancy, prolonged steroid use, long-term care or correctional inmate, immigrants from high prevalence area

> 15 mm: All other persons < 35 years old

New converters:

> 10 mm increase: All persons < 35 years old

> 15 mm increase: All persons > 35 years old

40. What is an empyema?

The presence of pus in the pleural space. It also includes an exudative pleural effusion with a positive Gram stain.

- Almost 60% of empyemas occur as a complication of parapneumonic effusion.
- 20% occur after thoracic surgical procedure
- 20% occur as a complication of thoracic trauma, esophageal perforation, or extension of subdiaphragmatic infection

41. What are the common pathogens responsible for empyema?

The most common pathogens causing empyema as complication of **pneumonia** are **anaerobes.** Empyema associated with **NP** may be caused by **enteric gram-negative bacilli.** Empyema that follows **trauma** or **hemothorax** is caused most commonly by *S. aureus.* Empyema that occurs **after surgery** such as lung resection or esophageal surgery may result from intraoperative contamination or postoperative extension of infection from a nearby focus. Such infections may be caused by *S. aureus,* **gram-negative bacilli,** and **anaerobes.**

42. What are the clinical manifestations of empyema?

Empyema resulting from:

Aerobic bacterial pneumonia
- Fever
- Cough
- Pleuritic chest pain
- Dyspnea
- Leukocytosis

Anaerobic infection, such as in alcoholics
- Weight loss
- Leukocytosis
- Anemia

Postsurgical
- Postoperative fever
- Dyspnea
- Chest pain
- Amount of pleural fluid excess for the surgical procedure associated with the presence of air in the pleural space arising from a bronchopleural leak

43. How is empyema diagnosed?

The presence of empyema can be recognized on the **chest radiograph,** particularly lateral decubitus views. **CT scan** of the chest is useful in the management of empyema because it can distinguish between loculations, lung abscess, or tumor and detect bronchopleural fistulae. **Thoracentesis** is almost always required, and the presence of gross pus confirms the diagnosis of empyema. Early empyema may appear similar to noninfectious pleural effusions. The **pH of the pleural fluid** can help differentiate empyema from other causes of pleural effusion. Patients with pleural fluid pH < 7.2 are at risk of evolution to empyema. Other factors that favor empyema are positive Gram stain, pleural fluid glucose < 40 mg/dL, and high lactate dehydrogenase (> 1,000 IU/L).

44. What is the initial treatment of empyema?

All patients with suspected empyema must receive appropriate antibiotics guided by Gram stain of the pleural fluid when positive. Tube thoracostomy should be performed without delay if any of the diagnostic factor for empyema (see question 43) are present on the pleural fluid because a delay for even a few hours can increase morbidity.

45. How does the clinician follow the course of empyema after the placement of a chest tube?

A large-bore chest tube, such as 28F, should be used to drain empyema and should be placed in the most dependent part of the pleural cavity to allow complete drainage. Appropriate antibiotics must be continued throughout the course of the drainage. With this approach, improvement in the patient's clinical status and the radiograph usually occurs in first 24–48 hours. The chest tube should be left in place until the volume of the drained fluid becomes < 50 mL in 24 hours and the fluid appears clear yellow in color. If the patient does not improve by 48 hours, either the chest tube drainage is inadequate or the antibiotic therapy is not effective. Such patients should undergo an ultrasound evaluation of the pleural space to assess the adequacy of the drainage and confirmation of pleural fluid culture and sensitivities.

46. Discuss treatment options that are available for inadequately drained or multiloculated empyema?

If the empyema cavity remains inadequately drained after placement of a chest tube, a **second chest tube** can be inserted in the area of fluid accumulation. If the patient has multiple loculations on chest radiograph or chest CT scan, this approach usually is not successful.

Because the pleural fluid loculations are caused by the membranes composed of fibrin, **fibrinolytic agents** are used intrapleurally to destroy these fibrin membranes and to facilitate drainage. Streptokinase in a dose of 250,000 U or urokinase, 100,000 U diluted in 100 mL of saline, is instilled through the chest tube. The tube is then clamped for 2–4 hours before draining spontaneously. The procedure can be repeated daily or twice a day for 14 days without causing systemic fibrinolysis. Fibrinolytic therapy is considered successful if there is an increase in the amount of pleural drainage accompanied by an improvement in the chest radiograph. The success rate with fibrinolytic therapy has been 70–90%. Streptokinase and urokinase appear to be equally effective. Fibrinolytic agents are less likely to be effective if the process has been going on for > 7 days or if the pleural fluid is purulent.

Video-assisted thoracoscopy is an alternative therapy for multiloculated empyema in early stages to allow minimally invasive drainage. Adequate pleural fluid drainage and lung reexpansion may not occur in about 30% of patients after video-assisted thoroscopy and require open decortication to permit immediate lung reexpansion.

Small trials have suggested that thoracoscopy may be superior to chest tube drainage plus fibrinolytic therapy to facilitate drainage of multiloculated empyema and results in an increased rate of complete pleural drainage, reduced chest tube duration, and diminished length of hospital stay.

47. When is decortication indicated?

In patients who remain clinically ill, have inadequate pleural drainage, and have failure of pleural apposition after chest tube placement, use of intrapleural fibrinolytic agents, and video-assisted thoracoscopy. This procedure requires a full thoracotomy and removal of all fibrous tissue from pleural surfaces and pus from the pleural space. It is a major thoracic surgery and should not be considered for markedly debilitated patients.

48. What procedure can be done in patients with empyema who cannot tolerate decortication?

Open drainage procedures such as **open thoracostomy,** which involves resection of one to three ribs to permit open drainage at the inferior border of the empyema cavity and placement of one or more large-bore tubes into the cavity. The cavity is irrigated daily with a mild antiseptic solution, and the drainage can be collected in a colostomy bag attached to the chest tube. The chest tube is advanced gradually outward as the tract closes, and it may take 60–90 days for healing of the drainage site.

49. Discuss the management of postpneumonectomy empyema.

Postpneumonectomy empyema presents with fever, a large amount of sputum, lethargy, weight loss, and purulent drainage from the thoracotomy wound. About 40% of the patients have a bronchopleural or an esophagopleural fistula, necessitating the performance of a barium swallow and a bronchoscopy. If the aforementioned tests are normal, the patient should receive appropriate antibiotics along with tube thoracostomy. Antibiotics effective against the offending organisms should be instilled through the double-lumen chest tube or a separate smaller tube inserted into the second or third intercostal space and the drainage tube clamped for several hours before it is drained. This sequence is repeated until the pleural fluid becomes clear and sterile, which may take 30 days. If a bronchopleural fistula is shown, surgical closure of the fistula with intrathoracic muscle transposition or a pedicle omental flap is required.

BIBLIOGRAPHY

1. American Thoracic Society guidelines for community-acquired pneumonia. Am Rev Respir Dis 148:1418, 1993.
2. Barlett JG, Breiman R, Mandell L, et al: Community-acquired pneumonia in adults: Guidelines for management. Clin Infect Dis 26:811–838, 1998.
3. Bates JH, Campbell GD, Barron AL, et al: Micobial etiology of acute pneumonia in hospitalized patients. Chest 101:1005, 1992.
4. Brook I, Frazier EH: Aerobic and anaerobic microbiology of empyema. Chest 103:1502, 1993.
5. Doller G, Schuy W, Tjhen KY, et al: Direct detection of influenza virus antigen in nasopharyngeal specimens by direct enzyme immunoassay in comparison with quantitating virus shedding. J Clin Micobiol 30:866, 1992.
6. Greenburg SB: Viral pneumonia. Infect Dis Clin North Am 5:615, 1991.
7. Murray J, Nadel J: Text Book of Respiratory Diseases. Philadelphia, W.B. Saunders, 1994.
8. Sahn SA: State of the art: The pleura. Am Rev Respir Dis 138:184, 1998.
9. Temes RT, Follis F, Kessler RM, et al: Intrapleural fibrinolytics in the management of empyema thoracis. Chest 110:102, 1996.

23. IDIOPATHIC PULMONARY FIBROSIS

William J. Gibbons, M.D.

1. What is idiopathic pulmonary fibrosis (IPF)?

A chronic progressive pulmonary disease, primarily involving the interstitium. IPF is estimated to occur in at least 5 in 100,000 people in the United States annually. IPF is a clinical syndrome characterized by the insidious onset of exertional dyspnea, usually in people in their 40s and 50s. Usual interstitial pneumonitis (UIP) is recognized as the specific histologic pattern on lung biopsy specimens that is associated with the clinical syndrome of IPF. Male gender predominates in patients with IPF, and a significant cigarette smoking exposure history is common.

2. List the physical signs of IPF.

- Tachypnea
- Increased use of accessory muscles of respiration
- **Velcro**-type inspiratory crackles
- Finger clubbing (70%)

In **advanced** cases:

- Signs of chronic cor pulmonale, with internal jugular venous distention, loud P_2 heart sounds and pitting peripheral edema

3. Describe the radiographic findings of IPF.

Plain chest radiographs typically show loss of lung volumes with chronic bibasilar reticular interstitial infiltrates. Later in the course of IPF, bilateral areas of **honeycombing** can be found commonly in subpleural locations and are thought to represent areas of well-established fibrosis.

4. Discuss the use of CT in IPF.

Chest CT scan by high-resolution technique has been used in IPF to:

1. Differentiate noninvasively other chronic interstitial lung diseases from IPF
2. Prognosticate
3. Assess response to therapy

In patients with IPF, patchy areas of **ground-glass opacification,** which are thought to represent areas of active alveolitis, as well as **honeycombing** can be seen to varying degrees on high-resolution CT. The sensitivity and specificity of high-resolution CT for the diagnosis of IPF are in the range of approximately 80%; false-positive results for IPF can come from other entities, such as **pulmonary sarcoidosis** and **hypersensitivity pneumonitis.**

5. How is IPF manifested physiologically?

By a fall in oxygen saturation during exertion, even before abnormalities are detectable in spirometry, static lung volume, or single-breath diffusion capacity (D_LCO) measurements. Well-established IPF has a characteristic pattern of pulmonary function test abnormalities:

1. A **restrictive** ventilatory defect suggested by the combination of reduced vital capacity and forced expiratory volume in 1 second (FEV_1) with an increased FEV_1-to-FVC ratio found on spirometry
2. **Restrictive** defect confirmed by reduced total lung capacity and other static lung volume measurements
3. Low D_LCO

Resting hypoxemia is typical with established IPF, often requiring supplemental oxygen. The reduced D_LCO at rest is more due to ventilation-perfusion disturbances (inequalities) than to **thickened** alveolar basement membranes.

6. Discuss the differential diagnosis of IPF.

- Because IPF is a diagnosis of exclusion, a careful environmental, occupational, and medication use history is important.
- **Hypersensitivity pneumonitis** can occur, for example, from exposure to a pet bird at home.
- **Asbestosis** and **silicosis** could be suspected from appropriate exposures at occupations engaged in several decades ago as well as recently.
- Questioning about administration of **medications,** such as certain antibiotics (e.g., nitrofurantoin), chemotherapeutic agents (e.g., methotrexate, cyclophosphamide), and antiarrhythmics (e.g., amiodarone), should occur.
- Certain **connective tissue diseases** (collagen-vascular diseases) are associated with chronic interstitial lung disease, which potentially could be mistaken radiographically for IPF, including rheumatoid arthritis, scleroderma, polymyositis-dermatomyositis, Sjögren's syndrome, and systemic lupus erythematosus.
- Sometimes confounding the differentiation of IPF from connective tissue disease–associated chronic interstitial lung disease is the finding of low-level positive antinuclear antibody, rheumatoid factor, and erythrocyte sedimentation rate titers found in a few patients with IPF.
- Certain idiopathic chronic interstitial lung diseases can be mistaken for IPF. For example, **pulmonary sarcoidosis** is located more often in the upper lung zones than IPF, has significant mediastinal lymphadenopathy more frequently than IPF, and has extrapulmonary involvement at times, whereas IPF does not.
- Although **eosinophilic granuloma (histiocytosis X)** shares finger clubbing as a frequent physical finding with IPF, radiographic infiltrates are located more often in upper lung zones, and costophrenic angles are spared compared with IPF.
- Other potential chronic interstitial lung disease radiographic mimickers of IPF include desquamative interstitial pneumonitis (**DIP**), bronchiolitis obliterans with organizing pneumonia (**BOOP**), nonspecific interstitial pneumonia (**NSIP**), respiratory bronchiolitis interstitial lung disease (**RSILD**), lymphocytic interstitial pneumonitis (**LIP**), and giant cell interstitial pneumonitis (**GIP**), all of which have different ages of onset, prognoses, and response rates to corticosteroid treatment than IPF.

7. What is the mortality in IPF?

Factors such as younger age (<50 years), female gender, predominantly ground-glass rather than fibrotic (or honeycomb) pattern on high-resolution CT, shorter duration of symptoms before presentation, and less severe grade of disease (i.e., fewer symptoms, better lung function test results, less infiltration on radiographic studies) seem to predict better survival in IPF. Mortality rates for UIP reported in the medical literature are 60–70%, and median survival has been reported at approximately 2.8 years. At 5 years after diagnosis, about 50% of patients with IPF are still alive. Death is most often due to hypoxemic respiratory failure.

8. Discuss the relative advantages and disadvantages of transbronchial versus open lung biopsy approaches for confirmation of diagnosis in IPF?

Advantages

- Bronchoscopy with bronchial lavage can help exclude an infectious cause of interstitial infiltrates on radiographic studies, such as mycobacterial and fungal infections, as well as certain presumably immunologically mediated diseases, such as pulmonary alveolar proteinosis.
- Transbronchial biopsies performed during the same procedure can help exclude alternative noninfectious diagnoses that cause chronic interstitial infiltrates on radiographs, specifically sarcoidosis, hypersensitivity pneumonitis, eosinophilic granuloma, and lymphangitic carcinomatosis.

Diadvantages
- Transbronchial biopsies should be avoided in patients with interstitial lung disease complicated by significant pulmonary hypertension because of increased risk of significant bleeding.
- Because of the small size of samples obtained by transbronchial biopsies and the patchy nature of lung involvement, the chance of confirming a histologic pattern compatible with IPF is relatively low (25%).

9. When is an open lung biopsy recommended?

To confirm a specific pathologic pattern associated with IPF. Taking three or more specimens from several areas is recommended, both from those areas grossly involved with disease as well as from areas grossly uninvolved (normal-appearing). Although readily obtained from a technical standpoint, lingular or right middle lobe tip biopsies are not desirable because these areas can contain patchy microscopic fibrosis even in the absence of lung disease.

10. List the types of histologic patterns found in the lung biopsy specimens of patients with IPF.

- UIP
- DIP
- Bronchiolitis obliterans with interstitial pneumonitis (BIP)
- LIP
- GIP

11. What is the clinical correlation and relevance of different histologic patterns found in patients suspected preoperatively of having IPF?

- When **DIP** is found in the lung biopsy specimen, mean patient age is younger (42 years), and both expected response to systemic corticosteroids and mortality rate (27%) are better than with UIP.
- When **NSIP** or **RBILD** are found in the lung biopsy specimen, mean patient age is younger (49 years or 36 years), and expected response to systemic corticosteroids and mortality rate (11% or 0%) are better than with UIP.
- When **acute interstitial pneumonitis** (Hamman-Rich syndrome) is found in the lung biopsy specimen, mean patient age is younger (49 years), but expected response to systemic corticosteroids and mortality rate (62%) are comparable with UIP.

12. Discuss common causes and presentations of clinical deterioration in IPF.

Patients with IPF typically have so-called **traction bronchiectasis** resulting from inhomogeneous distribution of fibrotic strands attached to outer walls of bronchi and noncartilaginous bronchioles. This complication can lead to chronic cough; inhaled topical corticosteroids sometimes can help diminish this symptom. Occasionally, infectious exacerbations of traction bronchiectasis occur, manifested by increased colored sputa production, dyspnea, and sometimes fever. At times, definite radiographic evidence of pneumonia can be encountered. As in other patients, sputum culture and appropriate antibiotic therapy are indicated.

All patients with chronic lung disease of any kind, including those with IPF, are at increased risk of **spontaneous pneumothorax.** Warning about increased risk of spontaneous pneumothorax during air travel (because of overdistention of subpleural alveoli from acutely developing pressure differentials) should be provided. Increased flow of nasal oxygen is advisable during air travel because cabins are pressurized only to 8,000 feet altitude, where ambient inhaled oxygen tension is lower than at sea level.

As a result of the development of chronic pulmonary hypertension from various factors, including chronic alveolar hypoxia and destruction of pulmonary capillary beds, **chronic cor pulmonale** can develop in patients with more advanced IPF. This is characterized by clinical signs of peripheral edema, hypoxemia, internal jugular venous distention, and auscultated S_3 gallop accentuated by inspiration. The electrocardiogram in chronic cor pulmonale can manifest changes, such as right-axis deviation, right ventricular hypertrophy, and **p pulmonale.** The magnitude of elevated pulmonary artery pressures and right ventricular function can be estimated from transthoracic echocardiography; this approach in patients with IPF does not suffer from the same limitations encountered in hyperinflated patients with chronic air flow obstruction. Supplemental oxygen therapy and diuretics are important components of treatment of chronic cor pulmonale in patients with IPF.

Patients with IPF are at increased risk of **pulmonary emboli,** particularly those with chronic peripheral edema related to chronic cor pulmonale. As in other patients, lung ventilation-perfusion (V/Q) scanning and lower extremity venous Doppler studies are essential first steps in excluding venous thromboembolism in patients with IPF. In contrast to patients with no preexisting chronic lung disease, interpretation of lung V/Q scans can be more challenging, and selective pulmonary angiogram may be required more often. Risks of worsening preexisting pulmonary hypertension and precipitating acute-on-chronic cor pulmonale are not increased with selective pulmonary angiography.

Since the original autopsy reports of coexistent **lung cancer** and IPF, several studies have noted an association between these two conditions. Adenocarcinoma cell type has been mentioned specifically in this context. Although the available evidence is partially flawed in some instances, it would seem prudent to monitor patients with IPF clinically and radiographically for the possible development of lung cancer during the course of follow-up.

13. List treatment options that are available for patients with IPF.
- Supportive care
- Immunosuppressive agents
- Antifibrotic agents
- Lung transplantation

14. Describe supportive care for patients with IPF.
Because of chronic progressive hypoxemia, **supplemental domiciliary oygen** by nasal cannula often is prescribed. Sometimes, innovative means of oxygen administration must be considered when oxygen therapy by nasal cannula is insufficient. Transtracheal oxygen can be considered in carefully selected patients who have a history of reliable adherence to treatment, have few if any chronic respiratory tract secretions, are nonsmokers, have no coagulopathy, and have sufficient learning skills to master daily routine care of the catheter. Other examples of supportive care include **vaccinations** (against influenza and pneumococcal infections) and participation in an **outpatient pulmonary rehabilitation** program.

15. Describe treatment with immunosuppressive medications.
Factors such as younger age, worse pulmonary function test results, more extensive ground-glass opacities on high-resolution CT, and more extensive cellular (e.g., lymphocytes) infiltration on biopsy specimen seem to predict a better response to immunosuppressive therapy. Prescription of systemic corticosteroids, such as prednisone, is the first step in immunosuppressive therapy. One approach starts dosing at 1.0–1.5 mg/kg/d of prednisone for 12 weeks, followed by a reduction to 0.5–0.75 mg/kg/d over the next 12 weeks if the patient appears stable or improved. Gradual tapering of prednisone dosage to 0.25 mg/kg/d is accomplished over the next 6 months, and reassessment of need for prednisone is judged at 1 year. Careful attention to expected side effects, such as gastrointestinal upset, hyperglycemia, systemic hypertension, and osteoporosis, is needed. Potential prophylactic measures against side effects might include consideration of daily histamine$_2$-receptor blocker (e.g., famotidine) and alendronate (e.g., 5 mg/d).

16. Describe cytotoxic therapy in IPF.
- Cytotoxic agents, specifically cyclophosphamide and azathioprine, have been traditionally considered in patients who are deemed to be failing systemic corticosteroids after 3–6 months therapy or who are intolerant of corticosteroid therapy.

- One dosing approach has been to use 2 mg/kg/day orally of **cyclophosphamide** in combination with 0.25 mg/kg/day of prednisone. Careful regular monitoring of complete blood counts and urinalyses is recommended because of risk of bone marrow suppression as well as small increased risk of urinary bladder cancer with prolonged use of cyclophosphamide. Cyclophosphamide occasionally may induce interstitial lung disease independent of IPF.
- An alternative to cyclophosphamide, **azathioprine,** is dosed at 2 mg/kg/d, not to exceed 200 mg/d. Combination of azathioprine and low-dose prednisone has improved survival in patients with IPF when compared with prednisone alone. Careful regular monitoring of complete blood counts is recommended for azathioprine because of risk of bone marrow suppression.
- A positive response to a cytotoxic agent may take 6 months to be apparent
- Only about 25–30% respond positively to cytotoxic agents.

17. How does one judge the response to systemic corticosteroids or cytotoxic agents?
- Clinical follow-up
- Repeat radiographic studies (plain chest radiographs)
- Repetitive performance of pulmonary function tests, including spirometry, single-breath diffusion capacity, static lung volume measurements by helium dilution or body plethysmographic methods, plus resting and ambulatory pulse oximetry

Repeat chest CT scan may provide follow-up information about areas of ground-glass opacity (alveolitis) representing active inflammation in subpleural locations, which, by inference, may be amenable to immunosuppressive therapy. With initiation of therapy, improvement in symptoms is sometimes not paralleled by changes in lung function tests or chest CT scan results, making assessment of response to therapy confusing at times. **Composite scores,** such as the **CRP score** from lung function test results, radiographic studies (chest CT scans), and symptoms, have been proposed as an alternative valid means of objectively weighing the respective changes in these parameters during treatment and follow-up of patients with IPF.

18. Which patients with IPF should be referred for consideration of lung transplantation?
Symptomatic progressive IPF with failure to improve or at least maintain lung function while under treatment with systemic corticosteroids or alternative immunosuppressive medications in appropriate doses is a common indication for referral. Referral to a transplant program should be considered if lung function tests are abnormal even though the patient with IPF is only mildly symptomatic. Appropriately selected patients should be <65 years old by the time of transplant operation. To ensure this, the patient should be listed by a transplant program by age 63 years because a wait of 2 years for a donor is possible. In patients with IPF, particular attention to excluding bronchogenic cancer, tuberculosis, and bacterial colonization of bronchiectatic areas should be paid preoperatively.

19. List relative contraindications for lung transplantation.
- Symptomatic osteoporosis confirmed by bone densitometry
- Severe musculoskeletal disease affecting the chest (e.g., kyphoscoliosis)
- Requirement for invasive ventilation
- Unresolved psychosocial problems (including nonadherence to prescribed medical care)
- Colonization with fungi or atypical mycobacteria if they cannot be eradicated with antibiotic therapy preoperatively
- Coexistent diabetes mellitus if severe dysfunction of other vital organs is present (e.g., diabetic nephropathy with renal failure)

20. List absolute contraindications for lung transplantation.
- Significant dysfunction of other vital organs (e.g., creatinine clearance <50 mg/mL/min)
- Infection with human immunodeficiency virus
- Active malignancy within the past 2 years (except basal cell and squamous cell skin carcinomas)

- Positive hepatitis B antigen status
- Positive hepatitis C status with biopsy-proven histologic evidence of associated liver disease
- Progressive neuromuscular disease

21. Describe further recommendations regarding lung transplantation in IPF.

- Candidates >130% ideal body weight or <70% ideal body weight need to lose or gain weight to become eligible for transplantation.
- Current systemic corticosteroid dosage needs to be <20 mg/d of prednisone or prednisolone.
- Candidates need to be free of substance abuse, including cigarette smoking, for at least 6 months before transplantation.

BIBLIOGRAPHY

1. American Thoracic Society: Idiopathic pulmonary fibrosis: Diagnosis and treatment. International Consensus Statement. Am J Respir Crit Care Med 161:646–664, 2000.
2. Chang J, Raghu G: Use of corticosteroids for treatment of interstitial lung disease. Clin Pulm Med 7:9–14, 2000.
3. Egan J: Pharmacologic therapy of idiopathic pulmonary fibrosis. J Heart Lung Transplant 17:1039–1044, 1998.
4. Hubbard R, Venn A, Lewis S, et al: Lung cancer and cryptogenic fibrosing alveolitis: A population-based cohort study. Am J Respir Crit Care Med 161:5–8, 2000.
5. Katzenstein ALA, Myers JL: Idiopathic pulmonary fibrosis: Clinical relevance of pathologic classification. Am J Respir Crit Care Med 157:1301–1315, 1998.
6. King TE: Idiopathic pulmonary fibrosis. In Schwarz MI, King TE (eds): Interstitial Lung Disease, 3rd ed. Hamilton, Ontario, B.C. Decker, 1998, pp 597–644.
7. Lynch JP, McCune WJ: Immunosuppressive and cytotoxic pharmacotherapy for pulmonary disorders. Am J Respir Crit Care Med 155:395–420, 1997.
8. Maurer JR, Frost AE, Estenne M, et al: International guidelines for the selection of lung transplant candidates. J Heart Lung Transplant 17:703–709, 1998.
9. Panos RJ, Mortenson RL, Niccoli SA, et al: Clinical deterioration in patients with idiopathic pulmonary fibrosis: Causes and assessment. Am J Med 88:396–404, 1990.
10. Reynolds HY: Diagnostic and management strategies for diffuse interstitial lung disease. Chest 113:192–202, 1998.
11. Tung KT, Wells AU, Rubens MB, et al: Accuracy of the typical computed tomographic appearances of fibrosing alveolitis. Thorax 48:334–338, 1993.

24. BULLOUS DISEASE OF THE LUNG

Raffy L. Karamanoukian, M.D., and Lisa Apfel, M.D.

1. What is the definition of a bleb and a bulla?

A bleb is a collection of air enclosed by visceral pleura caused by rupture of alveoli. Bullae are air-filled spaces within the lung parenchyma caused by alveolar destruction. They have thick, fibrous walls.

2. Where do blebs and bullae typically occur?

Blebs typically occur at the apices of the lung. Bullae most frequently occur in the upper lobes of the lung. They are almost always confined to a lung segment or lobe of the lung.

3. What is the pathophysiology of bullous formation?

Originally described by Cooke et al. in 1952, a threefold mechanism is thought to contribute to the pathophysiology of bullous formation: (1) progressive enlargement is caused by the bronchus entering the bullous airspace via a "ball-valve" mechanism; (2) an enlarging cystic space causes destruction of adjacent normal pulmonary tissue, further increasing the size of the bulla; and (3) inflammation of the smaller airways causes further enlargement of the bulla. Overall, progressive enlargement of the bulla results from continued inflation and intrinsic destruction of pulmonary tissue.

4. What is vanishing lung syndrome?

This is a radiographic term used to define bullous disease that completely replaces the normal ipsilateral lung. This process is visible on plain radiographs at the terminal stages of the disease.

5. What techniques are used to image bullous disease of the lung?

Perfusion scans and ventilation-perfusion scans are used to stage severity of bullous disease of the lung. Split lung function can be estimated by perfusion scanning. Ventilation-perfusion scanning can determine localized reduction in blood flow resulting from destruction of pulmonary vasculature and/or pulmonary parenchyma. CT scanning is the imaging technique of choice for assessing patients with bullous disease of the lung before surgery.

6. What are the indications for surgical intervention?

Bullae occupying more than one third of the ipsilateral lung in patients with moderate or severe symptoms of dyspnea.

7. What are the complications of bullous disease?

Pneumothorax, infection, or massive hemoptysis are complications of bullous disease of the lung. All are indications for surgical intervention.

8. What is the Monaldi procedure?

The Monaldi procedure was originally described for tuberculous cavities refractory to conventional therapy. Subperiosteal rib resection is performed overlying the bulla and a Foley catheter is placed through a purse string incorporating the parietal and visceral pleura and wall of the bulla. The balloon is inflated and placed under suction. This space is obliterated by instillation of sclerosing agents or talc for pleurodesis. It is an excellent technique to obliterate bullous spaces and improve lung function in debilitated patients.

9. How is standard bullectomy performed?

Via a thoracotomy incision, the bulla is opened and fibrous septa excised. The walls of the bulla are used to reinforce the staple line at the base of the resected bulla. This double layer of cyst wall (bullous wall) is an effective buttress for the stapler and prevents prolonged air leaks after staple resection. This technique has also been performed via video-assisted thoracoscopy.

10. Is there a role for lobectomy for bullous disease of the lung?

Yes, provided the bullous disease is limited to that lobe of the lung and the whole lobe is involved with bullous disease.

11. What procedure is required for patients with bullous disease who present with hemoptysis?

Bronchoscopy should be performed to rule out endobronchial lesions. Since hemoptysis in these patients is almost always associated with secondary infection of the bulla, they almost always resolve with antibiotic therapy and surgery is reserved for recurrent or massive hemoptysis.

12. What is the treatment for pneumothorax complication of bullous disease of the lung?

Resection of the lung parenchyma involving the bulla is the treatment of choice to prevent chronic bronchopleural fistula.

13. Is there a role for lung volume reduction surgery for bullous disease?

Only if the disease process is diffuse and noncompressive of the underlying lung. Lung volume reduction surgery is still investigational in nature.

BIBLIOGRAPHY

1. Cooke FN, et al: Cystic disease of the lungs. J Thorac Surg 23:546, 1952.
2. Goldberg M: Emphysema and bullous disease. In Pearson FG, Deslauriers J, Ginsberg RJ, et al (eds): Thoracic Surgery. New York, Churchill Livingstone, 1995.
3. Klingman RR, Angelillo VA, DeMeester TR: Cystic and bullous lung disease. Ann Thorac Surg 52:576, 1991.

25. MASSIVE HEMOPTYSIS

Jacob DeLaRosa, M.D.

1. What is massive hemoptysis?
Expectoration of blood from the lungs in quantities sufficient to be life-threatening. The arbitrary quantified amount is 200–1,000 mL of coughed blood over 24 hours. The consensus among clinicians is 600 mL over 24 hours.

2. How often does massive hemoptysis occur?
Rarely; 1–4% of patients with hemoptysis.

3. What is the mortality of massive hemoptysis?
80%

4. What is the blood supply of massive hemoptysis?
- Bronchial circulation   95%
- Pulmonary circulation   4%
- Systemic collateral circulation   1%

5. List the factors contributing to life-threatening massive hemoptysis.
- Rate of blood loss
- Baseline pulmonary function
- Antecedent disease states
- Mechanism of bleeding
- Volume of blood loss
- Efficacy of cough
- Anticoagulation

6. Name the most common precipitating factor for bronchial artery bleeding.
Inflammatory lung disease, particularly tuberculosis.

7. What is the most common cause of massive hemoptysis resulting from pulmonary circulation?
Flow-directed pulmonary artery catheterization (Swan-Ganz). Hemoptysis occurs in 1 of every 500 Swan-Ganz catheter insertions. Injury to the pulmonary artery is due to perforation by the tip of the catheter, which can be avoided by limiting advancement of the catheter from the insertion site.

8. How does collateral circulation cause massive hemoptysis?
Fistulization of the bronchial tree with a systemic artery can cause massive hemoptysis. Such an occurrence may be related to concurrent or preexisting vascular trauma, aneurysmal erosion of the airway, or inflammatory fistulization induced by surgical maneuvers (e.g., posttracheostomy tracheoinnominate artery fistula).

9. What is the acute treatment of massive hemoptysis?
Diagnostic modalities are the initial step in treatment: Localize the site of bleeding, and protect the other lung.

10. What is the most common history related by a patient with massive hemoptysis?
In >40% of patients, a previous episode of hemoptysis, usually within 3 months of presentation.

11. List the principles of managing massive hemoptysis.
- Maintenance of airway

- Preservation of ventilation in nonbleeding lung
- Identification of bleeding site
- Isolation of bleeding site
- Control of source of bleeding

12. How does endobronchial balloon tamponade work?
A Fogarty-type of embolectomy catheter is positioned in the main stem, lobar, or segmental bronchi, with subsequent inflation to occlude the bleeding bronchus.

13. How does endobronchial iced saline lavage work?
It is a technique used to control bleeding temporarily by the induction of hypothermic vasospasm of the likely bronchial artery source.

14. What is the definitive therapy in patients with massive hemoptysis?
Surgical resection of the site that is bleeding:
- Lobectomy
- Segmentectomy
- Pneumonectomy

15. Define transcatheter vessel embolization.
Occlusion of the bleeding vessel by transcatheter embolization from the bronchial artery or the pulmonary circulation.

16. List the causes of massive hemoptysis.
- Lung abscess
- Bronchiectasis
- Trauma
- Tumor

17. Do patients with massive hemoptysis die from hemorrhagic shock?
No. Patients commonly die from asphyxiation from airway obstruction.

18. Is massive hemoptysis seen in aortic dissections?
Yes, but it is more common in chronic dissections representing manifestations of bronchial erosion owing to an enlarging false lumen.

19. What is coital hemoptysis?
Hemoptysis associated with increased cardiovascular demands and left ventricular dysfunction brought on by sexual activity.

BIBLIOGRAPHY

1. Baue AE (ed): Glenn's Thoracic and Cardivascular Surgery, 6th ed. Stamford, CT, Appleton & Lange, 1996.
2. Grenvik A (ed): Textbook of Critical Care, 4th ed. Philadelphia, W.B. Saunders, 2000.
3. Sabiston DC Jr (ed): Textbook of Surgery, 15th ed. Philadelphia, W.B. Saunders, 1997.
4. Sabiston DC, Spencer FC: Gibbon's Surgery of the Chest, 5th ed. Philadelphia, W.B. Saunders, 1992.
5. Schwartz SI, Shires GT, Spencer FC (eds): Principles of Surgery, 7th ed. New York, McGraw-Hill, 1999.
6. Shields TW (ed): General Thoracic Surgery, 4th ed. Baltimore, Williams & Wilkins, 1994.
7. Turney SZ, Rodriguez A, Cowley RA (eds): Management of Cardiothoracic Trauma. Baltimore, Williams & Wilkins, 1990.

26. LUNG ABSCESS

Jacob DeLaRosa, M.D., and Raffy L. Karamanoukian, M.D.

1. What is a lung abscess?
A localized area of suppuration and cavitation in the lung caused by a foreign body or pyogenic organisms.

2. List the causes of lung abscess.
- Aspiration pneumonia (55%)
- Primary necrotizing pneumonia (15%)
- Bronchial obstruction secondary to neoplasm (20%)
- Septic emboli
- Infection of pulmonary infarction

3. What is a simple or primary lung abscess?
Pyogenic abscess secondary to aspiration pneumonitis as opposed to an abscess occurring in association with systemic diseases or malignancy.

4. List the primary risk factors for aspiration pneumonia.
- Altered mental status
- Poor dentition
- Periodontal infections
- Vocal cord paralysis

5. What are the most common organisms involved in primary abscess?
1. **Anaerobic bacteria** (most common)
2. Alpha-hemolytic streptococci
3. *Neisseria catarrhalis*
4. Pneumococci
5. *Pseudomonas*
6. *Proteus*
7. *Escherichia coli*
8. *Klebsiella*

6. What are the most common organisms causing primary necrotizing pneumonia?
- *Staphylococcus aureus*
- Gram-negative organisms (especially *Klebsiella*)

7. List the most common sites of primary lung abscess.
1. Superior segment of the right lower lobe
2. Posterior segment of the right upper lobe
3. Superior segment of the left lower lobe

8. Why are the aforementioned sites of primary lung abscess the most common?
Patients are usually in the supine or recumbent position, and these are the first dependent portions of the lung.

9. Describe the clinical presentation of lung abscess.
The presentation is relatively uniform. The patient appears ill, is likely to be febrile, and often describes recent onset of copious foul sputum production, reflecting decompression of the abscess into the airway.

10. In a febrile patient with copious production of foul sputum, the differential diagnosis can be reduced to what three entities?
1. Lung abscess
2. Bronchiectasis
3. Cavitating carcinoma

11. What is the treatment of primary lung abscess?
Prolonged antimicrobial therapy. **Penicillin G** has traditionally been the antibiotic of choice and can be initiated even before the results of sputum cultures are known. In one randomized controlled trial, **clindamycin** was found to be more effective in community-acquired putrid lung abscess.

12. What is the role of bronchoscopy in the treatment of lung abscess?
- Diagnosis
- Removal of foreign body if one is present
- Drainage of the abscess

13. Has surgical treatment for primary lung abscess increased or decreased in recent years?
The effectiveness of antibiotics in treating primary lung abscess has dramatically **decreased** surgical intervention.

14. List the complications of lung abscess.
- Empyema
- Septicemia
- Metastatic brain abscess
- Bronchogenic spread
- Hemoptysis

15. What is the mortality of aspiration-type lung abscess?
5–6%.

16. What is the mortality if surgical treatment is required for a primary lung abscess?
11%.

17. What is the reported mortality of children treated medically for primary lung abscess?
0%.

18. What is the distinction between a lung abscess and a consolidated pneumonia?
The distinction is made as areas of cavitation develop, and peripheral margins of the infection develop sharper definition. Dyspnea is not a prominent finding in lung abscess, and auscultatory findings are primarily seen in pneumonia.

19. Can a lung abscess hide a cancer?
Yes. A lung abscess can form distal to an obstructive lung carcinoma. Frequently a carcinoma becomes visible as the distal infection responds to antibiotic treatment.

20. Can parasites cause lung abscess?
Yes; in certain parts of the world, parasitic infections are common causes.

21. How does *Entamoeba histolytica* produce a lung abscess?
Hematogenous spread or direct extension from the liver, in which case it is almost always associated with an empyema.

22. What does the term anchovy paste denote?
When an amebic abscess of the liver ruptures through the diaphragm and into the lung, the abscess contents discharge into the bronchial tree, and a cough with expectoration of the classic **anchovy paste** sputum, which contains amebae and lysed liver tissue, is seen.

23. What color sputum is seen with an amebic abscess of the lung?
Creamy white and not anchovy.

24. What is the treatment for a parasitic lung abscess?
Metronidazole; operative intervention rarely is required.

25. Can sepsis lead to lung abscess?
Yes.

26. What is a pyopneumothorax?
When a lung abscess bursts into the pleural cavity.

27. Does a chest radiograph showing a well-delineated cavity with an air-fluid level confirm the diagnosis of lung abscess and exclude carcinoma?
No. **Bronchoscopy** and **biopsy** are essential in excluding carcinoma.

28. What is the duration of treatment with antibiotics for lung abscess?
8 weeks of antibiotics; some series report 3–4 months.

29. How effective is conservative treatment in lung abscess?
Successful in 95%.

30. Is there a role for percutaneous catheter drainage in lung abscess?
Yes. It was once thought that this type of drainage is inadequate, but more recent reports have shown efficacy with this treatment.

31. How is a percutaneous catheter drainage procedure done?
The technique involves insertion of a relatively small percutaneous drainage tube that is connected to a closed draining system or to a water seal or suction. Tube drainage was limited by the viscosity and particulate content of the pus, but with the introduction of thrombolytic therapy, such as urokinase, streptokinase, and tissue plasminogen activator, the viscosity can be reduced and the cavity drained.

32. Name the three options for operative treatment of lung abscess.
1. Pneumonostomy
2. Pneumonotomy
3. Pulmonary resection

33. What is the definitive operative treatment for lung abscess?
Pulmonary resection.

34. List the standard indications for pulmonary resection in the treatment of lung abscess.
- Failure of conservative treatment
- Serious hemorrhage
- Suspicion of associated carcinoma

35. List the advantages of pulmonary resection in the treatment of lung abscess.
- Removing the entire infection promptly
- Less hazardous than external drainage when the abscess is large or centrally located.

36. What is the most common cause of surgical intervention for lung abscess?
Bronchial obstruction resulting from carcinoma.

37. What kind of endotracheal tube should be used if surgical treatment is necessary for a lung abscess?
Double-lumen endotracheal tube to prevent spillage of pus into the contralateral lung.

BIBLIOGRAPHY

1. Cuschieri AI, Giles GR, Moossa AR (eds): Essential Surgical Practice, 3rd ed. Oxford, Butterworth-Heine-
     mann, 1995.
2. Sabiston DC Jr (ed): Textbook of Surgery, 15th ed. Philadelphia, W.B. Saunders, 1997.
3. Sabiston DC, Spencer FC: Gibbon's Surgery of the Chest, 5th ed. Philadelphia, W.B. Saunders, 1992.
4. Schwartz SI, Shires GT, Spencer FC (eds): Principles of Surgery, 7th ed. New York, McGraw-Hill, 1999.
5. Shields TW (ed): General Thoracic Surgery, 4th ed. Baltimore, Williams & Wilkins, 1994.
6. Turney SZ, Rodriguez A, Cowley RA (eds): Management of Cardiothoracic Trauma. Baltimore, Williams
     & Wilkins, 1990.

27. PRIMARY MALIGNANT NEOPLASMS OF THE LUNG

Chukwumere E. Nwogu, M.D.

1. Which are the most common histologic types of primary lung malignancies?
- **Adenocarcinoma** (most common) 50%
- Squamous cell tumors 30%
- Small cell carcinoma 20%
- Undifferentiated large cell carcinoma 10%

2. Does neoadjuvant or induction chemotherapy yield a survival advantage in the treatment of stage IIIA non–small cell lung carcinoma?

Yes, the role of neoadjuvant chemotherapy has been established in several trials. Significant improvement in median survival has been shown when neoadjuvant chemotherapy was combined with surgery.

3. Does chest CT provide adequate mediastinal lymph node staging?

No. Even with current CT scanners, sensitivity and specificity remain low. Several researchers have shown a marked increase in accuracy of mediastinal lymph node staging when mediastinoscopy is added to chest CT. In one such study, overall sensitivity and specificity of CT were 63% and 57%, vs. 89% and 100% when combined with mediastinoscopy.

4. In which population group is the incidence of lung carcinoma rising the fastest?

Reflecting the changing smoking habits in women that have occurred since the early 1950s and the long exposure required for the development of this malignancy, the rate in women is rising at an alarming pace. Lung cancer is currently the most common cause of cancer death in both men and women.

5. A percutaneous needle biopsy of a new, irregular, peripheral 2.5-cm right upper lobe lung mass in a 68-year-old medically fit woman shows no malignant cells. What should appropriate further management be?

Wedge resection of this lesion, preferably by video-assisted thoracoscopy (VATS), is indicated after appropriate workup. If frozen section analysis provides a malignant diagnosis, lobectomy is the therapy of choice. Percutaneous transthoracic needle biopsy has a significant false-negative rate — 15–25% — in indeterminate peripheral lesions. It is, however, useful in the patient with a clinically nonresectable tumor or in a patient who refuses resection or has medical contraindications to surgery.

6. How is VATS applicable to the management of lung carcinoma?

VATS provides a less invasive method of excising peripheral lung lesions than thoracotomy. Hilar and mediastinal lymph nodes can be sampled and pleural deposits biopsied. Invasion of surrounding structures may be observed. Complete drainage of malignant effusions followed by pleural sclerosis with various agents may be performed.

7. Is there a difference in the local control of lung cancer provided by either a lobectomy or segmentectomy?

Segmental and wedge resections are reserved for patients with extremely poor pulmonary function who cannot tolerate a lobectomy. It has been shown that these lesser resections carry a higher rate of local recurrence and decreased long-term survival, probably because of failure to remove occult intrapulmonary lymphatic spread.

8. Does external-beam radiation therapy, chemotherapy, or intrapleural BCG improve overall survival after complete resection of non–small cell lung carcinoma?

Probably not. Multiple randomized studies have failed to show an impact of strictly adjuvant therapies on overall patient survival after complete resection of non–small cell lung carcinoma.

9. What is the acceptable 30-day postoperative mortality after lobectomy for lung carcinoma?

2–3%, which is one half of that recorded for pneumonectomy. In patients ≥70 years old, the mortality may be increased.

10. What is the overall 5-year survival of all patients who present with lung carcinoma?

11–14%.

11. What factors affect overall 5-year survival?

Survival rate depends on stage of the disease, but only a few patients who present with lung cancer are considered potentially resectable. In only 30% of all non–small cell lung cancer patients is there a defined role for surgical resection; the other 70% have locally advanced or metastatic disease at presentation.

12. List the most likely causes of mortality after pneumonectomy.
- Pulmonary insufficiency
- Septic complications
- Cardiac arrhythmias
- Myocardial infarction
- Pulmonary embolus

13. What is the mortality rate for pneumonectomy in patients ≥70 years old?

6–30%; with proper preoperative selection and meticulous postoperative care, the rate may be kept at 6%.

14. Can improved survival after resection of solitary metastases from lung cancer to any organ be expected?

Aggressive treatment approaches have given encouraging results in carefully selected patients with solitary brain or adrenal metastasis.

15. On postoperative day 6 after a right pneumonectomy, a 62-year-old man develops a productive cough and has a drop in the air-fluid level on a chest radiograph. What should first-line therapy be?

This case scenario describes one mode of presentation of a **bronchopleural fistula.** The management of a clinically evident bronchopleural fistula depends on the time of its development postoperatively and its underlying cause. Early in the postoperative period, reoperation and repair of the bronchial stump may be indicated. Otherwise, initial evacuation of the fluid in the affected pleural space and institution of proper drainage are indicated. Additional measures to achieve closure of the fistula and to control the associated empyema can then be undertaken.

16. Name some effective therapeutic modalities for relief of obstruction from a left main stem lung carcinoma.
- Mechanical débridement
- Electrosurgery
- Cryosurgery
- CO_2 laser
- Nd:YAG laser

- Endobronchial brachytherapy
- Photodynamic therapy
- Endobronchial stenting
- External-beam radiation

17. Which histologic type of primary lung neoplasms has the most aggressive behavior?

Small cell lung cancer, accounting for approximately 20% of all lung cancer cases. More than other solid tumors, it behaves as a systemic disease.

18. Describe the therapy for small cell lung cancer.

Multimodality therapy, including effective chemotherapy, is required for locoregional control and systemic treatment of small cell lung cancer. Among patients with limited stage disease, thoracotomy for pulmonary resection is recommended as a component of therapy only in the small subset of stage I patients.

19. Describe some less common primary lung malignant neoplasms.

- **Carcinoid tumors** account for 0.5–1% of all tumors of bronchial origin. They represent a spectrum of neuroendocrine tumors of varying malignant potential, depending on their differentiation—typical versus atypical—and stage of presentation.
- **Adenoid cystic carcinoma** (cylindroma) and **mucoepidermoid** are the most common neoplasms arising from the bronchial glands. They constitute a small fraction of all lung neoplasms.
- **Carcinosarcomas** make up <1% of lung cancers and contain epithelial and mesenchymal types of tissue.

BIBLIOGRAPHY

1. Burt M, Wronski M, Arbit E, et al: Resection of brain metastases from non-small-cell lung carcinoma. J Thorac Cardiovasc Surg 103:399–411, 1992
2. D'Amico TA, Sabiston DC Jr: Carcinoma of the lung. In Sabiston DC Jr (ed): Textbook of Surgery, 15th ed. Philadelphia, W.B. Saunders, 1997, pp 1865–1876.
3. Gdeedo A, Van Schil P, Corthouts B, et al: Prospective evaluation of computed tomography and mediastinoscopy in mediastinal lymph node staging. Eur Respir J 10:1547–1551, 1997.
4. Ginsberg RJ: Carcinoid tumors. In Shields TW (ed): General Thoracic Surgery, 4th ed. Baltimore, Williams & Wilkins, 1994, pp 1287–1297.
5. Mentzer SJ: Mediastinoscopy, thoracoscopy, and video-assisted thoracic surgery in the diagnosis and staging of lung cancer. Hematol Oncol Clin North Am 11:435–447, 1997
6. Ponn RB, D'Agostino RS, Stern H: Adenoid cystic carcinoma, mucoepidermoid carcinoma and mixed salivary gland-type tumors. In Shields TW (ed): General Thoracic Surgery, 4th ed. Baltimore, Williams & Wilkins, 1994, pp 1298–1306.
7. Porte LP, Roumilhac D, Graziana J: Adrenalectomy for a solitary adrenal metastasis from lung cancer. Ann Thorac Surg 65:331–335, 1998.
8. Roberts JR : Trimodality therapy for non-small-cell lung cancer. Oncology (Huntingt) 13:101–106, 1999.
9. Rosell R, Gomez-Codina J, Camps C, et al: A randomized trial comparing preoperative chemotherapy plus surgery with surgery alone in patients with non-small-cell lung cancer. N Engl J Med 330:153–158, 1994.
10. Roth JA, Fossella F, Komaki R, et al: A randomized trial comparing perioperative chemotherapy and surgery with surgery alone in resectable IIIA non-small-cell lung cancer. J Natl Cancer Inst 86:673–680, 1994.
11. Rusch VW, Ginsberg RJ: Lung tumors. In Schwartz SI (ed): Principles of Surgery, 7th ed. New York, McGraw-Hill, 1999, pp 749–764.
12. Shields TW: Surgical treatment of non-small cell bronchial carcinoma. In Shields TW (ed): General Thoracic Surgery, 4th ed. Baltimore, Williams & Wilkins, 1994, pp 1159–1187.
13. Urschel JD, Finley RK, Takita H: Long-term survival after bilateral adrenalectomy for metastatic lung cancer: A case report. Chest 112:848–850, 1997.

28. LUNG CANCER STAGING

Timothy M. Anderson, M.D., and Mark S. Allen, M.D.

1. What factors are associated with improved survival in patients receiving neoadjuvant therapy for stage IIIA lung cancer?

The Sloan-Kettering experience reported that patients receiving neoadjuvant chemotherapy for N2 lung cancer who had **complete resections** after a major response to chemotherapy had longer survival (41% at 3 years). Survival was best (61% at 5 years) in a small subset of patients who had complete tumor sterilization. In a separate CALGB 8935 study, patients down-staged to N2 negative were more likely to benefit from surgical resection.

2. What is a negative prognostic factor in stage IIIA lung cancer patients receiving neoadjuvant therapy?

In the CALGB 8935 study evaluating induction therapy for stage IIIA non–small cell lung carcinoma (NSCLC), residual N2 disease after neoadjuvant therapy was a negative prognostic indicator.

3. Does the type of resection have any influence on results for stage I NSCLC?

Yes. The Lung Cancer Study Group (LCSG) compared lobectomy with limited resection (wedge or segment) for T1N0 and T2N0 NSCLC and found that patients undergoing limited resection had increased risk of local recurrence and a lesser chance of overall survival and disease-free survival compared with patients undergoing lobectomy. Earlier reports by Jensik et al. from Rush–Presbyterian proposed that segmental resection was equivalent to lobectomy in terms of survival and freedom from recurrence. More recent analysis by the Rush–Presbyterian group corroborates with the LCSG results in that higher local recurrence rates occurred for patients undergoing segmental resections.

4. Is M1 disease a contraindication to surgery in lung carcinoma?

In general, yes, but there are notable exceptions. According to the 1997 revisions in the International System for Staging Lung Cancer, intrapulmonary ipsilateral metastasis in a distant, non-primary tumor lobe is classified as M1 disease. Okada et al. in a Japanese series showed convincing data that patients with intrapulmonary metastasis in an ipsilateral lobe in which the primary lesion was not located who underwent surgical resection had a 23% 5-year survival after resection of the primary tumor and isolated metastasis. There are also data suggesting resection of the primary NSCLC after complete resection of brain metastasis results in improved survival. Long-term survival has been reported in selected patients resected for operable NSCLC combined with metastasectomy for solitary adrenal metastasis.

5. Has adjuvant radiation therapy been shown to improve survival in patients resected for NSCLC?

No. According to LCSG 773, resected stage II and III squamous cell carcinoma patients prospectively received radiotherapy postoperatively or no further treatment. Radiation significantly reduced the rate of local recurrence rates to the ipsilateral lung and mediastinum in patients with N2 disease but did not affect overall survival.

6. Does neoadjuvant therapy have a role in NSCLC?

Yes, in stage IIIA patients. Roth et al. reported a prospective, randomized trial of potentially resectable clinical stage IIIA NSCLC patients. Patients receiving preoperative chemotherapy and surgery had an estimated median survival of 64 months compared with 11 months for patients who had surgery alone ($P<.008$). Rosell reported similar results, in which stage IIIA NSCLC patients receiving chemotherapy followed by surgery had a median survival of 26 months compared with 8 months in surgery-alone patients ($P < .001$). These studies conclude that neoadjuvant chemotherapy followed by surgery in clinical stage IIIA patients increases survival. Neoadjuvant chemotherapy in early-stage NSCLC is currently an active area of investigation, and preliminary data from the Bimodality Lung Oncology Trial (BLOT) suggest that the bimodality approach to early-stage disease shows promise.

7. Which lymph node station is most likely involved when a patient with lung cancer presents with hoarseness?

The recurrent laryngeal nerve arises from the vagus nerve and wraps around the aorta at the level of the ligamentum arteriosum at lymph node station 5 (subaortic anteroposterior window, posterior to the ligamentum arteriosum). Lymph node involvement with tumor invading the recurrent nerve at this location is considered a contraindication to surgery. A direct laryngoscopy shows a paralyzed ipsilateral vocal cord on the left side.

8. Which lymph node stations are accessible by mediastinoscopy?

2R, 4R, and 7 anteriorly; 4L; and 2L.

9. How does one surgically approach lymph node levels 5 and 6?

Anterior or parasternal **mediastinotomy** as described by McNeill and Chamberlain permits exposure to the anterior mediastinum and aortopulmonary lymph nodes. **Thoracoscopy** from the left chest allows access to preaortic (level 6), subaortic (level 5), inferior pulmonary ligament (level 9), and paraesophageal (level 8) lymph nodes.

10. Compare the role of CT scanning versus mediastinoscopy in the evalution of patients with lung cancer.

CT scanning defines clinically the anatomic location, size, and extent of local invasion (T status); lymphadenopathy (N status); and possible metastasis into the liver, adrenal glands, and lung (M status). Gdeedo et al. reported CT scanning to have a sensitivity, specificity, and accuracy of 63%, 57%, and 59%. In contrast, **mediastinoscopy** had a much higher sensitivity, specificity, and accuracy of 89%, 100%, and 97%. Although CT scanning is routinely recommended to assess the clinical extent of disease initially, many advocate routine surgical staging of mediastinal lymph nodes for precise staging of NSCLC in patients considered potentially operable.

11. Discuss the approach to N2 disease that is encountered unexpectedly at thoracotomy for NSCLC.

Attempt at complete resection is recommended, particularly in young patients. Miller et al. reported on 167 patients with NSCLC with a clinically negative mediastinum that were found to have N2 disease at thoracotomy and were resected. Overall survival was 21%, which is superior to those undergoing surgery with known preoperative N2 disease. Multivariate analysis found that age, number of lymph node stations involved, postoperative radiation therapy, negative inferior mediastinal lymph nodes, and performance of a lobectomy significantly affected 5-year survival. Subcarinal N2 disease as noted by others was associated with a worse survival.

12. List 5 contraindications to lung resection in NSCLC, and explain each of their staging implications.

1. Phrenic nerve involvement, if the suprahilar nerve is involved secondary to cancerous N2 lymph node involvement invading the nerve.

2. Recurrent laryngeal nerve involvement because of lymph node invasion to the aortopulmonary window (level 5, N2).

3. Malignant pleural effusion (T4, stage IIIB disease).

4. Distant metastasis (M1, stage IV disease).

5. Superior vena cava syndrome secondary to mediastinal lymph node involvement invading the superior vena cava from the paratracheal region (N2).

CONTROVERSY

13. Discuss the role of positron emission tomography (PET) scanning in the staging of lung cancer.

As of January 1, 1999, the U.S. Food and Drug Administration approved PET scanning in the staging of lung cancer. Of patients considered resectable by conventional means, 18% are found to have more advanced disease on PET scan, rendering them inoperable. The poor spatial resolution of PET precludes precise anatomic definition of tumors. PET assessment of T status is interpreted as positive or negative for malignancies and is used in conjunction with CT scanning. PET scanning has been reported to have 100% sensitivity in detecting lung cancers; specificity ranges widely (52–88%), in part because of differences in the incidence of granulomatous disease among study populations. False-positive results can also occur with inflammation, hyperplasia, infection, and anthracotic nodes. Fludeoxyglucose (FDG)-PET has been shown to be more accurate than CT scanning in assessing nodal status (81–100% vs. 52–85%). Studies have shown that PET scanning has correctly increased or decreased nodal staging initially assessed by CT scanning in 21% of preoperative patients. Until the current specificity of PET scanning of 90% can be improved, however, surgical staging remains necessary. Combined PET and CT assessment of mediastinal lymph node metastasis has a greater negative predictive value (92–100%) compared with mediastinoscopy and in the future may obviate the need for mediastinoscopy in such instances. PET scanning has a higher sensitivity and specificity compared with CT scanning in detecting metastasis in adrenal, liver, and extrathoracic lymph nodes. Increased adrenal uptake by FDG in patients with NSCLC necessitates a biopsy specimen of the adrenal mass. Compared with bone scan, PET scanning has fewer false-positive results. The role of PET scanning in detecting CNS metastasis is currently unknown.

BIBLIOGRAPHY

1. Burt M, Wronski M, Arbit E, et al: Resection of brain metastases from non-small-cell lung carcinoma. J Thorac Cardiovasc Surg 103:399–411, 1992.
2. Foster ED, Munro DD, Dobell RC: Mediastinoscopy: A review of anatomical relationships and complications. Ann Thorac Surg 13:273–286, 1972.
3. Gdeedo A, Schil PV, Corthouts B, et al: Prospective evaluation of computed tomography and mediastinoscopy in mediastinal lymph node staging. Eur Respir J 10:1547–1551, 1997.
4. Lung Cancer Study Group: Effects of postoperative mediastinal radiation on completely resected stage II and stage III epidermoid cancer of the lung. N Engl J Med 315:1377–1381, 1986.
5. Lung Cancer Study Group: Randomized trial of lobectomy versus limited resection for T1N0 non-small cell lung cancer. Ann Thorac Surg 60:615–623, 1995.
6. Martini N, Kris MG, Flehinger BJ, et al: Preoperative chemotherapy for stage IIIa (N2) lung cancer: The Sloan-Kettering experience with 136 patients. Ann Thorac Surg 55:1365–1374, 1993.
7. Matin TA, Goldberg M: Surgical staging of lung cancer. Oncology 13:679–693, 1999.
8. Miller DL, McManus KG, Allen MS, et al: Results of surgical resection in patients with N2 non-small cell lung cancer. Ann Thorac Surg 57:1095–1101, 1994.
9. Mountain CF: Revisions in the International System for Staging Lung Cancer. Chest 11:1710–1717, 1997.
10. Okada M, Tsubota N, Yoshimura M, et al: Evaluation of TMN classification for lung carcinoma with ipsilateral intrapulmonary metastasis. Ann Thorac Surg 68:326–331, 1999.
11. Patz EF, Erasmus JJ: Positron emission tomography imaging in lung cancer. Clin Lung Cancer 1:42–48, 1999.
12. Pisters KMW: Phase II trial of induction paclitaxel/carboplatin in clinical stage T2N0, T-2N1, and selected T3N0-1 non-small cell lung cancer. Poster presentation at the Perugia International Cancer Conference IV, Chemotherapy of Non-Small Cell Lung Cancer: Ten Years Later, Perugia, Italy, October 11–13, 1998.
13. Porte HL, Roumilhac D, Graziana JP, et al: Adrenalectomy for a solitary adrenal metastasis from lung cancer. Ann Thorac Surg 65:331–335, 1998.
14. Rosell R, Gomez-Codina J, Camps C, et al: A randomized trial comparing preoperative chemotherapy plus surgery with surgery alone in patients with non-small-cell lung cancer. N Engl J Med 330:153–158, 1994.
15. Roth JA, Fossella F, Komaki R, et al: A randomized trial comparing perioperative chemotherapy and

surgery with surgery alone in resectable stage IIIA non-small-cell lung cancer. J Natl Cancer Inst 86:673–680, 1994.

16. Sugarbaker DJ, Herndon J, Decamp MM, et al: N2 status at resection predicts long-term outcome following induction therapy for stage IIIA non-small cell lung cancer: CALGB 8935. Proc ASCO 17:452a, 1998.

17. Warren WH, Faber LP: Segmentectomy versus lobectomy in patients with stage 1 pulmonary carcinoma: Five-year survival and patterns intrathoracic recurrence. J Thorac Cardiovasc Surg 107:1087–1094, 1994.

29. PULMONARY RESECTION

Reginald Abraham, M.D., and Hiroshi Takita, M.D., D.Sc.

1. What type of lung resection would you recommend for the patient with localized lung cancer?

The standard treatment of lung cancer whenever possible is lobectomy (or pneumonectomy) with hilar and mediastinal lymph node biopsy/dissection. The surgeon should review the chest x-ray and computed tomography (CT) scan carefully to determine what procedure may be done to completely remove the tumor.

2. How do you prepare the patient for lung surgery?

Place a catheter for the thoracic epidural anesthesia for the postoperative pain control (it needs to be done while the patient is conscious, but sedated). Secure adequate intravenous lines for administration of fluids, medications, and transfusion. Administer general anesthesia and insert a double-lumen endotracheal tube so that the gas exchange (ventilation) can be maintained by the contralateral lung during the surgery. Arterial catheter is inserted usually to the radial artery, so that blood pressure and arterial blood gasses can be monitored. Foley catheter is inserted for monitoring urinary output. Nasogastric tube is inserted to prevent gastric distention or regurgitation. An esophageal temperature probe is inserted. Usually sequential compression device stockings are applied to the legs to prevent deep venous thrombosis. Warming blanket is important if prolonged operating time is expected.

3. How is the patient positioned for lung surgery?

The posterolateral or lateral thoracotomy is usually performed; the patient is positioned in the lateral position.

4. How is the patient's condition monitored during surgery?

The status of the patient is constantly monitored by EKG, blood pressure, arterial O_2 saturation, and PCO_2 of expired breath. Body temperature, arterial blood gasses, hematocrit, urine output, IV fluid intake, and amount of blood loss are monitored closely.

5. Where do you make the incision?

The skin incision is made from one finger below the tip of the scapula and is extended forward to the skin crease of the breast (or 3–4 inches below the nipple in men). The latissimus dorsi muscle and the serratus anterior muscle are divided along the line of the skin incision. Recently, so-called muscle-sparing thoracotomy incision became popular, in which either latissimus dorsi or serratus anterior is not divided and the undivided muscle is instead retracted. Usually the chest cavity is entered at the 5th intercostal space. The intercostal muscles are divided by a cautery along the upper border of the 6th rib. At this time the surgeon requests the anesthetist to deflate the lung on which the operation is to be performed.

6. When the chest is opened, what do you see?

The presence of grossly visible implants of the tumor on the pleural surface is a contraindication to the curative surgery. In case of lung resection, there should be enough margin at the pulmonary artery, the pulmonary veins, and the bronchus. There should not be any involvement of adjacent vital structures such as heart, aorta, vena cava, esophagus, or vertebrae. Grossly obvious lymph node metastasis in the mediastinum is also contraindication for the resection.

7. What are the three important structures in performing the lung resection?

Pulmonary artery, pulmonary veins, and the bronchus. In order to perform a satisfactory anatomic resection, it is important to dissect out the above three structures at the beginning. By doing the above, one is able to easily control inadvertent bleeding.

8. How you remove the lung?

    A. Right lung resection

        I. Dissection of the hilar vessels (Fig. 1): The main pulmonary artery is found at the angle of the superior vena cava and the azygous vein. It is dissected with sharp and blunt dissections and a sling is applied. The superior pulmonary vein is identified just inferior and anterior to the main pulmonary artery and a sling is applied. In order to dissect out the inferior pulmonary vein, the inferior pulmonary ligament is separated and the lower lobe is retracted superiorly. After it is dissected, apply a sling.

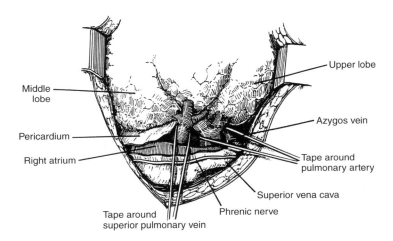

FIGURE 1. At the hilus of the right lung, the main pulmonary artery and the superior pulmonary vein are dissected and a sling is applied. (From Takita H: Surgery for cancer of the lung. In Bland KI, Karakousis CP, Copeland EM (eds): Atlas of Surgical Oncology. Philadelphia, W.B. Saunders, 1995, pp 259–282, with permission.)

        II. Lung resection (pneumonectomy or lobectomy): Usually the pulmonary artery is separated first and the vein is separated next. Then the bronchus is separated ant the lobe or the lung is removed. The lobar or segmental branches of the pulmonary vessels are usually ligated with 0-silk and cut. The main pulmonary vessels are usually separated after being stapled with a vascular stapler. The stump of the bronchus can be oversewn with stitches; however, most of the time it is closed by a stapler.

       III. Right upper lobectomy: At the hilus, the anterior trunk (apicoposterior and anterior branches of pulmonary artery) is separated. At the major fissure, branches of the pulmonary artery to the lower lobe are identified. The artery is dissected and followed up proximally. The middle lobe artery(ies) and the superior segmental branch of the lower lobe are identified. Finally, the ascending posterior segmental branch of the upper lobe is found and separated (Fig. 2). Following that, the upper lobe division of the superior pulmonary vein is stapled and separated. Finally, the right upper lobe bronchus is identified in the posterior part of the hilus and separated, completing the right upper lobectomy.

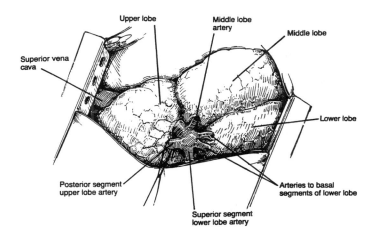

FIGURE 2. Any lobectomy on the right side requires dissection of branches of the pulmonary artery at the major fissure. (From Takita H: Surgery for cancer of the lung. In Bland KI, Karakousis CP, Copeland EM (eds): Atlas of Surgical Oncology. Philadelphia, W.B. Saunders, 1995, pp 259–282, with permission.)

     IV. In the similar fashion, other lobectomies and pneumonectomy are performed. Thus the most important dissection of the pulmonary artery is done at the hilus and at the major fissure. It is followed by identification of the pulmonary vein(s) (Fig. 3). Finally, identification of the bronchus becomes easy because it is the only structure remaining to be cut to remove the lung.

  B. On the left side, the lung resection is done in similar fashion as on the right side (Fig. 4). The procedure is relatively easier on the left because the hilar vessels are slightly longer on that side. Moreover, one can follow the pulmonary artery from its origin to the branches in the major

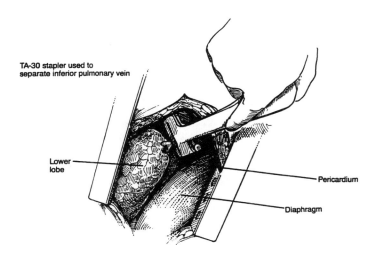

FIGURE 3. The right inferior pulmonary vein is stapled and separated. (From Takita H: Surgery for cancer of the lung. In Bland KI, Karakousis CP, Copeland EM (eds): Atlas of Surgical Oncology. Philadelphia, W.B. Saunders, 1995, pp 259–282, with permission.)

fissure in continuity (Fig. 5), while on the right side the pulmonary artery travels behind the superior pulmonary vein, which makes the dissection more tedious.

    C. Conservative lung resections

        I. Anatomic resection of the lung is called segmentectomy. Each lobe is anatomically subdivided to two or more segments. The technique was originally developed for the surgical therapy for tuberculosis. It is also used for removal of a small-cell lung cancer in high-risk patients. First, the segmental pulmonary artery branch is identified and is separated. The segmental branch of the bronchus is identified, usually just underneath the segmental pulmonary artery. It is separated and the proximal end is sewn with 3–0 stitches. Following this, the segment is removed either by blunt dissection or by staples.

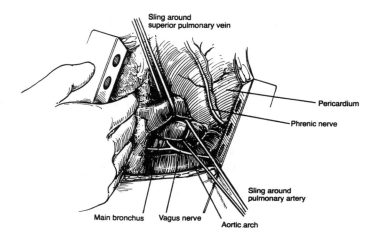

FIGURE 4. At the hilus of the left lung, the main pulmonary artery and the bronchus are dissected. (From Takita H: Surgery for cancer of the lung. In Bland KI, Karakousis CP, Copeland EM (eds): Atlas of Surgical Oncology. Philadelphia, W.B. Saunders, 1995, pp 259–282, with permission.)

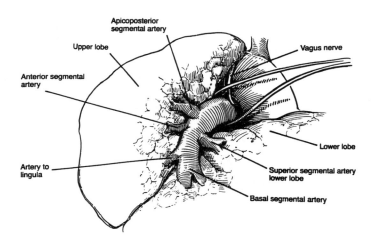

FIGURE 5. At the major fissure, all branches of the left pulmonary artery are dissected. (From Takita H: Surgery for cancer of the lung. In Bland KI, Karakousis CP, Copeland EM (eds): Atlas of Surgical Oncology. Philadelphia, W.B. Saunders, 1995, pp 259–282, with permission.)

II. Nonanatomic lung resection: Peripheral lung lesion, especially metastatic lung tumors, can be removed by the staplers. A wedge-shaped piece of the lung is removed, thus it is called the wedge resection.

D. Mediastinal node sampling (or dissection) (Fig. 6): In case of lung cancer surgery, biopsy or dissection of the hilar and mediastinal lymph nodes are routinely performed following lung resection. The paratracheal, subcarinal, hilar, interlobar, paraesophageal, and inferior pulmonary ligament nodes are separately submitted to the pathology department for the intraoperative (or surgical) staging.

E. After the lung resection and lymph node biopsy
   I. Hemostasis: Special attention should be given to the bleeding from small arteries such as bronchial artery and intercostal artery, because these are the most frequent causes of postoperative intrathoracic bleeding.
   II. Air leak control: Following the hemostasis, the chest cavity is filled with warm saline solution. Ask the anesthetist to inflate the lung and look for air leaks. Efforts should be made to close any air leaks identified because that will affect very much the postoperative recovery.

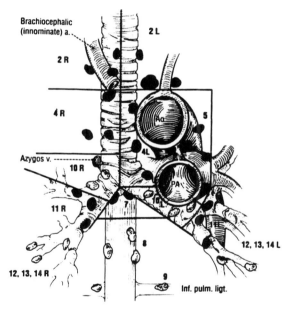

FIGURE 6. All removed lymph nodes are separately submitted according to the designated numbers. (From Takita H: Surgery for cancer of the lung. In Bland KI, Karakousis CP, Copeland EM (eds): Atlas of Surgical Oncology. Philadelphia, W.B. Saunders, 1995, pp 259–282, with permission.)

III. Chest tubes: In case of lobectomy or lesser procedures, usually two chest tubes are inserted before closing the chest. Tip of one of the tubes (anterior tube) is placed at the apex of the chest cavity in order to evacuate air. Tip of the other tube (posterior tube) is placed at the inferior-posterior part of the chest cavity in order to drain fluid (or blood). The tubes are connected to approximately -20 cmH$_2$O suction via the drainage system. Following a pneumonectomy, most of the surgeons close the chest without any chest tubes. However, some surgeons prefer inserting a chest tube. The advantage of putting a chest tube is to be able to monitor the amount of fluid or blood in the chest cavity. Also, the chest tube will prevent shift of the mediastinum toward the remaining lung side by excess build-up of the fluid. The disadvantage of the chest tube post-pneumonectomy is the possibility of infection of the chest cavity. Also, it can be dangerous if the chest tube is inadvertently connected to the suction—patient may die of cardiac arrest caused by sudden shift of the mediastinum.

  F. Closure of the chest incision: The first step is the closure of the intercostal space. We usually use 4–6 interrupted sutures of #1 or #2 synthetic absorbable sutures. Muscle layers are then closed with continuous suture of 0 absorbable sutures. Finally, the subcutaneous layer and skin are closed. Patient is then turned to the supine position, and when the patient begins to wake up and is out of effect of muscle paralysis, he/she is extubated. Portable monitor is attached and patient is sent to the intensive care unit.

BIBLIOGRAPHY

1. ATS Board of Directors: Official American Thoracic Society Statement: Clinical Staging of Primary Lung Cancer. Chicago, American Thoracic Society, 1981.
2. Bauer AE, Geha AS, Hammond GL, et al: Glenn's Thoracic and Cardiovascular Surgery, 6th ed. Stamford, CT, Appleton & Lange, 1996.
3. Franco KL, Putnum JB: Advanced Therapy in Thoracic Surgery. Hamilton, BC Decker, 1998.
4. Hood RM: Techniques in General Thoracic Surgery, 2nd ed. Philadelphia, Lea & Febiger, 1993.
5. Kaiser LR, Kron I, Spray TL: Mastery of Cardiothoracic Surgery. Philadelphia, Lippincott-Raven, 1998.
6. Pearson FG, Deslauriers J, Ginsberg RJ, et al: Thoracic Surgery. New York, Churchill-Livingstone, 1995.
7. Sabiston DC, Spencer FC: Surgery of the Chest. Philadelphia, W.B. Saunders, 1996.
8. Takita H: Surgery for cancer of the lung. In Bland KI, Karakousis CP, Copeland EM (eds): Atlas of Surgical Oncology. Philadelphia, W.B. Saunders, 1995, pp 259–282.

30. PULMONARY METASTASES

Colin J. Powers, M.D., and Hratch L. Karamanoukian, M.D.

1. Who performed the first pulmonary resection for metastatic disease?

Although the greatest growth in applicable techniques and indications has occurred since the 1950s and 1960s, the resection of metastatic cancer to the lungs has its beginnings in the late 19th century. In the 1880s, Weinlechner and Krolein removed pulmonary metastatic disease as part of en bloc chest wall resection. Divis, a European surgeon, performed the first true pulmonary metastasectomy in 1926. Two years later, the procedure of isolated pulmonary metastasectomy was performed in the U.S. by Torek. It was not until 1939 that pulmonary metastasectomy gained true acceptance and credibility at the hands of Barney and Churchill.

2. How did their patient fare?

The significance of Barney and Churchill's operation in 1939 was not only that a deliberate resection of an isolated pulmonary metastasis had been technically achieved, but that the patient then experienced postoperative survival of nearly 25 years! Their patient, a 55-year-old woman with renal cell carcinoma who underwent lobectomy and nephrectomy for local control of the disease process, went on to live to the age of 78 without further signs of recurrent cancer. She eventually died from coronary artery disease.

This series of events excited the surgical community in that the excision of metastatic cancer in the lung had been demonstrated to be technically feasible and became a treatment option offering the possibility of long-term remission or cure.

3. How are most pulmonary metastases detected?

Only approximately 15% of pulmonary metastases become symptomatic. Patients may complain of cough, hemoptysis, dyspnea or frank pain when these lesions involve either the central airways, pleura, or chest wall. Typically, however, pulmonary metastases are found within the periphery of the lung parenchyma in a subpleural location and remain asymptomatic. They are usually detected on radiographic evaluation of a patient with a known cancer or post-resection on surveillance chest x-ray or CT scan.

The standard chest x-ray can detect these nodules once they reach approximately 8–9 mm in size. CT scan will demonstrate metastases as small as 3 mm. The role of MRI and PET scanning is currently under investigation, yet any minimal increase in sensitivity is likely to be offset by markedly increased costs and decreased equipment and technician availability.

4. How is the identification of single vs. multiple pulmonary nodules interpreted in the setting of previous malignancy?

In a patient with a known history of malignancy, multiple pulmonary nodules represent metastases until proven otherwise. A single pulmonary lesion may signify either an additional primary tumor or metastatic disease. Three general rules of thumb in the latter situation include the following:

1. A diagnosis of sarcoma or melanoma increases the probability that the pulmonary lesion is a metastasis more than 10-fold.

2. A diagnosis of colorectal/genitourinary malignancy carries a 50% chance that the lesion represents a second primary tumor.

3. A diagnosis of squamous cell cancer of head or neck origin raises a probability that the pulmonary lesion is a second primary malignancy approximately twofold.

5. Outline a reasonable preoperative assessment for the patient with suspected pulmonary metastasis.

It must include three elements: (1) the site of a known or likely primary must be evaluated for disease; (2) sites other than the lung that are statistically likely to harbor further metastases should be investigated; and (3) the patient's pulmonary and cardiovascular reserve must be evaluated in regards to tolerating any considered operative intervention.

The above considerations can be further defined depending on the specific tumor histology. For sarcomas, which preferentially tend to metastasize to the lungs, CT scanning of the lungs and primary site with radionuclide bone scanning of the entire body is a reasonable radiographic evaluation. For carcinomas and melanomas, which tend to metastasize more diffusely and less predictably, CT scanning of the liver, adrenal glands, and brain is mandatory.

The role of mediastinoscopy and bronchoscopy prior to pulmonary resection is less well defined. Mediastinoscopy is warranted in instances of breast cancer and when the pulmonary lesion is particularly large and centrally located. In these cases, the additional risk and cost involved are balanced by a reasonable chance that nodal involvement within the mediastinum exists. Although some authors recommend bronchoscopy in every patient with pulmonary metastasis to rule out endoluminal involvement, the rate of positive findings is quite low. A more reasonable position might be that bronchoscopy is warranted in cases in which the lesion's size and location suggest airway invasion.

Finally, cardiovascular status and pulmonary function must be ascertained. The specifics of the cardiac testing must revolve around the patient's age, medical history, and any suggestive symptomatology. Pulmonary function testing should show an estimated residual postoperative FEV_1 of greater than 30% predicted. Most patients who demonstrate a postoperative FEV_1 of greater than 800 ml will not require prolonged ventilatory support following resection. An additional consideration is a history of preoperative chemotherapy. Agents such as bleomycin can cause pulmonary fibrosis. Also, doxorubicin is known to cause cardiomyopathy. Patients with known exposure to these drugs should receive particularly careful preoperative evaluation since these physiologic compromises not only affect the possibility of resection, but may dictate changes in the plan of anesthesia and intraoperative cardiopulmonary support.

6. Describe the criteria that all patients should meet prior to resection.

The original criteria as set forth by Ehrenhaft and coworkers in 1958 were based on assuring that operative intervention would occur in a setting in which a curative procedure is possible:

1. Preoperative radiographic evaluation should allow the possibility that all thoracic malignancy can be removed, i.e., **total resection is a necessity.**

2. The primary tumor site must be under control.

3. Preoperative evaluation must not demonstrate other sites of metastatic disease outside of the pulmonary parenchyma (this point is somewhat controversial).

4. The specific histologic type of malignancy must be one not likely to be cured with nonoperative treatment modalities.

5. The patient should have the necessary cardiopulmonary reserve to tolerate the resection.

7. Once the above criteria are met, are there additional prognostic indicators for these patients?

Prognostic factors such as disease-free interval, the number and anatomic location of metastases, the tumor-doubling time, and response to chemotherapy have all been investigated. The significance of these factors has been inconsistent between studies and may vary widely between different types of malignancies.

8. What prognostic indicator has been consistently shown to be of importance?

The only variable that has been shown consistently and across multiple malignancies to improve postoperative survival is the performance of **complete excision** of malignant tissue/metastasis from the patient.

9. List the various approaches for resection of pulmonary metastases and explain their advantages and disadvantages.

The resection of pulmonary metastases can be performed via thoracotomy, sternotomy, or staged bilateral thoracotomies when necessary. Posterolateral thoracotomy usually allows excellent exposure of the entire lung, but limits access to the one hemithorax and can generate significant postoperative pain. Sternotomy allows good exposure of both lungs, but may restrict access to the posterior thorax and especially the left lower lobe. Staged thoracotomies may be performed separately over a period of 1–2 weeks in patients with bilateral lesions. This provides excellent exposure but involves the time and complications associated with a second surgical procedure.

10. Review the general technique for the surgical resection of metastatic tissue from the pulmonary parenchyma.

The goal of intervention in pulmonary metastasectomy is the excision of all malignant tissue. Therefore, once the chest cavity is entered, a meticulous exploration is performed. The use of a double-lumen endotracheal tube allows selective deflation of the lung and thorough palpation for deeper lesions. While subpleural metastases can be removed via wedge resection, deeper lesions may require segmentectomy or lobectomy. In these cases, the careful determination of the most appropriate resection technique is crucial. The need to remove all malignant tissue also must be balanced with the goal of preserving as much healthy pulmonary tissue as possible.

When performed on an appropriately selected patient base and with reasonable technical proficiency, resection of pulmonary metastases offers a very generous degree of safety despite its invasive nature. Most experienced centers report mortality of less than 1–2% and associated morbidity substantially less than 10%.

11. Is video-assisted thoracic surgery an appropriate modality for the treatment of pulmonary metastatic disease?

In this approach, the hemithorax is visualized and operative intervention performed with the use of a camera and ports placed through the chest wall in a fashion similar to laparoscopic surgery. This less invasive technique offers the distinct advantage of obviating the need for thoracotomy/sternotomy. However, most surgical oncologists have concerns in performing video-assisted thoracic resections for several reasons: (1) there may be increased difficulty in visualizing lesions not originally suspected by preoperative CT scan; (2) the ability to fully palpate the lung parenchyma for nonvisible lesions is lost; and (3) a number of operative series have shown an increased rate of future line and chest wall recurrences following video-assisted thoracic resections.

12. Is there evidence that patient well-being is enhanced by resection of pulmonary metastases?

Yes. Much of the early work concerning the resection of pulmonary metastases analyzed reports that combined patients with pulmonary metastases from varied malignancies. This naturally led to different and sometimes contradictory results. More recent case series that defined outcomes specific to tumor histology suggested more positive results.

Soft tissue sarcomas, osteogenic sarcomas, and renal carcinoma patients demonstrate improved post-thoracotomy survival when complete excision is performed. The resection of metastases from non-seminomatous germ-cell tumors and head/neck primary tumors has been shown to have a positive effect on post-thoracotomy survival in many series, but not to the same marked extent as the previously listed malignancies. The benefits of pulmonary resection in breast and colorectal cancer are less certain. Since these cancers often present with systemic spread, isolated pulmonary metastases are unusual and evidence of increased survival following removal is less convincing. Outcomes in patients with melanoma remain poor. Multiple studies suggest no significant difference in survival rates between patients with resectable and unresectable disease.

BIBLIOGRAPHY

1. Chen P, Pass H: Indications for resection of pulmonary metastases. In Baue A (ed): Glenn's Thoracic and Cardiovascular Surgery, 6th ed. Stamford, CT, Appleton & Lange, 1996, pp 499–510.
2. D'Amico T, Sabiston D: Surgical management of pulmonary metastases. In Sabiston D (ed): Surgery of the Chest, 6th ed. Philadelphia, W.B. Saunders, 1995, pp 669–675.
3. Holmes E: Pulmonary metastases. In Pearson F, Deslauriers J, Hiebert C, et al (eds): Thoracic Surgery. New York, Churchill-Livingstone, 1995, pp 827–834.
4. Lanza L, Putnam J: Resection of pulmonary metastases. In Roth J (ed): Thoracic Oncology, 2nd ed. Philadelphia, W.B. Saunders, 1995, pp 569–589.
5. Mark J: Surgical treatment of pulmonary metastases: Where do we stand? Ann Surg 218:703–704, 1993.
6. McCormack P: Surgical resection of pulmonary metastases. Semin Surg Oncol 6:297–302, 1990.
7. Moores D: Pulmonary metastases revisited. Ann Thorac Surg 52:178–179, 1991.
8. Pogrebniak H, Pass H: Initial and reoperative pulmonary metastectomy: Indications, technique, and results. Semin Surg Oncol 9:142–149, 1993.
9. Rusch V: Pulmonary metastasectomy: Current indications. Chest 107:322S–332S, 1995.
10. Stewart J, Carey J, Merrill W, et al: Twenty years' experience with pulmonary metastasectomy. Am Surgeon 58:l00–103, 1992.
11. Todd T: Pulmonary metastectomy: Current indications for removing lung metastases. Chest 103:401S-403S, 1993.

31. NEOADJUVANT AND ADJUVANT TREATMENT OF NON–SMALL-CELL LUNG CARCINOMA

Lynn M. Steinbrenner, M.D.

1. What is the long-term survival in non–small-cell lung carcinoma (NSCLC) patients undergoing surgical resection alone according to stage?

STAGE	5-YEAR SURVIVAL (%)
1, T1N0	80
1, T2N0	50
2	25–30
3A	10

2. Discuss the role of postoperative chemotherapy in completely resected stage I and II NSCLC.

The first Lung Cancer Study Group (LCSG) trial of cyclophosphamide, doxorubicin, and cisplatin (CAP) versus bacillus Calmette–Guérin (BCG) in resected stage 2 and 3A patients showed no advantage of chemotherapy over the BCG arm. The next study of CAP versus observation showed no survival advantage for treatment, and the third trial of immediate versus delayed CAP showed no difference in the median time to recurrence or median survival in the immediate treatment group. Only a Finnish trial showed a survival advantage for CAP over observation, but there were 22 pneumonectomies in the surgery arm versus 11 in the chemotherapy arm, which may have had an influence on overall survival. Several new agents with activity against NSCLC include vinorelbine, paclitaxel, and gemcitabine. Phase II trials have shown the feasibility of giving these agents in the neoadjuvant and adjuvant setting. The Bimodality Lung Oncology Trial (BLOT) is a phase 3 trial currently under way looking at paclitaxel plus carboplatin preoperatively versus surgery alone in stage 1B, 2, and selected 3A patients. At present, there is no standard postoperative chemotherapy for resected stage 1 or 2 patients. All such patients should be considered for enrollment in ongoing trials.

3. Discuss the role of postoperative radiotherapy in patients with resected stage 1 and 2 NSCLC.

A trial by Patterson et al. looked only at pneumonectomy patients, and the field size was small by today's standards. A second trial by Bangma et al. had only 72 patients. The trial by Van Houtte et al. comprised all node-negative T1–T3 patients. The most often quoted trial was done by the LCSG and reported in 1986. It looked at squamous cell carcinoma with N1 or N2 disease and found no evidence for improved survival but a significant decrease in local recurrence. The final trial by the MRC looked at 308 patients with N1 and N2 disease and used 40 Gy. The overall survival was not improved, but subset analysis showed an improved survival for the T2N2 subset. A meta-analysis looked at nine randomized, controlled trials that included 2,128 patients. Radiation doses were 30–60 Gy in 10–30 fractions. All trials included patients with completely resected tumors with stage no greater than 3A. The results showed a detriment for survival in patients who received postoperative radiation therapy with a 13% relative increase in the risk of recurrence or death. Although one must exercise caution in interpreting a meta-analysis, these results indicate that postoperative radiotherapy should not be used routinely to treat patients with completely resected early-stage NSCLC.

4. What about combined chemotherapy and radiotherapy in stage 1 and 2 patients?

Few trials have addressed the role of both chemotherapy and radiotherapy in stage 2 patients.

Most studies involved stage 2 and resected 3A disease. The studies in stage 2 disease did not find an improvement in overall survival.

5. List the different patient groups that comprise clinical stage 3A disease.
- All mediastinal (N2)
- T3N1

CONTROVERSY

6. Discuss the optimal management for patients with stage 3A disease as derived from results of clinical trials.

Patients with **chest wall involvement** are often technically resectable. In patients with **Pancoast tumors**, preoperative radiation therapy followed by definitive surgery has yielded long-term survivals of 20–35%. N2 patients are patients who present with locally advanced stage 3 disease with **mediastinal lymph node involvement.** Neoadjuvant treatment is attractive in these patients for several reasons. Drug delivery to a tumor is better before blood supply is interrupted. Clinical and pathologic tumor response may indicate a population of patients who may benefit from postoperative therapy. Neoadjuvant treatment may convert an unresectable tumor into a resectable tumor. Martini et al. conducted an early phase 2 trial of preoperative mitomycin + vindesine or vinblastine + high-dose cisplatin (MVP) for 2 or 3 cycles in patients with N2 disease. In 136 patients, 105 had a major radiographic response and went on to surgery. 50% were resected. Three-year survival was 28% for all patients and 41% for resected patients. Many small, nonrandomized trials yielded similar results. Preoperative chemotherapy can be safely given and results in pathologic complete response in about 20%.

One of the earliest studies by Rosell et al. randomized patients to surgery and radiation therapy versus neoadjuvant chemotherapy with mitomycin C, ifosfamide, and cisplatin for 3 cycles followed by surgery and radiation therapy. The chemotherapy arm had a median survival of 26 months compared with 8 months for the control arm. Roth et al. conducted a similar trial using 3 cycles of cyclophosphamide, etoposide, and cisplatin. Both of these studies were flawed in that they accrued only 60 patients; however, results of both suggested the superiority of chemotherapy preoperatively in patients with stage 3A NSCLC. A large phase 3 trial completed in 1999 randomized 373 patients with stage 1, 2, and 3A NSCLC to surgery versus neoadjuvant chemotherapy with mitomycin, ifosfamide, and cisplatin. In both arms, T3 and N2 patients were given postoperative radiation therapy, and responders on the chemotherapy arm were given postoperative chemotherapy as well. There was a survival advantage for the neoadjuvant arm, but further maturation of the data is required to see if this result holds up.

Phase 2 trials of preoperative combination chemotherapy plus radiation therapy showed that this could be given safely. A Southwest Oncology Group (SWOG) trial reported in 1995 treated 156 stage 3A and B patients with 2 cycles of cisplatin and etoposide and concurrent radiation therapy of 45 Gy. Resectability was 85% in the stage 3A patients, and 3-year survival was 26%. Many modern trials are looking at split fractionation and newer chemotherapeutic agents to improve response rates and reduce toxicity. Although one might expect complication rates to be increased over that of chemotherapy alone, this does not appear to be the case. Whether surgery or radiotherapy should be used as the primary modality to achieve local control is now the subject of a North American phase 3 trial comparing chemoradiotherapy with chemoradiotherapy plus surgery in patients with stage 3A disease. An EORTC trial is looking at chemotherapy followed by either radiotherapy or surgery. The results of these studies should help answer the question of how to manage this heterogeneous group of patients.

BIBLIOGRAPHY

1. Albain KS, Rusch VW, Crowley JJ, et al: Concurrent cisplatin, etoposide plus chest radiotherapy followed by surgery for stages IIIA (N2) and IIIB non-small cell lung cancer: Mature results of SWOG Phase II Study 8805. J Clin Oncol 13:1880, 1995.
2. Bangma PJ: Postoperative radiotherapy. In Deeley TJ (ed): Carcinoma of the Bronchus: Modern Radiotherapy. New York, Appleton-Century-Crofts, 1972, p 163.
3. Bleehan NM, British Medical Research Council Lung Cancer Working Party: Randomized trial of surgical resection with or without postoperative radiotherapy in NSCCL. Lung Cancer 11(suppl 1):148, 1994.
4. Depierre A, et al, for the French Thoracic Cooperative Group: Phase III trial of neoadjuvant chemotherapy in resectable stage I, II and IIIA non-small cell carcinoma of the lung. ASCO Proc 18:1792, 1999.
5. Feld R, Rubinstein L, Thomas PA: Adjuvant chemotherapy with cyclophosphamide, Adriamycin and cisplatin in patients with completely resected stage I NSCCL. J Natl Cancer Inst 85:299, 1993.
6. Figlin RA, Piantadosi S: A phase III randomized trial of immediate combination chemotherapy versus delayed combination chemotherapy in patients with stage II and III NSCCL. Chest 106:310S, 1994.
7. Holmes EC, Gail M, for the LCSG: Surgical adjuvant therapy for stage II, stage III adenocarcinoma and large cell undifferentiated carcinoma. J Clin Oncol 4:710, 1986.
8. Martini N, Kris M, Flehinger BJ, et al: Preoperative chemotherapy for IIIA (N2) lung cancer: The Sloan-Kettering experience with 136 patients. Ann Thorac Surg 55:1365, 1993.
9. Niiranen A, Niitamo-Korhonen S, Karisi M, et al: Adjuvant chemotherapy after radical surgery for NSCCL: A randomized study. J Clin Oncol 10:1927, 1992.
10. Patterson R, Russell MH: Clinical trial in malignant disease: IV. Lung cancer: Value of postoperative radiotherapy. Clin Radiol 13:141, 1962.
11. PORT Meta-Analysis Trialists Group: Postoperative radiotherapy in non-small cell carcinoma of the lung: Systematic review and meta-analysis of individual patient data from nine randomized trials. Lancet 352:257, 1998.
12. Rosell R, Gomez-Codina J, Camps C, et al: A randomized trial comparing preoperative chemotherapy plus surgery with surgery alone in patients with non-small cell carcinoma of the lung. N Engl J Med 330:153, 1994.
13. Roth JA, Fossello F, Komaki R, et al: A randomized trial comparing perioperative chemotherapy and surgery with surgery alone in resectable stage III non-small cell carcinoma of the lung. J Natl Cancer Inst 86:673, 1994.
14. Ruckdeschel JC, Robinson LA: Non-small cell lung cancer: Surgery and postoperative adjuvant chemotherapy. In Pass H, et al (eds): Lung Cancer, Principles and Practice. Philadelphia, Lippincott-Raven, 1996, pp 839–849.
15. Van Houtte P, Rocmans P, Smets P, et al: Postoperative radiation therapy in lung cancer: A controlled trial after resection of curative design. Int J Radiat Oncol Biol Phys 6:983, 1980.
16. Van Houtte PJ: Non-small cell lung cancer: Surgery and postoperative radiotherapy. In Pass H, et al (eds): Lung Cancer, Principles and Practice. Philadelphia, Lippincott-Raven, 1996, pp 851–861.
17. Weisenberger TH, Gail M, for LCSG: Effects of post-operative mediastinal radiation on completely resected stage II and III epidermoid cancer of the lung. New Engl J Med 315:1377, 1986.

32. PANCOAST TUMOR

Timothy M. Anderson, M.D., and Kamal A. Mansour, M.D.

1. Who was Pancoast?

Henry K. Pancoast, M.D., was Chairman of Radiology at the University of Pennsylvania. In 1924, he described four cases of **superior sulcus tumors.** In 1932, he wrote another article establishing the Pancoast syndrome.

2. What is the difference between a Pancoast tumor and Pancoast syndrome?

Pancoast described a homogeneous, shadow-producing lesion in the extreme apex of the thoracic inlet (superior sulcus) with more or less local rib destruction and often vertebral infiltration. **Pancoast tumors** are synonymous with **superior sulcus tumors,** a term referring to the sulcus or groove created by the subclavian artery as it passes under the clavicle and above the first rib, on the pleural cupola and apices of the upper lobes. Pancoast tumor refers to the tumor's anatomic location and existence of a lung carcinoma that ultimately causes the syndrome. The lesion produces severe shoulder pain radiating down the arm and hand on the same side as the tumor, corresponding to C8 and T1 nerve roots or inferior trunk of brachial plexus with atrophy of the hand muscles, and may be associated with Horner's syndrome (ptosis, miosis, and anhydrosis). This symptom complex is the **Pancoast syndrome.**

3. Is tissue diagnosis necessary before treatment for Pancoast syndrome?

Yes, because in < 10% of the cases other lesions besides pulmonary tumors occur in the superior sulcus, including carcinoma of the thyroid, carcinoma of the pharynx, mesothelioma, tuberculosis, pulmonary abscess, hydatid cyst, actinomycosis, invasive aspergillosis, cryptococcosis, and *Staphylococcus aureus* infection.

4. How is histologic diagnosis of Pancoast syndrome obtained?

By **percutaneous fine-needle aspiration.** A few cases are defined by sputum examination, bronchoscopic aspirate or brushings, and rarely transcervical supraclavicular or supraclavicular thoracotomy techniques.

5. Discuss the preferred treatment for Pancoast tumors.

Pancoast tumors were once thought to be unresectable; however, neoadjuvant radiation therapy as first reported by Shaw has improved survival dramatically. Preoperative radiation modifies the extent of the lesion and sterilizes the periphery of the disease at the chest wall level. Preoperative irradiation dose is usually 4,500 rad followed by reevaluation. Two to three weeks after irradiation is complete, an extended en bloc resection of the chest wall and tumor is performed, including the upper two or three ribs, portions of thoracic vertebrae, the lower trunk of brachial plexus, stellate ganglion, the dorsal sympathetic chain, and lung resection. It is not known whether neoadjuvant chemoradiation plays a significant role in tumor management.

6. List contraindications to surgical resection for Pancoast tumor.

- Extensive brachial plexus involvement
- Intervertebral foramina involvement
- Vertebral body involvement with cortical bone erosion
- Mediastinal lymph node involvement (N2 disease)
- Distant metastasis
- Encasement of the great vessels
- Extension into the supraclavicular fossa

7. Are all the above-listed contraindications absolute?

Although several of the aforementioned contraindications are relative, some tertiary centers challenge the more advanced stages (IIIB) of tumor involvement. Great vessel involvement with resection and Gore-Tex reconstruction and extension into the vertebral bodies with vertebrectomy and spinal reconstruction are examples of more radical approaches.

8. List factors having a negative impact on survival after surgical resection.
- Mediastinal nodal involvement (N2 or N3).
- Vertebral body or subclavian vessel involvement (T4 disease).

9. What is the overall survival after irradiation and extended resection?
30–35%. In node-negative patients, survivals of 44% have been achieved.

10. Describe the Dartevelle procedure.

In some anterior apical tumors that may invade the clavicle and subclavian vessels, Dartevelle's large L-shaped anterior transcervical thoracic incision with division of the clavicle allows radical resection of upper lobe lesions and excellent exposure when only the first and second ribs are involved. Although considered aggressive and somewhat controversial by some, when the subclavian artery is also involved, it can be sacrificed and replaced with Gore-Tex graft. In such cases, preoperative Doppler studies of both internal carotid arteries to ensure integrity are mandatory.

11. What morbidity can be expected after resection of Pancoast tumor?

Although C8, T1, and T2 nerve roots are often sacrificed, the neurologic defects are not incapacitating. If the eighth cervical nerve is preserved, the defect is not as severe. Horner's syndrome develops secondary to resection of the dorsal sympathetic chain and stellate ganglion. Persistence of spinal fluid leaks and pleural drainage may occur, and meningitis is possible. Otherwise, complications are similar to those for lung resections.

12. What role does irradiation play in Pancoast tumor?

In the event that a patient is found inoperable or, according to Anderson et al. is found to have N2 disease at preoperative mediastinoscopy, definitive radiation (in addition to 4,500 rad given preoperately) to a total dose of 6,000 rad can be given. Palliation of pain can be achieved using radiation alone. When analyzing survival data, it is unclear in most studies whether irradiation was given for cure or simply palliation. Doses are usually 5,000 to 6,000 rad. Most series of patients receiving irradiation alone report low survivals. In studies in which selected patients had a reasonable chance of cure, 5-year survivals close to 20% have been reported.

13. What implications does Horner's syndrome have in patients with Pancoast tumor?

Horner's syndrome is the triad of (1) ptosis, (2) miosis, and (3) anhydrosis. It is secondary to tumor involvement of the stellate ganglion (T1). Horner's syndrome has been reported by some as a negative prognostic factor in resected patients. Sartori et al. reported a 5-year survival of 8% with Horner's syndrome compared with 35% without the syndrome. Ginsberg et al. found 5-year survivals of 13% with the syndrome compared with 26% for the overall population. Clinically, Horner's manifestations may revert to normal after irradiation.

CONTROVERSY

14. What role does chemotherapy play in the management of Pancoast tumor?

Limited data preclude meaningful interpretation concerning the role of chemotherapy in Pancoast tumor; however, considerable literature has been devoted to patients with stage IIIA or IIIB non-Pancoast disease that have set the stage for future trials with Pancoast tumor. Roth's and Rosell's randomized phase III trials involving patients with stage IIIA non–small cell lung cancer show a survival benefit with induction chemotherapy with or without radiation in the surgical setting. These results have led to the exploration of concurrent induction chemotherapy and radiation followed by surgical resection for Pancoast tumor in the Intergroup Study (INT-0160) and CALGB 9495.

BIBLIOGRAPHY

1. Anderson TM, Moy PM, Holmes EC: Factors affecting survival in superior sulcus tumors. J Clin Oncol 4:1598–1603, 1986.
2. Berrino F: Epidemiology of superior pulmonary sulcus syndrome (Pancoast syndrome). Adv Pain Res Ther 4:15–21, 1982.
3. Dartevelle PG, et al: Anterior transcervical-thoracic approach for radical resection of lung tumors invading the thoracic inlet. J Thorac Cardiovasc Surg 105:1025–1034, 1993.
4. Detterbeck FC: Pancoast (superior sulcus) tumors. Ann Thorac Surg 63:1810–1818, 1997.
5. Ginsberg RJ: Resection of a superior sulcus tumor. Chest Surg Clin North Am 5:315–331, 1995.
6. Ginsberg RJ, Martini N, Zaman M, et al: Influence of surgical resection and brachytherapy in the management of superior sulcus tumor. Ann Thorac Surg 57:1440–1445, 1994.
7. Mansour K: Extended resection of bronchial carcinoma in the superior pulmonary sulcus. In Shields T (ed): General Thoracic Surgery, 4th ed. Baltimore, Williams & Wilkins, 1994, pp 572–578.
8. Rosell R, Gomez-Codina J, Camps C, et al: A randomized trial comparing preoperative chemotherapy plus surgery with surgery alone in patients with non-small-cell lung cancer. N Engl J Med 330:153–158, 1994.
9. Roth JA, Fossella F, Komaki R, et al: A randomized trial comparing perioperative chemotherapy and surgery with surgery alone in resectable stage IIIA non-small-cell lung cancer. J Natl Cancer Inst 86:673–680, 1994.
10. Sartori F, Rea F, Calabri F, et al: Carcinoma of the superior pulmonary sulcus: Results of irradiation and radical resection. J Thorac Cardiovasc Surg 104:679–683, 1992.
11. Shaw RR. Pancoast's tumor. Ann Thorac Surg 37:343–345, 1984.
12. Shaw RR, Paulson DL, Kee JL: Treatment of the superior sulcus tumor by irradiation followed by resection. Ann Surg 154:29–40, 1961.
13. Van Houtte P, MacLennan I, Poulter C, et al: External radiation in the management of superior sulcus tumor. Cancer 54:223–227, 1984.
14. York JE, Walsh GL, Lang FF, et al: Combined chest wall resection with vertebrectomy and spinal reconstruction for the treatment of Pancoast tumors. J Neurosurg (Suppl 1) 1:74–80, 1999.

33. LUNG TRANSPLANTATION

Marco Ricci, M.D., Ph.D., and Eliot R. Rosenkranz, M.D.

1. Give a concise history of lung transplantation.

In the early 1950s, several investigators conclusively showed the feasibility of pulmonary transplantation in experimental models. In 1963 at the University of Mississippi, the first human lung transplant was performed. During the 2 decades that followed, lung transplantation was largely abandoned throughout the world as a result of early failures and discouraging mortality rates that characterized the initial attempts. In the early 1980s, a better understanding of mechanisms of graft rejection and bronchial healing favorably altered early survival after transplantation and ultimately led to the first successful lung transplant at the University of Toronto. Such advancements, in combination with those regarding better patient selection, graft procurement, and organ preservation, contributed to the progress in the field of pulmonary transplantation. The development of transplant immunology along with the introduction of new immunosuppressive agents, such as cyclosporine, during the mid-1980s decreased the need for high doses of steroids in the immediate postoperative period, diminishing their adverse effects on bronchial healing. The evolution of surgical techniques of lung graft implantation led to the popularization of single-lung, en-bloc double-lung, heart-lung, and bilateral sequential lung transplantation.

2. How many lung transplants are performed each year throughout the world and in the United States?

>1,200 worldwide; of these, approximately 800 are performed in the United States, in approximately 90 transplant centers.

3. List the indications for lung transplantation.

- **Chronic obstructive pulmonary disease (COPD)**
- Cystic fibrosis (CF)
- Fibrotic or restrictive lung disease (idiopathic pulmonary fibrosis)
- Pulmonary hypertension (primary pulmonary hypertension and Eisenmenger's syndrome)

4. Discuss COPD as an indication for lung transplantation.

COPD has been reported as the most common disorder requiring lung transplantation. It includes emphysema, which alone accounts for >50% of the transplants performed in the United States, and α_1-antitrypsin deficiency. Patients affected with end-stage COPD resulting from emphysema invariably display severe reduction of expiratory flow parameters (FEV_1), in combination with marked hypoxemia and hypercarbia. Despite the initial concerns regarding contralateral pulmonary hyperinflation after single-lung replacement, there is evidence that these patients may be treated successfully by single-lung transplantation.

α_1-antitrypsin deficiency represents a rare cause of COPD requiring transplantation. Patients affected with this disease rapidly develop severe bullous emphysema with a markedly reduced respiratory function. As a result of the severe bullous parenchymal degeneration, bilateral sequential lung transplantation has been advocated as the ideal treatment of this disease.

5. Discuss CF as an indication for lung transplantation.

CF is an inherited condition caused by a defect in the cAMP-dependent regulation of transmembrane chloride transport. As a result, sweat chloride levels >60 mEq/L are commonly found, in combination with pancreatic insufficiency and chronic pulmonary disease. Thick respiratory secretions invariably result in frequent pulmonary infections, bronchiectasis, and, ultimately, respiratory failure. Pulmonary function tests in patients affected with advanced CF are similar to those observed in patients with COPD. Bilateral lung replacement represents the only form of therapy for advanced stages of the disease because there is a high risk of reinfection of the transplanted

graft if only one lung is replaced. Although heart-lung transplantation has been advocated originally as the method of choice in the treatment of CF patients, these patients are currently managed by bilateral sequential lung transplantation. In contrast to en-bloc double-lung transplantation, this approach offers the advantages of avoiding cardiopulmonary bypass (CPB) in most
patients and of eliminating the tracheal anastomosis (at higher risk for ischemic dehiscence). Although bilateral sequential lung transplantation may be performed frequently without CPB in
adults, CPB is often required in children.

6. Discuss idiopathic pulmonary fibrosis as an indication for lung transplantation.
   This is a rare indication for lung transplantation. Patients commonly display features of restrictive lung disease, although various degrees of pulmonary hypertension may be present. Single-lung transplantation is the recommended form of treatment.

7. Discuss pulmonary hypertension as an indication for lung transplantation.
   Pulmonary hypertension includes primary pulmonary hypertension and Eisenmenger's syndrome. Although these patients were originally treated with heart-lung transplantation, reports
from the literature have shown good results after single-lung replacement.

8. What are the lung donor selection criteria?
   In addition to the **standard exclusion criteria for organ donation,** such as malignancy, active
infection, HIV disease, and hepatitis B and C infection, **specific criteria for lung donation** include:
   - Age <55 years old
   - Absence of pulmonary disease
   - Normal chest radiographs
   - History of cigarette smoking of <20-pack-years
   - Normal bronchoscopic findings
   - Absence of purulent respiratory secretions at bronchoscopy
   - PaO_2 >300 mm Hg on a FIO_2 of 1.0 and positive end-expiratory pressure of 5 cm H_2O
   - Matching for ABO blood group with recipient
   - Size matching with recipient
   - Matching donor and recipient cytomegalovirus (CMV) serology

9. Why is CMV serology an important criterion for lung donor selection?
   CMV infections in CMV-negative recipients receiving lung grafts from CMV-positive
donors are particularly severe. When matching for CMV serology cannot be accomplished, prophylaxis with ganciclovir is instituted.

10. Discuss the implications of size matching.
   Although size matching can be accomplished by comparing vertical lung measurements and
transverse thoracic diameters of donor and recipient on chest radiographs, more accurate matching can be obtained by comparing lung volumes. These are calculated most realiably by using
nomograms based on age, sex, height, and weight. **Undersizing** of a lung allograft may lead to
potentially serious complications, such as hyperinflation of the lung graft and overexpansion of
the residual opposite lung. Undersizing in the setting of single-lung transplantation for pulmonary
hypertension may affect right ventricular performance adversely by decreasing pulmonary vascular resistance only partially. Oversizing a lung allograft may result in compression and displacement of mediastinal structures. Similarly, oversizing in the setting of bilateral lung replacement may affect hemodynamics severely on closure of the chest. This problem can be dealt with
by stapled wedge resection of excessive lung parenchyma.

**11. Does the primary pathology for which lung transplantation is being performed have an
impact on size matching?**
   Yes. In single-lung transplantation for emphysema, lung allografts are slightly **oversized**
(15–20% greater volume) because recipients commonly have a larger than normal chest cavity.

12. List criteria for recipients of lung transplantation.
- End-stage lung disease (defined by clinical and physiologic parameters)
- Limited life expectancy (1–2 years) in the absence of alternative forms of treatment
- Potential for rehabilitation
- Appropriate psychologic profile

13. List the contraindications to lung replacement.

Absolute
- Acute illness or instability
- Significant disease of other organ systems (cardiac, renal, hepatic, CNS)
- Uncontrolled sepsis or neoplasm
- Psychologic problems

Relative
- Age >65 years old
- Systemic disease with involvement of nonpulmonary organs
- Cardiac disease
- High-dose steroid therapy
- Unsatisfactory nutritional status
- Ventilator-dependent respiratory failure

14. Is HLA matching necessary?
In general, no. Data from the literature have shown that the effect of HLA matching on graft survival is uncertain. HLA matching would invariably delay organ harvesting with the potential of jeopardizing parenchymal integrity of the lung graft. Crossmatching of recipient serum with donor lymphocytes is usually performed in highly sensitized recipients with a high panel reactivity assay.

15. How is graft preservation accomplished?
By administering 3 L of cold (4°C) pulmonary perfusate (modified Euro-Collins solution) directly into the pulmonary artery. Experimental studies have shown that the injection of cold perfusate directly into the pulmonary artery may result in unwanted pulmonary vasoconstriction, resulting in inhomogeneous distribution of the perfusate and suboptimal organ preservation; based on this, prostaglandin E_1 (PGE_1) is administered routinely into the pulmonary artery before delivering the cold perfusate. Then harvesting is performed with the lungs in a state of moderate inflation. Storage and transportation are accomplished by placing the graft in cold crystalloid solution, then packed in ice. In so doing, ischemic time can be extended to 6–8 hours.

16. How is the donor operation performed?
1. Harvesting of the thoracic organs is accomplished concomitantly with the extraction of the abdominal organs.
2. After sternotomy and laparotomy are performed, the superior and inferior vena cavae, ascending aorta, and pulmonary artery are exposed.
3. After heparinization is accomplished, a cannula for cardioplegia is inserted in the ascending aorta, and a second cannula is inserted into the pulmonary artery for injection of the pulmonary perfusate.
4. After administration of PGE_1 into the pulmonary artery, the inflow through the vena cavae is occluded, the aorta is cross-clamped, and cardioplegia is administered, then injection of the cold pulmonary perfusate is begun (3 L of modified Euro-Collins solution).
5. Distention of the heart is avoided by excising the left atrial appendage.
6. Subsequently the heart and lungs can be extracted simultaneously or sequentially by extracting the heart first.
7. The trachea is stapled and divided with the lungs moderately inflated.
8. The organs are removed and placed in cold crystalloid solution.

17. Which side is replaced in single-lung transplantation?
Usually the one that has the poorest function based on preoperative quantitative ventilation/perfusion scan. If use of CPB is expected, the right side is often chosen. Similarly, if a concomitant cardiac procedure is planned, a median sternotomy is commonly performed.

18. Which lung is transplanted first in bilateral sequential lung transplantation?

The one with the least function so that the best lung is more likely to support the circulation and maintain gas exchange during one-lung ventilation.

19. How is the recipient operation conducted?

1. After endotracheal intubation with a double-lumen tube, recipient pneumonectomy is performed through a standard posterolateral thoracotomy incision.

2. The implantation of the lung allograft is begun.

3. The bronchial anastomosis is performed first using a 4–0 absorbable suture, then the pulmonary artery and, lastly, the pulmonary vein of donor and recipient are anastomosed using 5–0 Prolene in a running fashion.

4. On completion of the anastomoses, the transplanted lung is de-aired, and PGE_1 is administered as a continuous infusion to minimize pulmonary vasoconstriction.

5. For bilateral sequential lung transplantation, a bilateral anterolateral thoracotomy (**clamshell** incision) is used.

6. The institution of CPB may be required during implantation of the first lung or, more frequently, when the second lung is implanted, if the newly transplanted lung does not maintain adequate gas exchange.

20. List drugs that are used to induce immunosuppression.
- Cyclosporine
- Azathioprine
- Methylprednisolone

21. List the postoperative complications associated with lung transplantation.
- Acute rejection
- Bacterial pneumonia
- CMV pneumonia
- Bronchial complications

22. Describe the clinical manifestations and treatment of acute rejection.

Occurring in every patient undergoing lung transplantation, it may appear from several days to several years after the operation. Although its mechanism is not entirely understood, rejection seems to involve cytotoxic T lymphocytes against major histocompatibility complex (MHC) antigens of the donor. **Clinical manifestations** of acute rejection may be subtle and generally include malaise, fever, appearance of a new infiltrate on chest radiograph, deterioration of pulmonary function tests (FEV_1 decreasing by $\geq 10\%$), and a fall in PaO_2 by ≥ 10 mm Hg. **Treatment** is often begun on clinical grounds, although the most accurate way to diagnose rejection is by bronchoscopy with transbronchial lung biopsy. Treatment is with high doses of methylprednisolone or, in patients who do not respond to steroids, the monoclonal antibody OKT3.

23. Discuss bacterial pneumonia as a postoperative complication of lung transplantation.

It represents the most common infection in lung transplant recipients. Its therapy routinely involves intravenous antibiotics, respiratory toilet, frequent bronchoscopy, and collection of infected secretions in an attempt to identify the responsible organism. *Pseudomonas* infections in CF patients may be particularly difficult to manage.

24. What are the clinical manifestations and treatment of CMV pneumonia?

This is associated with substantial mortality. **Clinical manifestations** may be difficult to differentiate from those of acute rejection. Similarly, the diagnosis is made most reliably by bronchoscopy with transbronchial lung biopsy. **Treatment** consists primarily of ganciclovir.

25. Discuss bronchial complications after lung transplantation.

Historically, dehiscence of the bronchial anastomosis was responsible for most of the failures in the early era of lung transplantation. Advancements in graft preservation, surgical techniques of implantation, perioperative management, and immunosoppression have contributed in reducing its occurrence. A better understanding of mechanisms of bronchial healing have suggested that most cases of dehiscence are due to ischemia. As a result, during implantation, the length of the donor bronchus is kept short because bronchial viability of this portion of the airway in the immediate postoperative period largely depends on pulmonary collaterals. Bronchial anastomotic dehiscence is best identified by bronchoscopy and CT scan of the chest. Early management is usually expectant and includes drainage of the chest and antibiotics. Periodic bronchoscopy and débridement are indicated. Patients who progress to anastomotic strictures are best managed by insertion of endobronchial stents.

26. Define bronchiolitis obliterans.

A devastating condition that develops in approximately 30% of patients undergoing lung transplantation and consists of progressive obstruction of the distal airways, obliteration of bronchioles, peribronchial and interstitial fibrosis, and perivascular mononuclear infiltrates that appear in the transplanted lung several months after transplantation. It represents a manifestation of chronic allograft dysfunction and rejection and is best diagnosed by bronchoscopy with transbronchial lung biopsy. It frequently manifests as a progressive deterioration of pulmonary function tests, dyspnea, and cough. Bronchiolitis obliterans currently is responsible for most late deaths after lung transplantation. The only cure is retransplantation.

27. How is follow-up of lung transplant patients performed?

Surveillance for graft dysfunction is essentially based on **pulmonary function tests** and **bronchoscopy** with transbronchial biopsy.
- Pulmonary function testing is performed weekly for the first 3 months after transplantation, then monthly from 3 months to 1 year, then every 1–2 months thereafter. A decrement of the FEV_1 compared with baseline values is frequently associated with graft dysfunction.
- Bronchoscopy and transbronchial biopsy specimens are obtained at 1 month, 3 months, 6 months, 1 year, then annually thereafter.

26. What survival rates can be expected after lung transplantation?

The overall **1-year** survival of patients undergoing lung transplantation is approximately **70%**, whereas the **5-year** survival is **43%**. A slight survival advantage may be seen in patients undergoing bilateral lung transplantation as well as in those in whom lung replacement is performed for emphysema. Those who undergo lung transplantation for pulmonary hypertension have the worst prognosis.

BIBLIOGRAPHY

1. Mendeloff EN: Lung transplantation for cystic fibrosis. Semin Thorac Cardiovasc Surg 10:202–212, 1998.
2. Meyers BF, Alexander Patterson G: Technical aspects of adult lung transplantation. Semin Thorac Cardiovasc Surg 10:213–220, 1998.
3. Novick RJ, Stitt L: Pulmonary retransplantation. Semin Thorac Cardiovasc Surg 10:227–236, 1998
4. Patterson GA: Adult lung transplantation: Introduction. Semin Thorac Cardiovasc Surg 10:190, 1998.
5. Sundaresan S: Bronchiolitis obliterans. Semin Thorac Cardiovasc Surg 10:221–226, 1998.
6. Sundaresan RS, Patterson GA: Lung transplantation. In Baue AE, Geha AS, et al (eds): Glenn's Thoracic and Cardiovascular Surgery. Stamford, CT, Appleton & Lange, 1996, pp 511–535.
7. Waddel KT, Keshavjee S: Lung transplantation for chronic obstructive pulmonary disease. Semin Thorac Cardiovasc Surg 10:191–201, 1998.

IV. The Pleura

34. ANATOMY AND PHYSIOLOGY OF THE PLEURA AND PLEURAL SPACE

Mark R. Jajkowski, M.D., and Hratch L. Karamanoukian, M.D.

1. What is the pleura?

An elastic, serous membrane with a smooth lubricating surface. It is divided into the visceral and parietal pleurae, which merge at the lung hilum.

- The **visceral pleura** covers the lung parenchyma and extends between the lobes, keeping them separate.
- The **parietal pleura** covers the inner surface of the thoracic cavity, diaphragm, and mediastinum.

2. What is the function of the pleura?

It gives flexibility to the organs of the thoracic cavity. The heart and lungs are allowed to expand, retract, and displace each other within the thorax. The pleura provides a smooth surface, which reduces friction as the intrathoracic organs move against each other.

3. Define pulmonary ligament.

During lung development, the dorsal and ventral parietal pleurae are pulled into the thorax along with the lung. They form a double-layered fold that extends from the hilum of the lung to the diaphragm.

4. How is a pneumothorax a possible complication of central venous catheter insertion into the internal jugular vein?

The apex of the pleura extends as far cranially as 2–3 cm superior to the first rib behind the sternocleidomastoid muscle.

5. Define pleural space.

A closed potential space that exists between the visceral and parietal pleurae. It normally contains a thin layer of fluid, which acts as a lubricant between the pleural layers during respiration.

6. How many distinct layers are identifiable in the pleura by light microscopy?

Five.

1. From the pleural surface, the first layer is the mesothelial cells. These cells are 0.001–0.004 mm thick.
2. Next is a thin connective tissue layer.
3. The next deepest layer is the superficial elastic layer.
4. The next layer is a loose connective tissue layer. This loose connective tissue layer contains the blood vessels, nerves, and lymphatics.
5. A fibroelastic layer is the deepest.

7. How do the visceral pleura and its mesothelial cells differ by location?

The visceral pleura is thinner in the cranial portion with flat mesothelial cells, which are covered with sparse microvilli. Caudally the pleura is thicker, and the mesothelial cells are more cuboidal in shape with increased microvilli. The thinner cranial pleura is responsible for the increased likelihood of spontaneous rupture of apical bullae.

8. What is the most important function of the mesothelial cells?
Secretion of hyaluronic acid. Glycoproteins rich in hyaluronic acid are enmeshed by the microvilli of the pleura. These microvilli reduce friction between the lung and the thorax. This function is most apparent in the lower thorax, where the density of the microvilli is the greatest.

9. What is the normal amount of fluid found in the pleural space?
< 1mL; this fluid forms a layer approximately 0.01 mm thick between the visceral and parietal pleurae.

10. What is the normal resting pressure in the pleural space relative to atmospheric pressure?
Pressure varies by the timing of the respiratory cycle and the level within the thorax. The pressure at **midlung height** and at **rest** is approximately − 5 cm H_2O. With **deep inspiration** this may decrease to −25 to −35 cm H_2O. There is a pressure gradient vertically within the thorax. The pressure is most negative at the apex and is the greatest at the base. The gradient is approximately 0.2 to 0.5 cm H_2O/cm of vertical distance.

11. List factors that contribute to the pressure gradient within the thorax.
- Change in the lung shape from the apex to the base
- Weight of the intrathoracic structures

12. What accounts for the unequal distribution of ventilation within the lung?
Because alveolar pressure is constant, alveoli at the apex are larger than at the base.

13. What factors establish the negative pressure in the pleural space?
The lung and thorax have natural recoils that are in opposing directions. The **thorax** has a natural outward pull at rest, and the **lung** tends to pull inward on the pleural space at rest, creating a negative pressure.

14. How are the visceral and parietal pleurae innervated?
The **visceral pleura** contains no pain fibers. It may be manipulated without causing pain. The **parietal pleura** overlying the thorax and diaphragm does contain sensory nerves. Intercostal nerves supply the costal pleura and the peripheral portion of the diaphragm. The central portion of the diaphragm is supplied by sensory nerve endings from the phrenic nerve.

15. What clinical correlations can be made based on the difference in sensory innervation in the visceral and parietal pleurae?
- Irritation of the parietal pleura causes referred pain to the level of its intercostal nerve supply.
- Painful stimulation of the central portion of the diaphragm is experienced as pain referred to the ipsilateral shoulder.
- Because the visceral pleura contains no sensory fibers, pleuritic chest pain indicates irritation of the parietal pleura.

16. What is the origin of the fluid normally found within the pleural space?
The capillaries of the parietal pleura as a result of **Starling's law of transcapillary exchange.** The hydrostatic pressure in the parietal pleura is approximately 30 cm H_2O and approximately −5 cm H_2O in the pleural space, creating a net hydrostatic pressure of 35 cm H_2O favoring the movement of fluid into the pleural space. Pleural fluid normally contains 1–1.5 g of protein / dL, creating an oncotic pressure of 5 cm H_2O. The oncotic pressure of plasma is normally 34 cm H_2O. This creates a net gradient of 6 cm H_2O favoring the movement of fluid from the parietal pleura capillaries into the pleural space. The net gradient across the visceral pleura is

approximately 0 because of the hydrostatic pressure of the visceral pleural capillaries being 6 cm H_2O less than the parietal pleura capillaries. This is secondary to the former being drained into the pulmonary veins.

17. If there is no gradient for the movement of fluid across the visceral pleura, how is the accumulation of pleural fluid prevented?
Although not accepted by all, there is evidence that most pleural fluid is removed by the parietal pleural lymphatics.

18. What is the approximate daily lymphatic drainage of fluid from the pleural space?
Approximately 300 mL/d.

19. What are the lymphatic drainage patterns of the visceral and parietal pleurae?
The lymphatics of the **visceral pleura** course over the surface of the lung and penetrate the parenchyma to join the bronchial lymphatics. All lymph flow from the visceral pleura eventually reaches the hilum of the lung.

Lymphatic drainage of the **parietal pleura** varies depending on the location. The costal pleura drains ventrally to the internal mammary artery and dorsally to intercostal lymph nodes. Mediastinal lymphatics drain to the tracheobronchial and mediastinal lymph nodes. Diaphragmatic pleural lymph vessels drain to the posterior mediastinum, parasternal, and middle phrenic lymph nodes.

20. What is the mechanism responsible for pleural fluid absorption and the removal of particulate matter and cellular debris through the parietal pleura?
The parietal pleura contains stomas that are round openings 0.002–0.006 mm in diameter. These stomas are found mostly on the parietal pleura of the lower anterior chest wall and mediastinum. No such stomas have been found on the visceral pleura. These stomas are found only overlying dilated lymphatic spaces known as **lacunae.** At the stoma, the mesothelial cells are continuous with the endothelial cells of the lymphatic channels. During inspiration, the movement of the chest wall opens the stomas. Particulate matter, cells, and fluid are taken into the stomas by the negative pressure created and physically pushed by the expanding lung. Once within the stoma, these materials are taken into the underlying lacuna. During expiration, the stomas close, and the contents of the lacunae are forced into the lymphatic ducts.

21. How is the retrograde flow of particles and fluid prevented in the parietal pleural lymphatics?
The lymphatics contain valves similar to those found in veins.

BIBLIOGRAPHY

1. Agostoni E, Zocchi L: Mechanical coupling and liquid exchanges in the pleural space. Clin Chest Med 19:241–260, 1998.
2. Light RW: Anatomy of the pleura. In: Pleural Diseases. Baltimore, Williams & Wilkins, 1995, pp 1–6.
3. Light RW: Physiology of the pleura. In: Pleural Diseases. Baltimore, Williams & Wilkins, 1995, pp 7–17.
4. LoCicero J: Benign and malignant disorders of the pleura. In: Glenn's Thoracic and Cardiovascular Surgery. Stamford, CT, Appleton & Lange, 1996, pp 537–555.
5. Wang NS: Anatomy of the pleura. Clin Chest Med 19:229–240, 1998.

35. IMAGING OF THE PLEURA

Timothy G. DeZastro, M.D.

1. What is the pleura?

A duplex structure composed of parietal and visceral layers that line the inner chest wall and diaphragm and the outer surface of the lungs. There is a morphologic difference between the two layers, with the visceral pleura, having more elastic components to accommodate pulmonary inflation and deflation and the parietal pleura having connective tissue, helping to add stability to the inner chest wall.

The blood supply to the parietal pleura is derived from the systemic chest wall vasculature, an important fact to remember when considering the possibility of chest wall and pleural metastasis from remote primary malignancies. The blood supply to the visceral pleura is controversial, with some theories suggesting a pulmonary artery origin and others a bronchial artery supply.

2. How is the pleura best imaged?

Cross-sectional imaging with **CT scan** or **MRI** offers significant advantages over plain film examinations. Although CT and MRI offer increases in detection and differentiation of disease when compared with radiographs, the modalities are not interchangeable. CT, with its higher spatial resolution, offers greater anatomic detail, whereas the ability of MRI to distinguish subtle variations in tissue free water concentration is far superior in assessing extent of possible chest wall and pleural involvement (CT for diagnosis; MRI for staging).

3. Describe the imaging characteristics of normal pleura.

The pleura generally is not visualized unless some pathology exists. With the advent of high-resolution CT, this is not always an absolute, and the parietal pleura can occasionally be seen if there is an abundant amount of extrapleural fat. The pleura can always be seen in the presence of a pneumothorax as a line of increased density, representing the visceral pleural reflection juxtaposed to the extrapulmonic air on CT scan and chest radiograph. The visceral pleura can also be seen on CT scan, as it invaginates into the fissures, where the two layers oppose each other. Normal pleura is always seen as a uniformly thin line of increased density when viewed against extrapleural fat or extrapulmonic air.

4. How is normal pleura distinguished from abnormal pleura?

Any deviation from the uniformly thin morphology represents pathology. Abnormal pleura presents with thickening, and this thickening can be widespread, as in cases of diffuse mesothelioma or diffuse pleural lymphatic dissemination with metastatic tumor cells. Nonneoplastic diffuse pleural thickening can be seen in inflammatory or infectious conditions and can be used as a diagnostic discriminator between infected and noninfected pleural effusion (thickened in the former, usually thin in the latter). Localized forms of pleural thickening are almost always neoplastic but can be benign (benign pleural fibroma, pleural lipoma, or fibrosis) or malignant (mesothelioma, metastasis deposits). Reactive pleura can be diffuse or localized as seen in cases of asbestos exposure, radiation injury, or reactive pleura in cases of empyema.

5 What are the most frequently encountered benign conditions of the pleura?

Reactive changes in the pleura include localized fibrosis representing a healed pleurisy secondary to pneumonia. Localized pleural fibrosis, also called **benign mesothelioma**, can occur as a focal thickening of the pleura and is relatively uncommon ($> 1,000$ cases in literature). The cause is unknown. Reactive changes to asbestos or talc can produce areas of focal pleural thickening often accompanied by effusions, calcifications, and subpleural pulmonary fibrosis—asbestosis. Calcification is not unique to asbestos plaques and can be seen in healed tuberculous empyema, also known as the **calcified fibrothorax,** which less frequently can be seen in nontuberculous empyemas. Pleural lipomas represent one condition in which a relatively easy and accurate diagnosis can be made by CT scan. Hounsfield attenuation values of < -20 are consistent with fat and permit an end to further diagnostic workup. Uremia and some connective tissue disorders (rheumatoid) are associated with focal and diffuse benign pleural thickening. Approximately 20% of patients with uremia develop fibrous pleurisy.

6. What are the most frequently encountered malignant conditions of the pleura?

Malignant mesothelioma and metastasis — lung, colon, breast, and thymus. With CT scan, the presence of calcified plaque with agressive behavior suggests mesothelioma over metastasis, especially in the presence of an asbestos exposure history. It is not always possible to differentiate the cause of a malignant condition (or even some benign conditions) without histologic or cytologic sampling. Malignant mesothelioma is seen radiographically as diffuse nodular plaques. These plaques may or may not be calcified. Generally, metastases to the pleura from carcinoma do not calcify (except in the case of metastatic mucinous adenocarcinoma) so that calcification in the presence of aggressive pleural masses, associated with calcification in a patient without a history of prior mucinous adenocarcinoma, virtually eliminates all other possibilities except malignant mesothelioma. MRI plays a role in assessing the degree of chest wall or mediastinal invasion. Malignant thymoma also frequently produces diffuse pleural metastatic thickening.

7. How can one differentiate benign from malignant pleural disease?

The most reliable way is by biopsy. There is great overlap in the radiographic appearance of pleural disease and in the absence of a histologically or cytologically proven benign entity, only long-term (> 5 years) radiographic stability can impart a prediction of benign disease. In at least one entity, pleural lipoma, the diagnosis can be made with complete confidence based in the CT attenuation values of fat. In the face of a convincing history, a prediction of a benign condition can be made in cases of reactive pleuritis after treated pneumonia, calcified fibrothorax after empyema (granulomatous or otherwise), and asbestos-related pleural disease without interval change over 5 years with documented history exposure.

8. How is pleural fluid differentiated from solid pleural processes?

There are two main imaging discriminators. The more common tool is measurement of the CT attenuation values. Hounsfield units (HU) of -20 to $+20$ are synonymous with fluid, although there is not a great deal of specificity as to the type of fluid. Generally the higher the HU, the thicker the fluid. HU can in some cases of chronic empyema or hemothorax exceed $+20$, and in those cases the use of intravenous contrast enhancement usually allows the fluid to be distinguished from a solid process. Fluid does not show an increase in HU attenuation enhancement, whereas most solid processes containing blood vessels enhance to some degree. Fine-needle aspiration can be used in cases that are still unclear even after these methods are used.

9. How are pleural processes differentiated from pulmonary parenchymal processes?

There is a general rule of thumb used to ascribe location to a peripheral intrathoracic mass. If the mass forms acute margins with the chest wall or pleural lining interface, the mass is thought to be intraparenchymal. If the mass forms obtuse margins with the chest wall and pleura–lungs interface, it is supposed to be intrapleural or pleural-based. The word *supposedly* was chosen because there is great overlap between conditions that cause acute and those that cause obtuse angled margins so far as the organ of origin is concerned. Biopsy is the only reliable discriminator of intraparenchymal versus pleural-based diseases.

10. What is the usefulness of imaging-guided pleural biopsy?

Except in cases in which there is diffuse pleural involvement, imaging guidance is essential in obtaining the most representative sample of the pathologic process possible. Imaging guidance should be used in almost all cases of pleural thickening in which a definitive diagnosis is required. Some cases with long-term radiographic stability do not come to biopsy.

11. How do malignancies involve the pleura?

1. Direct extension, which can be seen in cases of intrathoracic and extrathoracic sarcoma as well as primary lung cancer. Invasive thymoma also involves the pleura by contiguous spread.

2. Hematogenous dissemination, as in sarcomas and lung cancer.

3. Via the lymphatics, as in sarcomas and lung cancer, especially in cases of breast cancer metastatic to the chest wall.

12. List some of the postsurgical pleural manifestations.

• A syndrome characterized by pleuritis, pneumonitis, and pericarditis that can progress to pericardial and pleural thickening and trapped lung

• Chylothorax, a recognized but somewhat infrequent complication of cardiovascular surgical procedures

• Hemothorax after any transsternal thoracotomy

These complications can be recurrent and require multiple thoracenteses or progress to loculation, septation, and compartmentalization; surgical decortication occasionally requires pleurodesis.

BIBLIOGRAPHY

1. Fraser R, Pare JA: Synopsis of Disease of the Chest, 2nd ed. Philadelphia, W.B. Saunders, 1994.
2. Haaga J, Alfidi R: Computed Tomography of the Whole Body, 2nd ed., St. Louis, C.V. Mosby, 1988.
3. Naidich D, et al: Computed Tomography of the Thorax. New York, Raven Press, 1984.
4. Wechsler R: Cross-Sectional Analysis of the Chest and Abdominal Wall. St. Louis, C.V. Mosby, 1989.

36. PNEUMOTHORAX

Kurt VonFricken, M.D.

1. What is a pneumothorax?
Air within the pleural space.

2. What is the usual cause of a primary spontaneous pneumothorax?
The intrapleural rupture of a peripheral lung bleb.

3. How is a small pneumothorax with minimal symptoms managed?
Observation; the pneumothorax usually resolves spontaneously.

4. When should a chest tube be inserted?
- If the pneumothorax is > 25%
- If a tension pneumothorax is present
- If disease is present in the contralateral lung
- If significant persisting symptoms are present
- If progression of the pneumothorax is visible on serial radiographs

5. Is the actual size of a pneumothorax more likely to be larger or smaller than estimated by plain films?
Using rough estimation, usually **larger** because the plain films are two-dimensional (vs. the actual volume of the lung, which is three-dimensional). There are formulas that help to estimate the size using measurements taken from radiographs, but they assume a constant shape of the lung during collapse.

6. How is a tension pneumothorax diagnosed?
Clinically, never by radiograph. (If you see a significant tension pneumothorax on radiograph, you have missed the clinical diagnosis.)

7. List the signs that are present in a tension pneumothorax.
- Unilateral decreased breath sounds with tympany to percussion
- Hypotension and other signs of shock
- Jugular venous distention
- Tracheal deviation away from the involved side (late sign)

8. What is the treatment for tension pneumothorax?
Immediate decompression with a chest tube or a large-bore catheter, such as an angiocath.

9. Once initially treated, how is a tension pneumothorax treated?
Tube thoracostomy as with a simple pneumothorax.

10. Does intubation help a patient with a tension pneumothorax?
Only in that it secures the airway. The positive-pressure ventilation makes a tension pneumothorax worse (keep this in mind any time you see someone with sudden cardiopulmonary deterioration after intubation).

11. When do most air leaks resolve?
Usually within 1–2 days.

12. What is the significance of subcutaneous emphysema after chest tube placement for a pneumothorax? What is the treatment? Is it dangerous?

This is typically caused by a kinked or blocked chest tube. The air that leaks from the lung cannot go out through the tube, so it follows the path of least resistance and exits through the chest tube site. If it cannot escape through the skin, it dissects into the subcutaneous plane and can extend into the neck and face, sometimes even into the eyelids.

13. What is the treatment for subcutaneous emphysema?
- Check the chest tube for proper functioning
- Relieve the obstruction

14. Is subcutaneous emphysema after chest tube placement dangerous?

Athough it can often look dramatic, it is a benign process that will resolve, and it is important to let the patient, family members, and nurses know this.

15. When should surgery be considered?
- If an air leak persists for > 5–7 days (this is known as a **bronchopleural fistula**)
- If the lung fails to reexpand
- If there are bilateral pneumothoraces
- If there is contralateral pneumonectomy
- If the patient has a specialized occupation (pilot, diver)
- If the patient is isolated from medical care

16. Name the basic principles of surgery for a spontaneous pneumothorax.
- Removal of the blebs causing the pneumothorax
- Pleural symphysis

17. How are the blebs removed?

By thoracotomy or video-assisted thorascopic surgery. Blebs currently are typically removed using a stapling/cutting device.

18. How is pleural symphysis achieved?
- **Mechanical** means include direct abrasion or parietal pleurectomy.
- **Chemical** means include sterile talc, tetracycline, or doxycycline instilled into the pleural space.

19. What percentage of patients have a recurrence?

About 20%.

20. Are patients with recurrence managed differently than patients with a first occurrence?

Treatment is basically the same, although most practitioners are generally more likely to perform pleurodesis or operative treatment for a recurrence.

21. What is a secondary spontaneous pneumothorax?

A spontaneous pneumothorax that occurs in persons with known lung disease (mostly chronic obstructive pulmonary disease in older patients).

22. How is a secondary spontaneous pneumothorax unique?
- It presents more often with shortness of breath, not pain as with primary spontaneous pneumothorax.
- It has larger air leaks that take longer to heal. All should be treated with tube thoracostomy.
- The recurrence rate is much higher, about 50%.
- More definitive treatment usually is recommended.

23. What is often the earliest radiographic sign of barotrauma (ventilator-induced pneumothorax)?

Pneumomediastinum.

24. What is often the first sign of barotrauma?

An acute change in hemodynamics or oxygenation.

25. Name the ideal site for chest tube insertion.

The anterior or midaxillary line behind the pectoralis fold.

26. List techniques that can be used to prevent injury to chest or abdominal organs during chest tube insertion.

- High placement of the tube (especially in trauma cases in which there could be a diaphragmatic hernia)
- Finger exploration of the pleural space

27. Is there a safe way to treat patients with spontaneous pneumothorax that require a chest tube as an outpatient?

Yes; a one-way flutter valve (Heimlich valve) can be attached to the end of the chest tube.

BIBLIOGRAPHY

1. Beauchamp G: Spontaneous pneumothorax and pneumomediastinum. In Pearson FG, Deslauriers J, Ginsberg RJ (eds): Thoracic Surgery. New York, Churchill Livingstone, 1995, pp 1037–1054.
2. Chechani V: Tetracycline pleurodesis for persistent air leak. Ann Thorac Surg 49:166–167, 1990.
3. Engdahl O, Toft T, Boe J: Chest radiograph—a poor method for determining the size of a pneumothorax. Chest 103:26–29, 1993.
4. Granke K, Fischer CR, Gago O, et al: The efficacy and timing of operative intervention for spontaneous pneumothorax. Ann Thorac Surg 42:540–542, 1986.
5. LoCicero J: Benign and malignant disorders of the pleura. In Baue AE, Geha AS, Hammond GL, et al (eds): Glen's Thoracic and Cardiovascular Surgery, 6th ed. Stamford, CT, Appleton & Lange, 1996, pp 537–555.
6. Maunder RJ, Pierson DJ, Hudson LD: Subcutaneous and mediastinal emphysema: Pathophysiology, diagnosis and management. Arch Intern Med 144:1447–1453, 1984.
7. O'Rourke JP, Yee ES: Civilian spontaneous pneumothorax: Treatment options and long-term results. Chest 96:1302–1306, 1989.
8. Schoenenberger RA, Haefeli WE, Weiss P, et al: Timing of invasive procedures in therapy for primary and secondary spontaneous pneumothorax. Arch Surg 126:764–766, 1991.
9. Weeden D, Smith GH: Surgical experience in the management of spontaneous pneumothorax, 1972–82. Thorax 38:737–743, 1983.

37. PLEURAL EFFUSIONS

Kevin Broder, M.D.

1. How are pleural effusions diagnosed?

Effusions of >150 mL are usually seen as blunting of the costophrenic angle on an upright chest radiograph. Subpulmonic effusions may present with elevation of the hemithorax, lateral displacement of the dome of the diaphragm, or increased distance between the apparent left hemidiaphragm and air in the stomach. Lateral decubitus radiographs are more reliable in detecting pleural effusions than is the upright chest radiograph. Large unilateral effusions shift the mediastinum to the contralateral hemithorax. Bilateral effusions with associated cardiomegaly are usually caused by congestive heart failure. Radiographic evidence of pneumonia or malignancy may suggest these findings are the cause for the effusion.

2. What is the indication for performing diagnostic thoracentesis?

Effusion of unknown cause.

3. List relative contraindications for performing diagnostic thoracentesis.

- Coagulopathy or systemic anticoagulation
- < 1 cm thick pleural effusion on lateral decubitus chest radiograph
- Area of infected skin

4. List the indications for performing therapeutic thoracentesis.

- Relieve symptoms of dyspnea secondary to pleural effusion
- Remove fluid to enable status of underlying lung to be evaluated
- Large effusions with mediastinal shift
- Serial thoracentesis in malignant effusions with mediastinal shift when pleurodesis has failed

5. What are the relative contraindications for performing therapeutic thoracentesis?

Same as for diagnostic thoracentesis.

6. How much fluid should be drained at a single thoracentesis?

1,000–1,500 mL.

7. What happens if >1,500 mL of fluid is drained at a single thoracentesis?

Reexpansion pulmonary edema can occur; this poorly understood syndrome results in unilateral pulmonary edema of the lung on the side of the thoracentesis. Monitoring pleural pressures during drainage of large effusions and avoiding rapid fluctuations < −20 cm H_2O may help prevent this phenomenon.

8. What are Light's criteria?

Criteria used to distinguish transudative from exudative pleural effusions:

	TRANSUDATE*	EXUDATE[†]
Ratio of pleural fluid protein to serum protein	<0.5	>0.5
Ratio of pleural fluid LDH to serum LDH	<0.6	>0.6
Absolute pleural fluid LDH level	<2/3 upper limit of normal for serum	>2/3 upper limit of normal for serum

*For pleural fluid to be called a transudate, all of the above criteria must be satisfied.
[†]For pleural fluid to be called an exudate, only one of the above criteria must be satisfied.

9. **Name the various methods available for draining pleural effusions.**
   - **Therapeutic thoracentesis**—usually used with small free-flowing effusions.
   - **Tube thoracostomy**—indicated for hemothorax, empyema, malignant effusions, and pneumothorax.
   - **Thoracotomy with decortication**—reserved for organizing pleural peels, loculated hemothorax, or empyema.
   - **Video-assisted thoracoscopy**—produces less morbidity and shorter hospital stays than thoracotomy.

10. **What is the most common cause of pleural effusion?**
    Congestive heart failure.

11. **Describe the pathophysiology of pleural effusion formation caused by congestive heart failure.**
    Left ventricular heart failure leads to elevation of pulmonary capillary pressure. Fluid then extravasates and enters the interstitial space of the lung, which, in turn, leads to an increase in subpleural interstitial pressure, and fluid moves across the permeable visceral pleura into the pleural space. Normally, pleural fluid exits the pleural space by parietal pleura lymphatics. Pleural effusion occurs when the rate of fluid accumulation exceeds the rate of lymphatic drainage. An increase in systemic venous pressure associated with congestive heart failure may decrease lymphatic clearance.

12. **Describe the mechanism for the formation of hepatic hydrothorax.**
    Hepatic hydrothorax is seen in cirrhotics with ascites. It most commonly results in right-sided pleural effusion. Increased intra-abdominal pressure associated with tense ascites causes stretching of the diaphragm, which results in the formation of microscopic defects in the diaphragm. Ascitic fluid in the peritoneal cavity then moves through these defects into the pleural space. Diagnosing hepatic hydrothorax usually involves performing thoracentesis and paracentesis and finding that the pleural fluid protein level is greater than that of the ascitic fluid but still <3 g/dL. The mainstay of treatment involves treating the underlying ascites.

13. **What percentage of patients with pulmonary emboli have associated pleural effusions?**
    30–50%.

14. **What percentage of pleural effusions are caused by pulmonary emboli?**
    5%.

15. **What percentage of effusions are malignant?**
    25% of all pleural effusions and 70% of exudative effusions.

16. **Describe direct causes of malignant effusions.**
    - **Pleural metastasis** results in increased permeability of pleural surfaces and can obstruct pleural lymphatic vessels.
    - **Mediastinal nodal involvement** can lead to decreased lymphatic drainage of the parietal pleura.
    - **Chylothorax** may develop if there is interruption of the thoracic duct.
    - **Bronchial obstruction** leads to more negative pleural pressures and accumulation of fluid.
    - **Pericardial involvement** with pericardial effusion leads to increased hydrostatic pressure and resultant transudation into the pleural space.

17. **Describe indirect causes of malignant effusions.**
    - **Hypoproteinemia** causes decreased oncotic pressure and movement of fluid into the pleural space.

- **Post-obstructive pneumonitis** leads to parapneumonic effusion.
- **Pulmonary embolus** results in right-sided heart failure, increased parietal pleural capillary pressure and pleural fluid accumulation. Another mechanism by which pulmonary emboli may cause effusions is release of inflammatory mediators from platelet-rich thrombi, which cause an increase in the permeability of lung capillaries and increased interstitial and pleural fluid.

18. List the most common sites of primary malignancy that give rise to malignant effusions.
- Lung   36%
- Lymph nodes   16%
- Breast   15%
- Ovary   8%

19. Discuss the treatment options for malignant effusions.
- When definitive chemotherapy is used for treatment of the primary tumor, **thoracentesis** should be performed because antineoplastic drugs may accumulate in the pleural space and lead to systemic toxicity.
- **Repeated thoracenteses** may be performed; however, reaccumulation and loculation limit utility. Tube thoracostomy is another option.
- **Chemical pleurodesis** is indicated when the patient is symptomatic with dyspnea and when there are no indications for chemotherapy, when chemotherapy or radiation therapy has failed, and when there is no chylothorax present.
- **Mediastinal radiation** is indicated for chylothorax secondary to lymphoma or metastatic carcinoma.
- **Pleurectomy** and decortication may be performed at the time of diagnostic thoracotomy and with trapped lung when chemical pleurodesis cannot be performed.
- Permanent catheters, such as the **pleuroperitoneal shunt** or indwelling **Tenckhoff catheter,** may be inserted when the patient becomes symptomatic.
- **No treatment** is indicated when life expectancy is only a few days.

20. What are advantages and disadvantages of permanent catheters over pleurodesis?
Advantages
- Less pain
- Shorter hospital stay

Disadvantages
- Obstruction of the catheter
- Risks of anesthesia
- Requirement of most catheters to be pumped >400 times per day

21. List therapeutic options for recurrent malignant effusions.
- Pleurectomy
- Mechanical pleurodesis
- Chemical pleurodesis
- Pleuroperitoneal shunts
- Tube thoracostomy with sclerosis

22. What agent has proved to be the most successful in accomplishing chemical pleurodesis?
Talc, which can be administered by a thoracostomy tube in the form of a slurry, or it may be insufflated throughout the pleural space with the aid of thoracoscopy.

23. List other agents that are used for chemical pleurodesis.
- Quinacrine   • Doxycycline   • Bleomycin

24. What diagnostic modalities are recommended if negative cytology is obtained after therapeutic thoracentesis?

A **repeat thoracentesis** should be performed along with a **pleural biopsy** and a **perfusion lung scan** to look for pulmonary embolus.

25. What is the recommended diagnostic workup for a malignant effusion with an unknown primary malignancy?

CT scan of the chest, abdomen, and pelvis. If the chest CT scan is positive, **bronchoscopy** is indicated to obtain a tissue diagnosis. In female patients, a thorough **pelvic examination** is warranted.

BIBLIOGRAPHY

1. Colice GL, Rubins JB: Practical management of pleural effusions: When and how should fluid accumulations be drained? Postgrad Med 105:67–77, 1999.
2. Light RW: Pleural Diseases, 3rd ed. Baltimore, Williams & Wilkins, 1995, pp 83–116.
3. LoCicero J: Benign and malignant disorders of the pleura. In Baue AE (ed): Glenn's Thoracic and Cardiovascular Surgery, 6th ed. Stamford, CT, Appleton & Lange, 1996, pp 547–548.
4. Rubins JB, Colice GL: Evaluating pleural effusions: How should you go about finding the cause? Postgrad Med 105:39–48, 1999.

38. EMPYEMA

Vivian Lindfield, M.D., and Hratch L. Karamanoukian, M.D.

1. What is a pleural empyema?

A collection of infected fluid in the pleural space. The empyema may be encapsulated (localized) or may be diffuse and involve the entire pleural cavity. Empyemas may be acute or chronic depending on duration of time present and pathologic response.

2. Describe the different stages of empyema.

- **Exudative empyemas** are characterized by thin fluid and low cell content. The underlying lung readily reexpands once the fluid is removed.
- **Fibropurulent empyemas** are characterized by a lot of polymorphonuclear leukocytes and deposition of fibrin on the visceral and parietal pleural surfaces. In the stage between acute and chronic infection, there is a tendency toward loculation and fixation of the lung.
- In **organizing empyemas,** fibroblasts appear in the coating of the pleural membranes. The exudate at this point is thick in consistency.

3. What is the most common cause of empyema?

Pneumonia is the most common primary process in the underlying lung. Empyema occurs less commonly now because of improved antibiotic therapies.

4. What are other causes of empyema?

- Trauma, especially penetrating trauma of the chest with a nonsterile object.
- Systemic sepsis in the immunocompromised or trauma patient.

5. How does infection spread from the pneumonic process to the pleura?

1. Direct extension from the infiltrate
2. Lymphatic spread from neighboring lung, mediastinal, or chest wall infection
3. Hematogenous spread from remote areas
4. Direct inoculation by penetrating trauma
5. From ruptured thoracic viscera (i.e., esophageal)
6. Extension of a subdiaphragmatic infection

6. List organisms that are commonly involved in empyema formation.

Staphylococcus aureus (most common), *Streptococcus, Pseudomonas, Klebsiella pneumoniae, Escherichia coli, Proteus,* and *Bacteroides* (tend to be present with a mixed flora of organisms).

7. How is empyema diagnosed?

Diagnosis depends on signs and symptoms associated with the underlying infectious process. Many symptoms are similar to those of pleural effusions.

- Radiograph of the chest shows fluid, fluid and air combined, or a pleural opacification.
- Needle aspiration can confirm the diagnosis by showing pus.

8. List complications that can occur as a result of empyema.

- **Empyema necessitatis** (invasion of chest wall by empyema)
- Bronchopleural fistula
- Extension to the pericardium
- Osteomyelitis of the ribs
- Generalized sepsis

9. List the objectives of treatment of empyema.

1. Control of the primary infection and any secondary manifestations.
2. Removal of pleural contents and the empyema sac. Removal of the sac helps prevent chronicity of the empyema.
3. Reexpansion of the underlying lung to restore function.

10. What treatment modalities are used for empyema?

- Appropriate antibiotics based on the causative organism
- Prompt drainage of the pleural space

11. What is the role of needle aspiration in the treatment of empyema?

It may be the only treatment necessary for drainage if the fluid is thin and easily removed by the small-gauge needle that is used. This is usually the case with streptococcal infections.

12. Are there any problems associated with needle aspiration?

- Longer hospital stay compared with the tube drainage
- Increased risk of loculation of the fluid with needle aspiration

13. Describe the preferred method of drainage of an empyema.

An underwater-seal closed tube drain should be placed promptly, especially if the pus is thick and cannot be evacuated by thoracentesis. A tube should be placed if the infection is unresponsive to antibiotic therapy or if fluid reaccumulates after needle drainage. The chest tube should be a generous size to prevent occlusion. The tube is placed in the most dependent portion of the empyema. Negative pressure may be applied to the tube to help increase reexpansion of the lung.

14. Discuss surgical measures that are used in the treatment of empyema.

- **Resection of a rib segment** may be necessary to obtain adequate drainage if the pus is thick and loculated or if the patient remains toxic after tube drainage. The purpose is to increase exposure for better evacuation of the purulent fluid and to increase the ability to break up loculations that may be present.
- **Open drainage** may be needed, which involves the placement of a large-bore tube in the empyema, which is left open to the atmosphere.
- The **Eloesser skin flap** is a variation that was used originally in the treatment of tuberculous empyemas. This technique combines open and closed drainage but eliminates the need for wide-bore tubes. In this procedure, a flap of skin is sutured to the pleura, creating an epithelium-lined sinus into the empyema sac to assist in drainage.

15. What percent of empyemas result from thoracic surgical procedures?

About 25%, especially after pneumonectomy. These empyemas may be associated with bronchopleural fistulas. If this occurs in the first week postoperatively, it may be due to a technical cause.

16. How are empyemas resulting from thoracic surgeries treated?

Closure of the fistula should be attempted early. A fistula that occurs later is usually due to residual tumor or a condition that predisposes the patient to poor wound healing. The pleural space needs to be irrigated with antibiotics. The **Clagget technique** includes open drainage, irrigation of the pleural cavity with antibiotics for several months, and later surgical closure of the chest wall.

BIBLIOGRAPHY

1. King TC, Smith CR: Chest wall, pleura, lung and mediastinum. In Schwartz SI, Shires GT, Spencer FC (eds): Principles of Surgery, 6th ed. New York, McGraw-Hill, 1994.
2. Scott SM, Takaro T: The pleura and empyema. In Sabiston DC (ed): Textbook of Surgery: The Biologic Basis of Modern Surgical Practice, 15th ed. Philadelphia, W.B. Saunders, 1997.
3. Turley K: Thoracic wall, pleura, mediastinum and lung. In Way LW (ed): Current Surgical Diagnosis and Treatment, 10th ed. Norwalk, CT, Appleton & Lange, 1994.

39. PLEURAL NEOPLASMS

Reginald Abraham, M.D., and Hiroshi Takita, M.D., D.Sc.

1. What are the different types of tumors of the pleura?

The most common primary tumors of the pleura are benign and malignant pleural mesothelioma. Other less common malignant tumors known to originate from the pleura are soft tissue sarcoma, lymphoma, desmoplastic small cell tumor, and thymoma.

Virtually all cancers metastasize to the pleura. Lung cancer is the most common cause that occurs in 25% of patients with malignant pleural effusions. Ovarian and gastric cancers also commonly metastasize to the pleura. Seven percent of patients with malignant effusions have unknown primary site.

2. What causes malignant pleural mesothelioma?

In 1960, Wagner et al. reported 33 cases of diffuse malignant pleural mesothelioma (MPM) in asbestos mine workers from South Africa. Subsequently, it was confirmed that inhalation of asbestos fibers was the major risk factor for MPM. The latent period of developing MPM following asbestos exposure is 20–40 years. Besides asbestos, erionite is known to cause mesothelioma. It is a zeolite fiber that is found in volcanic deposits of central Turkey and is the major building material of homes in that area. Radiation is also implicated in the etiology. Recently, SV40 virus has been isolated in MPM.

3. What is the incidence of MPM?

In the U.S., 2,000 to 3,000 new cases per year are reported. The majority of patients are over 55 years of age at presentation. The disease is more common in men (male:female ratio 3:1).

4. How is the diagnosis of MPM made?

Symptoms and signs: The majority of patients present with dyspnea and chest pain. Other symptoms are cough, weakness, and weight loss.

Radiologic findings: Chest x-ray demonstrates a pleural effusion or pleura-based mass lesion. Irregular thickening of the pleura and loss of volume of the lung are seen in later stages. Following the above x-ray findings, CT scan is usually obtained and suspicion of MPM is established (see figure below).

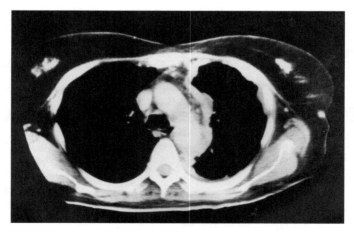

A 61-year-old female presented with left-sided chest pain and shortness of breath. CT scan showed irregular thickening of the pleura. A diagnosis of the epithelial-type mesothelioma localized to one hemithorax was made by thoracoscopy and biopsy. She was treated with pleurectomy and intracavitary photodynamic therapy. Pathologically it was staged as T3N0M0 (stage III). The patient expired of locally advanced disease in 8 months.

Confirmation of the diagnosis by microscopy: Thoracentesis and microscopic examination of pleural effusion is usually unsatisfactory. The cytologic examination correctly diagnosed the MPM only in 30% of cases. Presently the recommended method of diagnosis is the thoracoscopy and biopsy of the pleura. Thoracoscopy is also useful for the staging of the disease. Bronchoscopy is used to rule out possibility of lung cancer.

5. Describe cytopathologic diagnosis of MPM.

There are three types of MPM: epithelial type, sarcomatous (fibrous) type, and mixed type. The **epithelial type** is the most common and accounts for 50–60% of all MPM cases. It can have papillary, tubular, cord-like, or sheet-like pattern. The papillary and tubular forms are often extremely difficult to differentiate from adenocarcinoma of the lung. In the **fibrous type,** the cells are spindle-shaped and have an ovoid or elongated nucleus with well developed nucleoli. It accounts for about 20% of MPM cases. In the **mixed type,** epithelial and fibrous types are mixed and it is seen in 30–40% of MPM cases. Presence of obvious droplets of mucicarmine-positive or periodic acid schiff (PAS)-positive material in cytoplasm of the tumor cells make the diagnosis of MPM very likely. MPMs usually produce large amounts of hyaluronic acid, which can be demonstrated with alcian blue or colloidal iron stains. MPM is usually negative for CEA, Leu-M1 (CD15), and B 72.3.

6. How is MPM staged?

Numerous staging systems have been proposed; however, the staging recently proposed by the American Joint Committee for Cancer Staging, UICC, and/or the International Mesothelioma Interest Group (IMIG) are used most commonly (see table on next page).

7. What is the prognosis of MPM?

The median survival from the time of diagnosis is 7–12 months. The median duration of the symptoms prior to diagnosis is 3 months. The natural history of MPM involves a diffuse local process affecting the pleura, lung, diaphragm, and mediastinum. Patients develop progressive symptoms of the chest and death occurs usually from respiratory failure. Up to two thirds of patients with MPM die of locally advanced disease without distant metastasis.

8. What treatments are available for MPM?

There is no known effective curative therapy. However, because up to two thirds of patients die of locally advanced disease, the feasibility of the surgical therapy has been explored.

Surgical therapy alone: Pleuro-pneumonectomy or pleurectomy alone did not produce improvement in survival and can be associated with significant mortality.

Radiation therapy: As a single-modality therapy, radiation also had disappointing results and there was no advantage in the survival of treated patients noted. However, radiation therapy appears to be a good palliative therapy, e.g., for pain caused by MPM.

Chemotherapy: Some chemotherapeutic agents were found to produce temporary shrinkage of MPM; however, there has been no effect in prolonging the survival.

Biologic therapy: Cytokines (interferons and interleukins) have been given intrapleurally and some beneficial results have been reported. Also, gene therapy in preliminary clinical studies is being carried out.

Photodynamic therapy: It has been clinically investigated, mostly in combination with the surgery.

Combined-modality therapy: Pleurectomy or pleuro-pneumonectomy in combination with radiation and/or chemotherapy or photodynamic therapy have been investigated clinically. Results of the largest clinical trial (183 patients) of extrapleural pneumonectomy, radiation, and chemotherapy have been reported; the overall median survival was 17 months, yielding the overall 2- and 5-year survival of 38% and 15%, respectively. In the patients with earlier stages, 5-year survival of 46% was reported.

9. What are metastatic tumors of the pleura?

As mentioned before, virtually all cancers can metastasize to the pleura and cause malignant pleural effusion. Most frequently, lung, ovarian, gastric cancer, and lymphoma are involved.

New International Staging System for Diffuse MPM

T1	
T1a	Tumor limited to the ipsilateral pleura, including mediastinal and diaphragmatic pleura
T1b	Tumor involving the ipsilateral parietal pleura, including mediastinal and diaphragmatic pleura. Scattered foci of tumor also involve the visceral pleura.
T2	Tumor involving each of the ipsilateral pleural surfaces (parietal, mediastinal, diaphragmatic, and visceral) with at least one of the following features: involvement of diaphragmatic muscle; confluent visceral pleural tumor (including the fissure); or extension of tumor from visceral pleura into the underlying pulmonary parenchyma.
T3	Describes locally advanced but potentially resectable tumor
	Tumor involves all of the ipsilateral pleural surfaces (parietal, mediastinal, diaphragmatic, and visceral) with at least one of the following features: involvement of the endothoracic fascia; extension into the mediastinal fat; solitary, completely resectable focus of tumor extending into the soft tissue of the chest wall; or nontransmural involvement of the pericardium.
T4	Describes locally advanced technically unresectable tumor
	Tumor involving all of the ipsilateral pleural surfaces (parietal, mediastinal, diaphragmatic, and visceral) with at least one of the following features: diffuse extension or multifocal masses of tumor in the chest wall, with or without associated rib destruction; direct transdiaphragmatic extension of tumor to the peritoneum; direct extension of tumor to one or more mediastinal organs; direct extension of tumor into the spine; tumor extending through to the internal surface of the pericardium with or without a pericardial effusion; or tumor involving the myocardium.
N	Lymph nodes
NX	Regional lymph node cannot be assessed
N0	No regional lymph node metastases
N1	Metastases in the ipsilateral bronchopulmonary or hilar lymph nodes
N2	Metastases in the subcarinal or the ipsilateral mediastinal lymph nodes, including the ipsilateral internal mammary nodes
N3	Metastases in the contralateral mediastinal, contralateral internal mammary, ipsilateral, or contralateral supraclavicular lymph nodes
M	Metastases
MX	Presence of distant metastases cannot be assessed
M0	No distant metastasis
M1	Distant metastasis present
Stage Description	
Stage I	
Ia	T1a N0 M0
Ib	T1b N0 M0
Stage II	T2 N0 M0
Stage III	Any T3 M0
	Any N1 M0
	Any N2 M0
Stage IV	Any T4
	Any N3
	Any M1

Adapted from Rusch VW: A proposed new international TNM staging system for malignant pleural mesothelioma. Chest 108:1122–1128, 1995, with permission.

10. What is the prognosis in malignant pleural effusion?

The diagnosis of malignant pleural effusion portends a poor prognosis. Patients generally survive only a few months, whereas patients with breast cancer and lymphomas may survive several months to years.

11. How is malignant pleural effusion treated?

Generally, the treatment is aimed at palliation. For most patients, the most effective and least morbid method for controlling a symptomatic malignant effusion is chest tube drainage with instillation of a sclerosing agent to cause adhesion between visceral and parietal pleura and abolish accumulation of fluid in the pleural space. Usually the procedure is performed in the operating room with the monitored anesthesia care. A chest tube is inserted and the pleural effusion is completely drained. Following this, a sclerosing agent is instilled into the pleural cavity by the chest tube. As the sclerosing agent, doxycycline, bleomycin, or sterile talc powder are used.

BIBLIOGRAPHY

1. Boutin C, Rey F: Thoracoscopy in pleural malignant mesothelioma: A prospective study of 188 consecutive patients. Cancer 72:389–393, 1993.
2. Hilaris B, Nori D, Kwong E, et al: Pleurectomy and intraoperative brachytherapy and postoperative radiation in the treatment of malignant pleural mesothelioma. Int J Radiat Oncol 10:325–331, 1984.
3. Pass H, Temeck B, Kranda K, et al: Phase III randomized trial of surgery with or without intraoperative photodynamic therapy and postoperative immunochemotherapy for malignant pleural mesothelioma. Ann Surg Oncol 4:628–633, 1997.
4. Price B: Analysis of current trends in the United States mesothelioma incidence. Am J Epidemiol 145:211–218, 1997.
5. Rice TW, Adelstein DJ, Kirby TJ, et al: Aggressive multimodality therapy for malignant pleural mesothelioma. Ann Thor Surg 58:24–29, 1994.
6. Ruffie P, Cormier M, Boutan-Laroze A, et al: Diffuse malignant mesothelioma of the pleura in Ontario and Quebec: A retrospective study of 332 patients. J Clin Oncol 7:1157–1168, 1989.
7. Rusch VW, Piantadosi S, Holms EC: The role of extrapleural pneumonectomy in malignant pleural mesothelioma. J Thor Cardiovasc Surg 54:941–946, 1991.
8. Rusch VW: Diffuse Malignant Mesothelioma. In Shields TW (ed): General Thoracic Surgery, 4th ed. Baltimore. Williams & Wilkins, 1994, pp 731–747.
9. Rusch VW: A proposed new international TNM staging system for malignant pleural mesothelioma. Chest 108:1122–1128, 1995.
10. Sahn SA.: Malignant pleural effusions. In Shields TW (ed): General Thoracic Surgery, 4th ed. Baltimore. Williams & Wilkins, 1994, pp 757–764.
11. Takita H, Dougherty T: Intracavitary photodynamic therapy for malignant pleural mesothelioma. Semin Surg Oncol 11:368–371, 1995.

40. CHYLOTHORAX

Marco Ricci, M.D., Ph.D., and Eliot R. Rosenkranz, M.D.

1. What is chylothorax?
An accumulation of lymphatic fluid within the pleural space.

2. List the causes of chylothorax.
- **Iatrogenic chylothorax**—inadvertent injury to the thoracic duct during surgical proce-dures involving the esophagus, thoracic aorta, or epiaortic vessels (most common cause).
- **Posttraumatic chylothorax**—may occur after blunt or penetrating trauma to the chest. Hyperextension of the vertebral column may result in injury to the thoracic duct, which is located anterior to the thoracic vertebral bodies. Penetrating chest trauma with injuries to the intrathoracic organs located in the posterior mediastinum (esophagus, aorta) may in-volve the thoracic duct.
- **Nontraumatic chylothorax**—various benign and malignant tumors, along with infectious diseases involving the intrathoracic structures, as a result of obstruction of the lymphatic channels or direct destruction of the lymphatic pathways by malignant tumors.
- **Congenital chylothorax**—complete absence or abnormal development of the lymphatic channels constituting the thoracic duct (rare). Trauma at birth has been recognized as a pos-sible pathogenetic mechanism of chylothorax in neonates.
- **Rare causes**—thrombosis of the jugular and subclavian veins, increased central venous pressure resulting from various causes (i.e., after Fontan procedure), liver cirrhosis, and tu-berculosis.

3. Where is the thoracic duct located?
The thoracic duct originates in the right posterior mediastinum from the abdominal chylifer-ous channels and the cisterna chyli as they traverse the diaphragm with the aorta through the aor-tic hiatus. At its origin in the right posterior mediastinum, just above the diaphragm, the duct lies just to the right of the descending thoracic aorta, between the esophagus anteriorly and the azy-gos vein posteriorly. As it courses cephalad, the duct crosses the posterior mediastinum from the right to the left, approximately at the level of the tracheal bifurcation. It then continues superi-orly, joining the confluence between the left internal jugular vein and the left subclavian vein.

4. Does thoracic duct injury result in right or left pleural effusion?
- As a result of its anatomic location, injuries of the thoracic duct in the **lower chest** often result in a **right-sided pleural effusion.**
- Injuries to the **upper** portion of the duct are commonly accompanied by a **left-sided pleural effusion.**
- In some patients, bilateral spillage of chylous fluid in both pleural spaces may occur.

5. Describe the initial clinical manifestations of chylothorax.
The clinical manifestations are determined by the underlying pathology leading to chylotho-rax. In the case of iatrogenic injuries to the thoracic duct and in posttraumatic injuries, clinical manifestations may be subtle. In this setting, chylothorax may not be recognized until 7–10 days after the primary insult, as signs and symptoms of a pleural effusion become manifest. These in-clude **shortness of breath, chest discomfort,** and **various degrees of respiratory distress.**

6. How is the diagnosis of chylothorax usually made?
In the setting of traumatic or iatrogenic injuries to the thoracic duct, thoracentesis performed for persistent pleural effusion yields a whitish, milky fluid in the pleural aspirate. Fat globules,

which stain with Sudan III on microscopic examination, are a distinctive feature of this fluid. Chemical analysis of the pleural fluid classically reveals a high content in triglycerides (0.4–6 g/100 mL). This is usually accompanied by negligible levels of cholesterol so that a cholesterol-to-triglycerides ratio of <1 is indicative of chylothorax. Additional **laboratory data** consistent with chylous fluid are a total protein content of approximately half that of the plasma (2.2–5.9 g/100 mL) and a high content in lymphocytes, predominantly T lymphocytes (400–6,800 cells/mm^3). This peculiar fluid composition allows one to differentiate chylous fluid from **pseudochyle**, a milky fluid occasionally found in the presence of malignancies or infections of the pleura. Despite its similarity in appearance, pseudochyle characteristically has a lower content in triglycerides, a higher level of cholesterol, and a lower content of proteins and lymphocytes.

7. How much lymphatic fluid can accumulate daily in the pleural space?

1,500–2,500 mL/d. This represents the daily amount of chylous fluid that commonly flows through the thoracic duct each day. The daily amount and composition of lymphatic fluid are influenced by dietary intake. Lymphatic flows as high as 200 mL/h may be observed when high-fat meals are ingested. Rates of accumulation >400–500 mL/d are usually considered clinically significant.

8. Discuss conservative management of chylothorax.

Most cases initially can be managed expectantly, regardless of cause, unless surgical intervention is required for other coexisting conditions. A trial of conservative management includes tube thoracostomy and avoidance of oral alimentation in conjunction with total parenteral nutrition. Occasionally, special preparations, such as those containing medium-chain triglycerides, may be used orally because they are absorbed directly into the enterohepatic circulation, bypassing the lymphatic system. Electrolyte imbalances should be corrected as required. In approximately 50% of cases, conservative management results in closure of the lymphatic fistula. Enteral nutrition can be restarted and the pleural drain removed if chylothorax does not recur.

9. Discuss surgical treatment of chylothorax.

Patients with continued chest drainage after at least 2 weeks of conservative management or patients in whom the chylous leak is >1,000 mL/d should be considered for surgical intervention because spontaneous closure of the leak is unlikely. If these patients are left untreated, the clinical manifestations of severe metabolic and immunologic derangement owing to the loss of triglycerides, vitamins, proteins, and lymphocytes may become manifest. Surgical candidates are best explored through a right thoracotomy. Occasionally the leaking thoracic duct or its branches may be identified intraoperatively and ligated. This may be facilitated by injection of methylene blue in the lower extremities or by introducing fatty substances (milk, cream, or olive oil) in the stomach through a nasogastric tube 2–3 hours before surgery. The right pleural space is entered, and the right lower lobe of the lung is displaced anteriorly by dissecting the inferior pulmonary ligament. The mediastinal pleura is opened posteriorly, just above the diaphragm. If the leaking duct cannot be identified, supradiaphragmatic ligation of the duct is required. This is performed by **mass ligation** of all the mediastinal tissues located between the esophagus, the azygos vein, and the descending thoracic aorta, and it leads to interruption of the lymphatic channels, including the thoracic duct, with prompt resolution of the chylous fistula.

BIBLIOGRAPHY

1. Higgins CB, Molder DG: Chylothorax after surgery for congenital heart disease. J Thorac Cardiovasc Surg 61:411, 1971.
2. Miller JI: Chylothorax. In Shields TW (ed): General Thoracic Surgery. Baltimore, Williams & Wilkins, 1994.
3. Milson JW: Chylothorax: An assessment of current surgical management. J Thorac Cardiovasc Surg 89:221, 1985.
4. Murphy TO, Piper CA: Surgical management of chylothorax. Ann Surg 43:719, 1977.

V. The Mediastinum

41. ANATOMY OF THE MEDIASTINUM

Colin J. Powers, M.D., and Hratch L. Karamanoukian, M.D.

1. Outline the anatomic boundaries of the mediastinum.

The mediastinum extends between the two pleural cavities from the thoracic inlet most superiorly to the diaphragm inferiorly. The anterior boundary is defined as the posterior surface of the sternum, whereas the posterior boundary is the anterior surface of the vertebral bodies.

2. Name the four compartments of the mediastinum.

Anterior, middle, posterior, and superior mediastinum.

3. What are the anatomic boundaries of the four compartments of the mediastinum?

Anterior mediastinum	The anatomic boundaries consist of the posterior aspect of the sternum and the most ventral surface of the pericardium. The cephalad limit is designated as a line drawn from the sternomanubrial joint to the lower edge of the T4 vertebral body. The caudad limit is the diaphragm. The lateral borders are designated by the pleural sacs.
Middle mediastinum	The area comprised within the pericardium and its most closely associated structures.
Posterior mediastinum	Extends from the most dorsal surface of the pericardium to the ventral surface of the vertebral bodies. The lateral borders are designated by the pleural sacs.
Superior mediastinum	Originates at the thoracic inlet and extends distally to the horizontal plane established between the sternomanubrial joint and the lower border of the T4 vertebral body (the transition point to the anterior and posterior mediastinum). The left and right pleural surfaces define the lateral borders.

4. Which clinically important structures reside within the four compartments of the mediastinum?

Anterior mediastinum	Contains the thymus and an extensive network of lymphatics. The thymus extends from the superior mediastinum into the more inferiorly located anterior mediastinum. This is most noticeable in childhood before the natural regression and involution of the thymus occurs.
Middle mediastinum	Contains the heart and surrounding pericardium along with closely adherent portions of the great arteries and the tracheal bifurcation with the origins of the pulmonary bronchi.
Posterior mediastinum	Holds the esophagus and the descending aorta, both of which have arisen in the superior mediastinum. The thoracic duct, azygos veins, sympathetic chains, and splanchnic nerves course through it.
Superior mediastinum	The thymus, the great thoracic vessels, the esophagus, the trachea, and the thoracic duct.

5. Are there alternatives to the four-compartment model of the mediastinum?

Yes, both six-compartment and three-compartment models of the mediastinum have been described in the literature. While the six-compartment model is seldom used clinically, the three-compartment model as described by Shields has proven to be more functional. It encompasses the same total area, but divides the mediastinum into anterior, visceral, and paravertebral sulci compartments.

6. Which side of the mediastinum is known as the blue side? Why?
    The right side of the mediastinum is referred to as the blue side because of the presence of the right atrium, the vena cava, and the azygos vein.

7. Which side of the mediastinum is known as the red side? Why?
    The left side of the mediastinum is referred to as the red side, because of the presence of the aorta, the left common carotid, and the subclavian arteries.

BIBLIOGRAPHY

1. Dresler C: Anatomy and classification [of the mediastinum]. In Pearson F, Deslauriers J, Hiebert C, et al (eds): Thoracic Surgery. New York, Churchill Livingstone, 1995, pp 1325–1332.
2. Moore K: Clinically Oriented Anatomy, 3rd ed. Baltimore, Williams & Wilkins, 1992, pp 79–120.
3. Ronson R, Duarte J, Miller J: Embryology and surgical anatomy of the mediastinum with clinical implications. Surg Clin North Am 80:157–169, 2000.

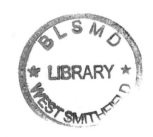

42. IMAGING OF THE MEDIASTINUM

Timothy G. DeZastro, M.D.

1. What is the mediastinum?

The central portion of the chest that contains the vascular organs that separate the two lungs.

2. What are the radiographic boundaries of the mediastinal compartments?

Radiographically the mediastinal compartments are classically defined on the basis of a lateral chest radiograph by Dr. Ben Felson (see figure).

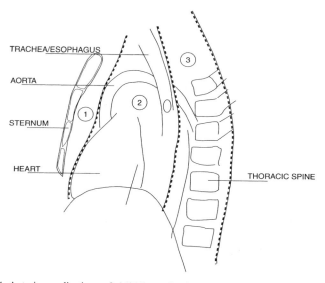

1, Anterior mediastinum; 2, Middle mediastinum; 3, Posterior mediastinum.

- The **anterior mediastinum** is defined as the space between the sternum anteriorly and a line drawn anterior to the great vessels and pericardium of the heart.
- The **middle mediastinum** lies between this line along the anterior border of the heart and the anterior border of the aorta and a line drawn posterior to the tracheoesophogeal shadow and along the posterior aspect of the heart silhouette.
- The **posterior mediastinum** includes structures between the posterior aspect of the tracheoesophageal line, along the posterior pericardium and the spine.
- Heitzman further subdivides the mediastinum into right and left and superior and inferior subdivisions, which are not as commonly used radiologically as Dr. Felson's classic division.

3. List the structures that lie within the anterior mediastinum.

- Thymus
- Retrosternal space
- Lymph nodes
- Internal mammary vessels

4. **List the structures that lie within the middle mediastinum.**
    - Heart and pericardium
    - Great vessels
    - Trachea and esophagus
    - Central pulmonary vessels
    - Hilar lymph nodes

    There is some controversy over placement of the esophagus in the middle mediastinum. Some authors (Fraser and Pare) place it in the posterior mediastinum, and others place it in the middle mediastinum as classically defined by Dr. Felson. I personally feel that it more properly belongs in the middle mediastinum with the other embryologic derivatives of the foregut.

5. **List the structures that lie within the posterior mediastinum.**
    - Paraspinal spaces
    - Spinal nerves
    - Descending thoracic aorta
    - Azygos and hemiazygos veins
    - Thoracic spine

6. **What are the most common conditions affecting the anterior mediastinum?**
    Neoplastic
    Thymoma is the most common neoplasm in the anterior mediastinum. Its imaging characteristics are not specific. It generally presents as a smoothly marginated mass in the anterior mediastinum not typically associated with calcification. It can be associated with myasthenia gravis; 50% of patients with thymoma have myasthenia gravis, and 15% of patients with myasthenia gravis have thymoma. Other neoplastic entities include **lymphoma** (usually seen as bulky conglomerate mediastinum masses, **teratomas** (which demonstrate derivatives of the embryologic components—teeth, calcification, fat), and **substernal thyroid goiters** (almost invariably presenting with heterogeneous attenuation, cystic and calcified components, and continuity with the cervical thyroid gland). Less frequent neoplastic masses include thymolipoma and thymic carcinoid.
    Posttraumatic
    Posttraumatic conditions include **hematomas** from aortic tear or internal mammary vessel lacerations from blunt chest wall trauma. This is readily diagnosed by contrast-enhanced CT.
    Postoperative
    Postoperative causes of anterior mediastinal pathology are seen most frequently in **post-sternotomy** patients. Substernal abscesses and other postoperative fluid collections can be seen in the anterior mediastinum.

7. **Describe the specific imaging characteristics of the anterior mediastinal processes.**
    The imaging features frequently overlap. The commonly recited differential of anterior mediastinal masses consists of **the four Ts:** thymus, teratoma, thyroid, and T-cell Hodgkin's lymphoma occasionally can be differentiated but many times cannot.
    - Classic teratomas demonstrate calcification, possible fat-fluid levels, and other mesodermal derivatives.
    - Substernal thyroid goiter in the anterior mediastinum looks identical to thyroid goiters in the neck with calcification and heterogeneous attenuation.
    - Anterior mediastinal fluid collections usually can be differentiated more by history than by imaging characteristics. The presence of air in a retrosternal fluid collection >2 weeks after sternotomy is a strong indication of a retrosternal abscess. Anterior mediastinal fluid should have Hounsfield unit (HU) attenuation values between −20 and +20.
    - History is key in the case of treated lymphoma. Treated lymphoma frequently calcifies, and in conjunction with the proper history, calcified mediastinal masses can be given the correct diagnosis of treated burned-out lymphoma rather than the diagnosis of another calcified mediastinal mass.

- Fatty thymic tumors (thymolipoma) usually contain enough fat to allow a definite diagnosis based on HU attenuation of -20.

8. What are the most common conditions affecting the middle mediastinum?

Neoplastic lymphadenopathy is the most frequently seen abnormality. Ninety percent of all masses in the middle mediastinum are malignant. **Lesions** or **masses** of the **foregut derivatives** are the most frequently encountered nonneoplastic masses. These include bronchogenic foregut duplication and pericardial cysts as well as primary esophageal disease (diverticula, dilation, or tumor).

9. Describe the imaging characteristics of middle mediastinal masses.

The imaging characteristics can occasionally be diagnostic, especially in cases in which well-defined cystic masses are seen in typical locations for foregut duplication cysts.

- Typical patterns of calcification, such as **eggshell calcification** in silicosis, sarcoid, or tuberculosis, frequently can differentiate nodal disease in these entities from metastatic lymphadenpathy.
- **Vascular lesions** such as aberrant vessels and aneurysms can be differentiated by their continuity with other vascular structures and by their pattern of enhancement on contrast-enhanced CT.
- **Foregut duplication** and vascular anomalies frequently can be demonstrated and differentiated better by MRI or magnetic resonance angiography (MRA) than CT because of the occasional artifactual increase in CT Hounsfield attenuation units in cysts containing fluid with high protein content or in fluid collections in which there is hemosiderin from previous hemorrhage.

10. What are the most frequently encountered conditions of the posterior mediastinum?

Conditions are related to anatomic structures occupying the posterior mediastinum and include:

- Neurogenic/neuroenteric tumors
- Diseases of the spine
- Extramedullary hematopoiesis
- Conditions of the descending thoracic aorta (aneurysm or dissection)

11. Describe the imaging characteristics of posterior mediastinal masses.

Imaging characteristics are specific to the organ of origin.

- Lesions of the **aorta** show marked vascular enhancement on contrast-enhanced CT. Type II and type III thoracic aorta dissections demonstrate a uniformly thin line with flowing enhanced blood on both sides indicating flow in the true and false lumens of a dissected aorta.
- **Neurogenic/neuroenteric cysts** are best demonstrated on MRI, which can document exquisitely the connection to the spinal cord or spinal nerves as well as any bone changes in the vertebral column. Neuroenteric cysts frequently are associated with hemivertebra or butterfly vertebra.
- **Extramedullary hematopoiesis**, because of its increased hemoglobin, is quite distinctly visualized on MRI, although its characteristic location with the supporting history of splenomegaly and chronic anemia allow the diagnosis to be made by CT as well.

12. How can benign processes be differentiated from malignant disease in the mediastinum by imaging?

Benign processes can be differentiated on the basis of contrast enhancement, fat content, calcification, water content, or position.

- The presence of **vascular enhancement** as well as the ability to trace on multiple slices a vascular entity allows for confident diagnosis of varices or an aberrant vessel from a soft tissue mass.
- The presence of **fat** in a lesion in the anterior mediastinum can allow for a fairly confident diagnosis of thymolipoma or mature teratoma. Exquisite CT or MRI demonstration of

diffuse fat in the mediastinum allows for a diagnosis of mediastinal lipomatosis and excludes other more ominous diagnoses.
- The presence of **calcification** in an intramediastinal mass would fairly limit the differential to a mature teratoma or an intrathoracic thyroid. The position and continuity of the intrathoracic portion of the thyroid to the thyroid gland in the neck allows for a confident diagnosis of the substernal calcified thyroid goiter from other causes.
- **Water content** in mediastinal cysts can allow for a more limited differential diagnosis.
- The differential diagnosis of cystic mediastinal masses occasionally can be narrowed based on **position** in the mediastinum, whether anterior, middle, or posterior. This allows for a differentiation of thymic cysts (anterior mediastinum) versus foregut or middle mediastinal duplication cysts (middle mediastinum) versus neuroenteric cysts, which most frequently occur in the posterior mediastinum.

13. Discuss the role of imaging in guiding interventional procedures in the mediastinum.

Imaging-guided techniques allow for biopsy of almost all parts of the mediastinum. Primary mediastinal lesions require tissue biopsy. Few lesions are inaccessible to current techniques, including **transsternal biopsy** and even **transvenous fine-needle aspiration (FNA) through large mediastinal veins.**

Solid mediastinal masses, enlarged lymph nodes, thymic masses, and mediastinal germ cell malignancies all are usually approachable by CT-guided techniques. The type of lesion to be biopsied and the intervening structures determine if a core biopsy or FNA is used.

FNA (22 gauge) is employed where other structures (i.e., the vena cava) have to be traversed to reach the suspected area to avoid collateral trauma. FNA technique is used if the lung must be traversed to reach the desired lesion. Whenever possible, core biopsies of any mediastinal mass suspected to be lymphatic in origin are recommended because most pathologists favor architecture for lymphatic tissue over cytology obtained by FNA.

14. Discuss the role of positron emission tomography (PET) scanning in evaluation and staging of mediastinal disease.

PET combines the principles of axial CT with the photon emission techniques of nuclear single-photon emission CT. It uses metabolic differences to concentrate the radiopharmaceuticals in tissues and to display these differences in an anatomic mapping technique similar to CT. The spatial resolution is less with PET than with standard CT. Spatial resolution with PET scanning is on the order of 5 mm in the mediastinum, while spatial resolution in conventional CT is submillimeter.

PET's role is one of **differentiation of metabolic activity** of a particular structure rather than the anatomic characterization of that structure. PET is useful in staging mediastinal masses that may not be diagnostically apparent on the basis of CT. For example, by CT criteria, a mediastinal lymph node is considered abnormal if maximal cross-sectional diameter is >1.5 cm. In staging of lung cancer with mediastinum adenopathy, a ≥1.5 cm lymph node is considered evidence of metastatic lymphadenopathy. With PET scanning, nodes below this diameter also can be diagnosed as being metastatic on the basis of their metabolic activity and alter the surgical resectability of a lesion. PET scanning can, by virtue of differential metabolic activity, fairly accurately distinguish malignant from reactive adenopathy.

15. Discuss the relative advantages and disadvantages of CT versus MRI in the mediastinum.

CT of the mediastinum is **universally available.** There are **no contraindications to CT** as there are with MRI. Patients with pacemakers, with known ferromagnetic bodies, or who are unstable without non–MRI-compatible interventional life support devices cannot be scanned with MRI. MRI is usually of longer duration than a CT examination of the mediastinum, especially using state-of-the-art helical or spiral CT scanners.

CT demonstrates **better spatial resolution** than MRI in the mediastinum, although with newer MRI scanners, spatial resolution approaches but does not quite match a CT scan. This is a significant improvement over previous generations of MR scanners.

MRI is superior to CT in the mediastinum of patients who cannot receive intravenous contrast material. MRI with its vascular techniques such as time-of-flight imaging, does not need administration of **intravascular contrast material** because these techniques provide an inherent vascular contrast. This is especially useful in the evaluation of thyroid masses in the mediastinum. The use of iodinated contrast material may preclude imaging or therapy with radioiodine if the patient's thyroid or thyroid mass has been saturated with exogenous iodinated contrast material. The direct acquisition multiplanar capabilities of MRI are more useful for the evaluation of the vascular anatomy, especially for possible venous vascular invasion from mediastinal tumor. Spiral CT has multiplanar reconstruction capabilities but requires the use of intravenous contrast material, which MRI does not, and it is reconstructed rather than directly acquired imaging data, decreasing resolution.

One area in which CT surpasses MRI is in the **duration of the examination.** A spiral CT scan usually can complete an examination in <5 minutes. MRI, with its varying sequence acquisitions, even with multiplanar, echoplanar, and gradient echo sequences, would still exceed that time. For patients in extremis requiring emergent imaging in the mediastinum, spiral CT may be preferable to MRI.

MRI is superior to CT in **evaluation of cystic masses.** Cystic masses that have hemorrhaged or have increased proteinaceous content frequently appear solid by CT. With specific appearances on various MR sequences, these lesions can be characterized appropriately and accurately as cystic.

MRI is far superior to CT in **evaluation of the heart** and with the latest MRI sequences, cardiac MRI will soon rival cardiac angiography as a noninvasive way of evaluating cardiovascular anatomy. Cardiac MRI will perform the same function as intracranial magnetic resonance angiography in routine screening, having replaced the more invasive intracranial catheter angiography. Cardiac magnetic resonance imaging has the potential to do the same. The role of CT in the evaluation of the heart, pericardium, and pericardial space is limited, whereas the potential for MRI is unlimited in these regions. CT has no role in evaluation of the major coronary arteries except to determine the presence or absence of gross calcification. Cardiac magnetic resonance angiography, still in its infancy, shows great promise in its potential for noninvasive evaluation of cardiovascular anatomy.

MRI is superior to CT in the evaluation of **neurogenic tumors** because MRI can evaluate and display the relationships to the central and peripheral nervous system and extension into or from the spinal canal better with its multiplanar capability than CT can.

BIBLIOGRAPHY

1. Cohen AJ, et al: Primary cysts and tumors of the mediastinum. Ann Thorac Surg 51:378–386, 1991.
2. Dewan NA, et al: Diagnostic efficacy of PET-FDG imaging in solitary pulmonary nodules. Chest 104:997–1002, 1993.
3. Felson B: Chest Roentgenology. Philadelphia, W. B. Saunders, 1973.
4. Fraser R, Paré JA: Synopsis of Diseases of the Chest, 2nd ed. Philadelphia, W. B. Saunders, 1994.
5. Heitzman ER: The Mediastinum: Radiologic Correlations with Anatomy and Pathology. St. Louis, C. V. Mosby, 1977.
6. Kubota K, et al: Differential diagnosis of lung tumor with positron emission tomography: A prospective study. J Nucl Med 31:1927–32, 1990.
7. Naidich D, et al: Computed Tomography and Magnetic Resonance of the Thorax, 2nd ed. New York, Raven Press, 1991.
8. Oldham NH: Mediastinal tumors and cysts. Ann Thorac Surg 2:246–275, 1971.

43. MEDIASTINOSCOPY AND MEDIASTINOTOMY

Marco Ricci, M.D., Ph.D., and Raffy L. Karamanoukian, M.D.

1. What is the rationale of mediastinoscopy?

Mediastinoscopy is frequently employed in the management of patients with lung cancer to confirm or exclude metastatic involvement of mediastinal nodes (N2 disease).

2. Why is it important to stage mediastinal lymph nodes accurately in lung cancer patients?

Approximately 45% of the patients with non–small cell lung cancer present with N2 disease. The presence of lymph node metastases in the mediastinum from lung cancer (N2 disease) classically has been considered a contraindication to surgical therapy. Although pulmonary resection may be performed in the presence of N2 disease, 5-year survival in most of these patients is dismal (7–34%). The concept that N2 invariably contraindicates surgical resection has been challenged. There has been evidence to suggest that patients with mediastinal involvement limited to aortopulmonary lymph nodes or limited to ipsilateral tracheobronchial nodes have better survival rates and may benefit from pulmonary resection. Similarly, improved outcomes after resection have been reported in patients with microscopic metastases and localized invasion of mediastinal nodes as well as in patients whose N2 disease is discovered at surgery, in contrast to those who display evidence of N2 disease preoperatively. Various protocols of nonadjuvant chemotherapy and radiation therapy followed by surgical resection have been employed in the management of lung cancer with N2 involvement. Although their role remains under investigation, preliminary evidence suggests that survival of patients with N2 disease may be improved.

3. What is the role of CT scan of the chest in detecting mediastinal lymph node metastases in lung cancer patients?

Although CT scan probably represents the most valuable test for preoperative staging of lung cancer patients, its role in defining lymphatic mediastinal invasion is **limited**. Studies from the literature have shown that lymph node metastases are more likely to be found at the time of surgery in patients with evidence of mediastinal lymphadenopathy on preoperative CT scan (nodes > 10 mm). This radiographic finding is associated with a 15–20% rate of false-positive results. Similarly, false-negative results by CT scan are observed in 20% of patients with metastatic mediastinal involvement.

4. In which patients should mediastinoscopy be performed?

Although some surgeons believe that all patients who are candidates for pulmonary resection should be subjected to this procedure, others believe that mediastinoscopy should be used selectively. Those who use mediastinoscopy liberally in all patients base their strategy on the fact that noninvasive techniques of preoperative staging (i.e., CT scan of the chest) do not predict reliably involvement of mediastinal nodes and that preoperative assessment of mediastinal nodes is important because N2 patients should be excluded from surgical therapy. They claim that mediastinoscopy can be performed at a limited cost and carries only minimal operative risks.

Those who advocate the use of mediastinoscopy selectively employ this modality mainly to stage accurately patients with the appearance of mediastinal lymph nodes > 10 mm on CT scan. This strategy eliminates the risk of excluding lung cancer patients from resection in the presence of false-positive CT results (nodes appearing > 10 mm on CT but free from metastases), although it may lead to performing pulmonary resection in patients with preoperatively unrecognized N2 disease. Five-year survival of patients in whom mediastinal involvement is discovered at surgery is reported to be significantly better than that of patients in whom mediastinal involvement is recognized preoperatively. As a result, patients with preoperatively unidentified N2 disease may still benefit from resection.

5. How is mediastinoscopy performed?

1. The operation is carried out under general anesthesia, through a 2-cm transverse neck incision above the sternal notch.

2. After the platysma is transected, the strap muscles are divided in the midline.

3. Then the pretracheal plane is reached, and, by blunt finger dissection, a tunnel is created along the anterior surface of the trachea, between this structure posteriorly and the innominate artery anteriorly.

4. The mediastinoscope is inserted in this space, and the presence of lymphadenopathy is assessed carefully.

5. Nodes are biopsied after needle aspiration has excluded a vascular structure.

6. Hemostasis is usually accomplished using a long electrocautery or simply by packing the wound for several minutes. Alternatively, small hemoclips may be used.

6. What is a modified mediastinoscopy?

A technique that can be employed to biopsy lymph nodes in the anterior mediastinum as well as subaortic and para-aortic nodes, which could not be otherwise reached by standard cervical mediastinoscopy. In contrast to standard cervical mediastinoscopy, the mediastinoscope is inserted along a retrosternal, prevascular plane. This method also can be used to biopsy tumors located in the anterior mediastinum.

7. Which patients are candidates for mediastinotomy?

Patients affected with cancer of the left upper lobe of the lung, in which lymphatic drainage often involves stations that cannot be biopsied through a standard cervical mediastinoscopy (stations 5 and 6; aortopulmonary window and para-aortic nodes).

8. How is mediastinotomy performed?

The classic Chamberlain mediastinotomy is performed through an incision over the second intercostal cartilage, on the left side of the chest. The anterior mediastinum is entered by subperichondrially removing the second cartilage. The left internal mammary artery and veins are ligated and divided. Lymph nodes of the anterior mediastinum and aortopulmonary window can then be approached.

BIBLIOGRAPHY

1. Ginsberg RJ, Rice TW, Goldberg M, et al: Extended cervical mediastinoscopy: A single staging procedure for bronchogenic carcinoma of the left upper lobe. J Thorac Cardiovasc Surg 94:673, 1987.
2. Mackenzie JW, Riley DJ: Diagnostic and staging procedures: Mediastinal evaluation, scalene lymph node biopsy, mediastinoscopy, and mediastinotomy. In Baue AE, et al (eds): Glenn's Thoracic and Cardiovascular Surgery. Stamford, CT, Appleton & Lange, 1996, p 181.
3. Pearson FG: Staging of the mediastinum: Role of mediastinoscopy and computed tomography. Chest 103:346, 1993.
4. Shields TS: The significance of ipsilateral mediastinal lymph node metastases (N2 disease) in non-small cell carcinoma of the lung. J Thorac Cardiovasc Surg 99:48, 1990.
5. Van Klavaren RJ, Festen J, Otten HJ, et al: Prognosis of unsuspected but completely resectable N2 non-small cell lung cancer. Ann Thorac Surg 56:300, 1993.

44. MEDIASTINITIS

Paul G. Ruff IV, M.D.

1. What is the mediastinum?

The mediastinum is the central compartment of the chest. It is bounded by the thoracic inlet superiorly, the diaphragmatic hiatus inferiorly, the sternum anteriorly, the vertebral bodies posteriorly, and the pleura and lungs laterally. The major contents of the mediastinum are the heart and great vessels, the trachea and main bronchi, the esophagus, the vagus and phrenic nerves, the thymus, and the thoracic duct.

2. What is mediastinitis?

Mediastinitis is an acute or chronic inflammatory process that may be associated with suppuration, fibrosis, or sclerosis. The primary etiologies include post-sternotomy infection (most commonly associated with open-heart procedures), esophageal perforation, odontogenic infections, orofacial surgery, transmediastinal gunshot wound, and tuberculosis. Post-cardiac surgery mediastinitis is by far the most common etiology.

3. What is the eponym sometimes given to mediastinitis after cardiac surgery?

Hanuman syndrome is the eponym used to denote post-cardiac surgery mediastinitis. The name is derived from Hindu mythology and the monkey god who opened his chest to show his heart to Rama.

4. What is the incidence of mediastinitis after cardiac surgery?

Currently the incidence of mediastinitis after cardiac surgery is 0.4–5.0%.

5. What is the mortality of post-cardiac surgery mediastinitis?

Before the use of debridement and muscle flap closure of the mediastinum, the mortality was as high as 79%. Current mortality rates are 5–50%.

6. Can mediastinitis be treated nonsurgically?

Mediastinitis is considered a surgical emergency. Although isolated case reports exist of nonsurgical management of mediastinitis, debridement with muscle flap closure remains the mainstay of treatment. Debridement with closed-system irrigation using iodine-based solutions has been used with moderate success. In conjunction with surgery, broad-spectrum antibiotics must be started immediately.

7. Should treatment be staged?

This remains an area of controversy. Many surgeons prefer to perform an initial debridement followed by dressing changes and staged closure of the wound within 24–72 hours of the diagnosis of mediastinitis. However, there are many series reporting single-stage debridement and muscle flap closure of the wounds. Commonly cited is the Nahai et al. report on 211 consecutive cases, 95% of which underwent successful single-stage closure.

8. How does the use of the internal mammary artery (IMA) affect sternal wound infections?

In an excellent cadaver study by Arnold, the branches of the IMA were fully elucidated. Sternal branches that arise opposite each interchondral space supply the sternum. These branches bifurcate approximately 0.5 cm from the lateral border of the sternum and pass anteriorly and posteriorly into the periosteum. A periosteal plexus exists on the anterior and posterior aspect of the sternum, being denser on the posterior surface. There are very few communications between the sternal periosteal plexus and muscular or cutaneous branches. Therefore, once an IMA is used in a sternum that has been split, the blood supply is severely limited.

9. What are the risk factors for mediastinitis?

These include prolonged pump time in emergency operation, transfusion of more than 3 units of packed red blood cells (PRBC), reoperation for any reason, diabetes, intra-aortic balloon pump, obesity, use of both IMAs, hypertension, recent history of smoking, postoperative need for vasopressors, and chronic obstructive pulmonary disease.

10. What are the most commonly isolated organisms?

The type of isolate is dependent upon the etiology. Most infections are polymicrobial. Anaerobic species are found more commonly when the etiology is esophageal perforation, odontogenic infection, orofacial surgery, or transmediastinal gunshot wound. The most common isolates are *Staphylococcus aureus, Staphylococcus epidermidis,* alpha-hemolytic streptococci, *Pseudomonas* sp., fungi, *Enterobacter* sp., diphtheroids, *Morganella* sp., *Serratia marcescens, Escherichia coli, Proteus* sp., *Enterococcus* sp., *Acinetobacter* sp., *Bacteroides fragilis,* and *Klebsiella pneumoniae.* Rarely, *Mycobacterium tuberculosis* is isolated as a cause.

11. Describe the classification of sternotomy wound infections.

The most commonly cited classification system is that by Pairolero, who divides these wounds into three types:

1. Type I infected sternotomy wounds occur within the first 1–3 days following surgery. The initial drainage is serosanguinous in nature without concomitant cellulitis and cultures are frequently negative. Treatment consists of focused debridement and sternal rewiring.

2. Type II infected sternotomy wounds occur approximately 2–3 weeks postoperatively. These have purulent drainage with associated cellulitis, chondritis, and osteomyelitis. Aggressive debridement and flap reconstruction are required.

3. Type III infected sternotomy wounds occur months to years after cardiac surgery. These surface as a draining sinus tract from a focus of chondritis or osteomyelitis. Treatment is as for type II wounds.

12. What are the commonly used muscles for sternal reconstruction?

Because of its proximity to the sternum, the pectoralis major muscle is the first choice in the reconstructive armamentarium. The pectoralis major originates from the clavicle, sternum, upper six ribs, anterior chest wall, and the external oblique aponeurosis. It inserts on the intertubercular sulcus of the humerus. The blood supply is a Mathes-Nahai type V with the dominant pedicle from the thoracoacromial artery and multiple medial perforators from the IMA. It can be advanced or used as an island flap based on the dominant pedicle or turned over based on the secondary perforators. Most often, bilateral pectoralis major muscles are used to fully cover the defect. The rectus abdominis muscle is also employed, specifically for closure of difficult distal third of sternal wounds, or when the pectoralis major muscles are unavailable or inadequate. This muscle is a Mathes-Nahai type III, with two dominant pedicles. When the left IMA has been used during cardiac surgery, the contralateral rectus abdominis is harvested and turned over in a cephalad direction based on the terminal branch of the IMA, the deep superior epigastric artery. The latissimus dorsi muscle, a type V muscle based on the thoracodorsal artery (the dominant pedicle), may be rotated into the sternal wound for coverage and closure. The latissimus dorsi originates from the spinous processes of T7–T12 and L1–L5, the sacrum, posterior superior iliac crest, and ribs 9–12. It inserts on the intertubercular groove of the humerus. If the thoracodorsal artery is ligated, it may be able to survive based on the branch from the serratus anterior muscle.

13. Can the rectus abdominis muscle be used if the ipsilateral IMA has been used for by-pass grafting?

Although it is unreliable, the ipsilateral rectus abdominis muscle may be used based on a large perforator from the eighth intercostal artery.

14. Are other tissues used for reconstruction of the sternum?
The omentum may be harvested based on the right or left gastroepiploic vessels. It can be transposed into the sternal wound defect to close the space and bring generous blood flow and lymphatic drainage to an infected area. A small hiatus in the diaphragm is created just posterior to the sternal attachments. Care must be taken not to place too much tension on the omentum or the stomach. Further length may be obtained by "unraveling" the omentum on the omental arterial arcade.

15. What is the most common cause of sternal wound reconstruction failure?
Failure of a sternal wound reconstruction most commonly occurs due to inadequate debridement of the sternum and involved costal cartilages.

16. How well does the chest wall function after sternal reconstruction?
Even in the absence of the sternum that must be resected due to infection, most patients do not require permanent ventilatory support after reconstruction. Once the wound has healed and scarring has occurred, chest wall function is adequate for normal respiration.

BIBLIOGRAPHY

1. Arnold M: The surgical anatomy of sternal blood supply. J Thorac Cardiovasc Surg 64:596, 1972.
2. Brook I, Frazier EH: Microbiology of mediastinitis. Arch Intern Med 156:333, 1996.
3. Bryant LR, Spencer FC, Trinkle JK: Treatment of median sternotomy infection by mediastinal irrigation with an antibiotic solution. Ann Surg 169:914, 1969.
4. Cohen M, Silverman N, Goldfaden D, Levitsky S: Reconstruction of infected median sternotomy wounds. Arch Surg 122:323, 1987.
5. Fix RJ, Vasconez L: Use of the omentum in chest wall reconstruction. Surg Clin North Am 69:1029, 1989.
6. Hugo NE, Sultan MR, Ascherman JA, et al: Single-stage management of 74 consecutive sternal wound complications with pectoralis major myocutaneous advancement flaps. Plast Reconstr Surg 93:1433, 1994.
7. Jones G, Jurkiewicz MJ, Bostwick J, et al: Management of the infected median sternotomy wound with muscle flaps: The Emory 20-year experience. Ann Surg 225:766, 1997.
8. Nahai F, Rand RP, Hester TR, et al: Primary treatment of the infected median sternotomy wound with muscle flaps: A review of 211 consecutive cases. Plast Reconstr Surg 84:434, 1989.
9. Thurer RJ, Bognolo D, Vargas A, et al: The management of mediastinal infection following cardiac surgery. J Thorac Cardiovasc Surg 68:962, 1974.
10. Tizian C, Borst HG, Berger A: Treatment of total sternal necrosis using the latissimus dorsi muscle flap. Plast Reconstr Surg 76:703, 1985.

45. TUMORS OF THE MEDIASTINUM

Paula Michele Flummerfelt, M.D.

1. List mediastinal masses in order of decreasing frequency.
1. Neurogenic tumors
2. Primary cysts
3. Thymomas
4. Lymphomas
5. Germ cell tumors

2. Rank the incidences of mediastinal tumors by location and age.

LOCATION	CHILDREN	ADULTS
Anterosuperior	42%	54%
Posterior	40%	20%
Middle	18%	20%

3. Name the three most common tumors that arise in each part of the mediastinum.

ANTEROSUPERIOR	MIDDLE	POSTERIOR
Thymic neolplams (31%)	Cysts (pericardial and bronchogenic) (35%)	Neurogenic tumors (52%)
Lymphomas (23%)	Lymphomas (21%)	Cysts
Germ cell tumors (17%)	Mesenchymal tumors	Mesenchymal tumors

4. List common clinical syndromes described by the location of the mass.
- Anterosuperior mediastinum   Superior vena cava syndrome
- Middle mediastinum   Pericardial tamponade
- Posterior mediastinum   Spinal cord compression

5. Are most medistinal masses malignant?
No; 25–42% are malignant.

6. List the most common malignant neoplasms.
- Lymphomas
- Thymomas
- Germ cell tumors
- Primary carcinomas
- Neurogenic tumors

7. Does the frequency of mediastinal mass malignancy vary with the anatomic site in the mediastinum?
Yes. **Anterosuperior mediastinal tumors** are most likely malignant, followed by tumors of the middle mediastinum and posterior mediastinum.

8. Does the incidence of malignancy vary with age?
Yes. Patients in their **teens** through **30s** have a greater proportion of malignant mediastinal masses. In the first decade of life, a mediastinal mass is most likely benign.

9. Are most patients with a mediastinal mass symptomatic at the time of presentation?
Yes; 56–65% are symptomatic.

10. Are patients with a benign lesion more often symptomatic or asymptomatic?
  Asymptomatic (54% vs. 15%).

11. Is the correct histologic diagnosis made by CT scan in most patients?
  Yes. (68%).

12. List characteristic ultrastructural features of some mediastinal tumors.
  Neuroblastoma
    Neurosecretory granules and synaptic endings
  Germ cell tumor
    Prominent nucleoli and chromatin with scant desmosomes
  Thymoma
    Well-formed desmosomes, bundles of tonofilaments
  Lymphoma
    Absence of junctional attachments and epithelial features
  Carcinoid
    Dense core granules

13. What is the best incision to use to reach a mediastinal tumor, depending on the region?
  • Anterosuperior mediastinum—either a median sternotomy or anterolateral thoracotomy.
  • Superior aspect of the anterosuperior mediastinum—transcervical approach.
  • Middle and posterior mediastinum—posterolateral thoracotomy.

14. Name the tissues from which neurogenic tumors arise.
  • Sympathetic ganglia
  • Intercostal nerves
  • Paraganglia cells

15. Are most neurogenic tumors benign or malignant?
  Most are benign in adults, but most are malignant in children.

16. What are dumbbell tumors?
  The type of extension into the spinal column seen with approximately 10% of neurogenic tumors. They are called **dumbbell tumors** because of their shape, with relatively large paraspinal and intraspinal portions connected by a narrow isthmus of tissue traversing the intervertebral foramen.

17. How does knowledge of the behavior of dumbbell tumors affect clinical practice?
  All patients with a posterior mediastinal mass should be evaluated for possible intraspinal extension with CT, MRI, and vertebral tomography.

18. For adults, name the most common mass in each region of the mediastinum.
  • Anterosuperior mediastinum—thymic neoplasms.
  • Middle mediastinum—cystic lesions.
  • Posterior mediastinum—neurogenic tumors.

19. List some mediastinal tumors in order of decreasing incidence for adults and children.

Adults	Children
1. Thymic neoplasms	1. Neurogenic tumors
2. Lymphoma	2. Thymic neoplasms
3. Neurogenic tumors	3. Lymphoma
4. Germ cell tumor	4. Germ cell tumor

20. List the symptoms described most commonly among patients with mediastinal tumors.
- Chest pain
- Cough
- Dyspnea

21. Is it true that asymptomatic patients are commonly found to have benign lesions, whereas symptomatic patients more often harbor malignancies?

Yes. In a study of 400 patients, 85% of the patients with a malignant neoplasm were symptomatic, but only 46% of patients with benign neoplasms were symptomatic.

22. List some paraneoplastic syndromes that are associated with mediastinal tumors.
- Pel-Ebstein fever
- Erythrocyte abnormalities
- Peptic ulcer
- Myasthenia gravis, red cell aplasia
- Multiple endocrine neoplasia
- Von Recklinghausen's disease
- Hodgkin's lymphoma
- Neuroblastoma
- Neurilemoma
- Thymoma
- Thymic carcinoid
- Neurofibroma

BIBLIOGRAPHY

1. Blossom GB, et al: Neoplasms of the mediastinum. In De Vita V Jr (ed): Cancer: Principles and Practice, 5th ed. Philadelphia, Lippincott-Raven, 1997, pp 951–971.

46. MYASTHENIA GRAVIS

Harry W. Donias, M.D.

1. What is myasthenia gravis?

Myasthenia gravis (MG) is a neuromuscular disease caused by an antibody-mediated autoimmune attack directed against postsynaptic nicotinic acetylcholine receptors (AChRs) of voluntary muscles. The basic abnormality in MG is a decrease in the number of AChRs at the neuromuscular junctions. The decreased number of AChRs results in end-plate potentials of diminished amplitude, which fail to trigger action potentials in some muscle fibers. When transmission fails at many junctions, the power of the whole muscle is reduced, which is clinically manifested as weakness.

MG has a prevalence of 0.5–1.0 per 100,000 population, affecting approximately 25,000 people in the United States. There is a biphasic mode of distribution, with one peak in the second and third decades affecting mostly women and another peak in the sixth and seventh decades affecting mostly men. Women are affected twice as often as men. The mean age of onset is 26 years.

2. What clinical features are associated with MG?

Characteristic findings of MG are weakness and fatigue of skeletal muscles. Almost any muscle group in the body may be involved, and fluctuation in strength daily and even hourly is common. The weakness tends to increase with repeated activity and improve with rest. Ptosis and diplopia occur early in the majority of patients. The ocular muscles are the most frequently affected muscle group, being the presenting feature in 50–60% of patients, and they are ultimately involved in 90% of patients. Generalized weakness develops in approximately 85% of patients, affecting the muscles that control facial movement, mastication, swallowing, neck movement, ventilation, and the limb muscles. Symptoms of dysphonia, dysphagia, difficulty chewing, ventilatory fatigue, dyspnea, and proximal muscle wasting are common. In the extremities there is generally symmetric weakness involving proximal muscles more than distal groups of the arms more than the legs. Life-threatening myasthenic crisis occurs if weakness of respiratory muscles becomes severe enough to require mechanical ventilation. The findings are limited to the motor system, without loss of reflexes or alteration of sensation or coordination.

3. Describe the Osserman classification of MG.

The clinical severity of MG is usually graded by quantifying muscular strength and the variation that occurs in myasthenic patients. The most widely used scale is the Osserman classification: grade I involves focal disease restricted to ocular muscles; grade II is a generalized disease that is either mild (IIa) or moderate (IIb); grade III represents severe generalized disease; and grade IV is a crisis with life-threatening impairment of respiration. Criticism of this classification system is related to its failure to consider dependency on medication or to reflect subtle clinical improvement, creating difficulty in monitoring response to treatment.

4. What is the Tensilon test?

When the diagnosis of MG is suspected, the first study usually employed is the patient's response to anticholinesterase agents. These drugs block the hydrolysis of acetylcholine (ACh) in the synaptic cleft, prolonging its action and increasing the likelihood of an interaction between ACh and the postsynaptic AChR. These agents may reverse or improve the clinical and electrical abnormalities in MG. Edrophonium (Tensilon) is the most widely used because of the rapid onset (30 seconds) and short duration (5 minutes) of its effect. If there is unequivocal improvement in an objectively weak muscle, the test is positive.

5. What other tests are used to diagnose MG?

Further studies are required to confirm the diagnosis of MG. The Jolly test consists of repetitive stimulation of a peripheral nerve. Electrophysiologic demonstration of a rapid reduction in the amplitude of an evoked muscle action potential (decremental response of 15%) in response to repetitive nerve stimulation with electrical shocks delivered to the nerve at a rate of 3 per second is considered a positive test.

Single-fiber electromyography is sometimes helpful in difficult diagnostic situations. A single-fiber needle electrode is placed between two muscle fibers innervated by the same motor unit. The variation of neuromuscular transmission in MG leads to increased jitter or blocking of one of the action potentials in severe cases. It is positive in 88–95% of patients with MG. Assay of serum for elevated levels of circulating AChR antibodies is another approach that is becoming increasingly used to diagnose MG. A positive assay for AChR antibodies is specific for MG, but antibodies are detectable in only 80–90% of all patients, and in an even lower proportion (approximately 50%) of patients with purely ocular muscle weakness.

6. What is the role of the thymus in MG?

One of the unsolved problems in MG concerns the origin of the autoimmune response. For reasons that are not fully understood, the thymus is thought to play an integral role in its pathogenesis. About 70–80% of patients with MG have thymic abnormalities. Of these, 85% of patients have hyperplasia (germinal center formation) and 15% have thymomas. In addition, since the beginning of the 20th century it has been recognized that elective resection of the thymus influences the clinical course of MG in most patients; however, the exact role of the thymus still remains to be defined. The thymus is the site of T-lymphocyte education, with resultant self-tolerance. One hypothesis states that certain cells within the thymus gland, the myoid cells, which have a striking similarity to embryonic muscle and bear surface AChR, are the cause of MG. Because of the unique location of myoid cells in immediate proximity to maturing lymphocytes, an autoimmune reaction may develop directed against the AChR on myoid cells that later cross-reacts with AChR at the neuromuscular junction.

7. How is MG treated?

In general, four methods of treatment are currently in use: enhancement of neuromuscular transmission with anticholinesterase agents, surgical thymectomy, immunosuppression, and short-term immunotherapies, including plasmapheresis and intravenous immunoglobulin. However, variations in the natural history and the lack of prospective controlled studies of the different treatment modalities prevent an absolute determination of the preferred form of treatment for a particular patient at the present time. In recent years, uncontrolled data seem to clearly indicate that thymectomy gives much better results than medical treatment alone; thus, few patients with MG now are treated for long without surgery. In addition, a review of most published articles did not find any reported series in which patients treated medically fared better than those treated surgically. The closest thing to a prospective controlled trial comparing medical to surgical therapy comes from a retrospective Mayo Clinic series reported in 1976. This study showed a dramatically better clinical course for patients who underwent thymectomy when they were compared to a computer-matched historic control group treated medically. Although the use of historic control subjects, particularly in studies older than 20 years, is subject to confounding factors, it is unlikely that a prospective controlled trial comparing surgery with medical therapy alone will be conducted today, given the dramatic benefit seen in patients treated surgically.

8. What is the role of anticholinesterase agents in the treatment of MG?

Anticholinesterase agents have been the standard form of medical treatment for MG since their introduction in the mid-1930s. They act by preventing the hydrolysis of ACh and increase the likelihood of interactions between ACh and the AChR by increasing the duration of activity of ACh in the neuromuscular junction. However, these agents only provide symptomatic benefit without influencing the course of the disease. Neostigmine (Prostigmin), pyridostigmine (Mestinon), or both can be used, the dose being determined on an individual basis. Pyridostigmine is the most widely used anticholinesterase agent in the United States because it is thought to have a smoother effect and to be longer-acting, with a less abrupt loss of efficacy. It is generally given at a dose of 60 mg every 3–6 hours, and the extended-release form of 180 mg is available for more prolonged use, such as at night. These agents may produce considerable improvement with restoration of muscle strength, but the improvement is usually incomplete and often wanes after weeks or months of treatment.

9. What are the side effects of anticholinesterase agents?

Although these agents may produce considerable improvement, this response is only symptomatic, and these drugs in and of themselves do not lead to remission. Side effects include abdominal colic, diarrhea, nausea, salivation, and lacrimation as a result of smooth muscle and glandular stimulation. These symptoms may be controlled with atropine, but this is not recommended because the symptoms may indicate a developing cholinergic crisis. Cholinergic crisis is the result of excessive stimulation of AChR with prolonged depolarization of receptors and consequent muscle weakness not directly related to MG. More importantly, the symptomatic benefits provided by these agents may delay the introduction of early thymectomy, which is believed to be the preferred form of therapy. These agents, which increase bronchial and oropharyngeal secretions, may lead to respiratory compromise, particularly at the time of operation. Furthermore, after thymectomy there appears to be an increased sensitivity to anticholinesterase agents, which may lead to cholinergic weakness, complicating the postoperative management.

10. What is the role of immunosuppressive treatment?

Immunosuppressive therapy is indicated when weakness is not adequately controlled by anticholinesterase agents and is sufficiently distressing to outweigh the risks of possible side effects of immunosuppressive drugs. Corticosteroids, azathioprine (Imuran), and cyclosporine (Sandimmune) are the agents currently used for the long-term immunosuppression in MG. Of these, steroids are the most commonly used and most consistently effective. The clinical response may be dramatic with total remission of symptoms, but it is important to recognize that the introduction of steroids may be associated with a transient deterioration in up to 48% of patients, usually between the forth and eighth days of treatment. Therefore, it is recommended that they be initiated in the hospital setting, where provisions for respiratory support are available. Once weakness has stabilized after 2–3 weeks or any improvement is sustained, further management can be on an outpatient basis. The endpoint of steroid therapy is either a satisfactory clinical response or a dose of 50–60 mg/day. Improvement usually begins in 2–4 weeks with a maximal benefit realized after 6–12 months or more. After about 3 months of daily high-dose treatment, the schedule is gradually modified to an alternate-day regimen and tapered slowly to minimize the side effects of long-term steroid use. Azathioprine and cyclosporine are generally reserved for patients who are refractory to thymectomy and steroids.

11. What is the mechanism of action of corticosteroids in MG?

The exact mechanism of action of corticosteroids is not understood, but it is believed that steroid treatment may reduce AChR antibody levels and decrease the anti-AChR reactivity of peripheral blood lymphocytes. However, studies of thymectomy as the sole treatment modality have failed to confirm a direct correlation between the clinical status of patients with MG and the AChR antibody titer. Corticosteroids may also have a certain direct neuromuscular action, which has been suggested by the transient deterioration during the off day reported by patients on alternate-day steroid schedules. Experimentally, steroids increase the synthesis of AChR in cultured muscle cells and may enhance neuromuscular transmission, but the clinical relevance of such effects in MG has not been established.

12. How is plasmapheresis used in MG?

Plasmapheresis is a technique that permits the selective removal of plasma and plasma components by a centrifugal method. The remaining red blood cells are then suspended in a solution such as Ringer's lactate and reintroduced to the patient. Plasmapheresis removes antibodies from the circulation and produces a rapid, short-term clinical improvement in patients with MG. It is used primarily to stabilize the condition of patients in myasthenic crisis or to optimize the medical condition of patients prior to undergoing thymectomy. Typically, 4–6 exchange treatments of 3–4 liters each are carried out over a period of 2 weeks until the maximal clinical benefit is reached. The clinical improvement facilitates the perioperative period without the need for additional medications, especially corticosteroids that must be tapered slowly over months. Hypocalcemia and hypoalbuminemia may result from repeated runs and need to be identified and treated appropriately. To minimize the risk of bleeding and infection due to removal of clotting factors and immunoglobulins, surgical intervention is not recommended within 48 hours of the last run of plasmapheresis. Additional drawbacks include problems with venous access, the risk of infection of the indwelling catheter, hypotension, and pulmonary embolus.

13. When is intravenous immunoglobulin indicated in MG?

Indications for intravenous immunoglobulin (IVIg) are the same for plasmapheresis: to produce rapid improvement to help a patient through a myasthenic crisis or to prepare for thymectomy. It differs from plasmapheresis in that it does not require special equipment or large-bore vascular access. However, it is very expensive and side effects (occurring in less than 10% of patients) include headache, fluid overload, and, rarely, renal failure. The usual dose of IVIg is 400 mg/kg/day for 5 successive days. Published improvement rates after IVIg therapy average 73%. In patients who respond, improvement begins within 4–5 days. The effect is temporary but may be sustained for weeks to months, allowing intermittent long-term therapy in patients with otherwise refractory disease.

14. Which patients with MG should undergo thymectomy?

Surgical thymectomy is indicated for its therapeutic effect in MG or to prevent the spread of thymoma. The goal of thymectomy is to induce remission, or at least improvement, permitting a reduction of immunosuppressive medication. Patients with generalized MG who are between the ages of puberty and about 60 years should be considered for thymectomy as soon as possible. Although no adverse effects have been reported as a consequence of thymectomy in children, it is preferable to delay thymectomy until puberty, if possible, because of the established role of the thymus in development of the immune system. Thymectomy has also been advocated for elderly patients with MG, but there is uncertainty about the persistence of thymic tissue in patients older than 60 years. Thymic tumors must be removed surgically due to their tendency to spread locally and become invasive, even though they rarely metastasize. When thymectomy is performed at institutions with an experienced treatment team, consisting of surgeons, neurologists, anesthesiologists, and intensive care unit personnel, the operative mortality should be below 1%, with death occuring only in high-risk patients with profound clinical weakness.

15. What surgical approaches are available for thymectomy?

Various surgical techniques are available for thymectomy. Standard surgical approaches include the transsternal via a median sternotomy or partial median sternotomy, transcervical thymectomy, the "maximum" thymectomy, which combines the transsternal and transcervical approaches, and, most recently, video-assisted thymectomy. There is much debate as to which technique offers the best results, and the choice is usually based on the personal preference of the surgeon performing the procedure. The data to date suggest that a maximal thymectomy or an extended cervicomediastinal thymectomy allow the most exposure and resection of all the thymic tissue, leading to a better response rate than the transcervical or traditional transsternal approaches. The video-assisted approach, while allowing adequate exposure, has thus far had a lower response rate, but long-term follow-up is still needed. A prospective randomized trial comparing the various approaches is still needed to demonstrate a particular advantage of one technique over the others.

16. Where is the thymus located?

The thymus overlies the pericardium and great vessels at the base of the heart and is close to the left innominate vein. The gland has an H-shaped configuration, with variable fusion of the

right and left lobes at about the mid-portion of the gland. The upper portion of the gland attenu-
ates into the thyrothymic ligament connecting the thymus to the thyroid. There are many variations in the regional anatomy. It may lie posterior or anterior to the left innominate vein, and the
superior pole of the gland may extend along the pretracheal fascia into the root of the neck. At the
lateral extent of the gland there is a fine capsule that separates it from the pleura and parapleural
mediastinal fat that lies proximal to the phrenic nerve. However, thymic tissue is now documented
to be a normal component of perithymic fat outside the capsule. Furthermore, residual thymic tissue is present in 64–70% of patients showing partial improvement or no response after thymectomy. The ectopic thymic tissue can usually be located on reexploration in the pretracheal fat, under the phrenic nerves, behind the innominate vein, in the aortic pulmonary window, in the
aorto-caval groove, in the mediastinal fat, or in the cardiophrenic fat. Due to its great variability
in position and the fact that ectopic thymic tissue is frequently recovered, most surgeons try to remove not only the encapsulated gland but also all the perithymic fat at initial operation.

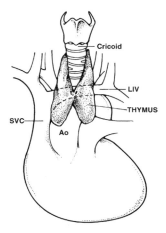

The thymus gland, showing the
H shape. (From Brumback RA,
James EC: Myasthenia gravis.
In James EC, Corry RJ, Perry JF
Jr (eds): Basic Surgical Practice.
Philadelphia, Hanley & Belfus,
1987, p 405, with permission).

17. What are the advantages of a transcervical thymectomy?
    Proponents of the transcervical approach maintain that their results of remission and clinical
improvement are comparable to those of the cervicomediastinal thymectomy. The advantages are
a more cosmetic incision, lower morbidity and complication rates, shorter operative time, and a
minimal postoperative hospital stay, with patients returning to unrestricted activity within 3–4
days after surgery. They also feel that the exposure afforded via the transverse collar incision is
adequate to perform a complete thymectomy. However, critics cite the fact that residual mediastinal thymic tissue has been found in up to 60% of patients after transcervical thymectomy, and
that recurrent MG associated with significant amounts of residual thymic tissue and even thymomas have been reported after the transcervical approach. Although the importance of total
thymectomy is unknown, there is concern that incomplete removal of the thymus may be associated with a higher recurrence rate of MG.

18. What are the results of thymectomy?
    Analysis of published data is complicated by differences in patient selection, timing of
thymectomy, choice of approach, underlying pathologic conditions, and perioperative care. Furthermore, even without treatment spontaneous remission of MG may occasionally occur. Clinical improvement after thymectomy has been reported in 57–97% of patients and permanent remission in 20–52%. However, clinical improvement after thymectomy may not be realized for as
long as 3–5 years after operation. Although these results come from many studies with many confounding variables, it is evident that patients treated with thymectomy fare much better than those

treated with medical management alone. Thymectomy is the only current therapy that offers a potential cure to this disabling and potentially fatal disease. Nonetheless, further studies to define which approach to thymectomy yields the best results are still needed.

BIBLIOGRAPHY

1. Aminoff MJ: Nervous system. In Tierney LM, McPhee SJ, Papadakis MA (eds): Current Medical Diagnosis and Treatment 2000, 39th ed. New York, McGraw-Hill, 2000.
2. Bulkley GB, Bass KN, Stephenson GR, et al: Extended cervicomediastinal thymectomy in the integrated management of myasthenia gravis. Ann Surg 226:324–335, 1997.
3. Calhoun RF, Ritter JH, Guthrie TJ, et al: Results of transcervical thymectomy for myasthenia gravis in 100 consecutive patients. Ann Surg 230:555–561, 1999.
4. Drachman DB: Myasthenia gravis. N Engl J Med 330:1797–1810, 1994.
5. Jaretzki A, Bethea M, Wolff M, et al: A rational approach to total thymectomy in the treatment of myasthenia gravis. Ann Thorac Surg 24:120–130, 1977.
6. Krendel DA: Neuromuscular diseases. In Lubin MF, Walker HK, Smith RB (eds): Medical Management of the Surgical Patient, 3rd ed. Philadelphia, J.B. Lippincott, 1995.
7. Mack MJ, Landreneau RJ, Yim AP, et al: Results of video-assisted thymectomy in patients with myasthenia gravis. J Thorac Cardiovasc Surg 112:1352–1360, 1996.
8. Mineo TC, Pompeo E, Ambrogi V, et al: Video-assisted completion thymectomy in refractory myasthenia gravis. J Thorac Cardiovasc Surg 115:252–254, 1998.
9. Wechsler AS: Surgical management of myasthenia gravis. In Sabiston DC, Spencer FC (eds): Surgery of the Chest, 6th ed. Philadelphia. W.B. Saunders, 1995.
10. Wittbrodt ET: Drugs and myasthenia gravis: An update. Arch Intern Med 157:399–408, 1997.

47. CHEST WALL TUMORS

Constantine P. Karakousis, M.D., Ph.D.

1. What is the meaning of the word "tumor"?

The word "tumor" was originally applied to any swelling or protuberance arising from a variety of causes such as a hematoma, an ecchymosis, or abscess formation. In medical terminology, however, the word tumor has been restricted to the meaning of a growth. Growths are causes of swellings that may be appreciated by the patients or their physicians or may cause pain or coughing, leading to radiologic investigation. In surgical oncology the term is used in its restricted meaning of a neoplastic growth. There are two major categories of growths, benign and malignant.

2. What is the frequency of chest wall tumors?

Tumors of the chest wall comprise about 2% of all the tumors of the body and in addition to being benign or malignant they also can be primary or metastatic. Benign tumors of the chest wall are by definition primary tumors, while a malignant tumor of the chest wall may be primary, i.e., arising from the tissues encountered in the chest wall, or metastatic, in which case the tumor cells have been carried through the blood stream from another site.

3. What are the signs and symptoms of a chest wall tumor?

The symptoms are related to an enlarging chest wall mass. Many of these tumors, because they grow slowly, are basically asymptomatic and as many as 75% of the patients present with a palpable chest wall mass. In these cases of slow, insidious growth, the pain is usually a late symptom. However, there are rib lesions that may manifest pain early on, particularly in association with a pathologic fracture, before a palpable mass has occurred. On physical examination, one is able to palpate a mass or elicit pain with palpation of a specific area. The mass, when it is identifiable on physical examination, should be examined to assess its mobility and firmness. This also provides an indication of anatomic structures involved by the mass. A mobile, well circumscribed mass will more likely be benign, while a fixed, more diffuse and less well defined mass will more likely be malignant. There are exceptions to this rule, since a benign rib lesion will certainly be firm and immobile and thus may provide an erroneous impression. The physical examination simply provides a general impression as to the possibility of the underlying pathology. The history is an important component of the initial evaluation of a chest wall mass since patients with metastatic tumors to the chest wall often have a history of a prior diagnosis or treatment of a malignant tumor and may have symptoms related to the tumor growing in other sites. A mass that has been present for years will more likely be benign, whereas one of recent onset and rapid growth is more likely malignant.

4. How is the diagnosis of a chest wall tumor made?

After taking the history and performing a physical examination, a simple posteroanterior and lateral radiograph of the chest provides further information. Even on a plain film, a soft tissue mass is often delineated, and lytic or blastic lesion(s) in the ribs are readily seen. The plain radiograph also provides information as to whether there is involvement of the lung parenchyma or any pleural effusion. A CT scan of the chest provides more information about the extent of a tumor mass in the chest wall and further information on the lung parenchyma and the mediastinum. Bronchoscopy is not generally indicated unless there is a primary lung lesion extending through the pleura into the chest wall. The definitive step, however, in the diagnosis of a chest wall tumor is a biopsy.

5. How is the biopsy obtained?

There are several basic biopsy techniques:

1. **Core needle biopsy.** Under local anesthesia, a small nick in the skin is made over the most protuberant area of the tumor mass, if it is palpable. Through that nick, a Tru-cut or other core nee-

dle is passed several times into the tumor mass and cores of tissue are obtained for pathologic evaluation. If the mass is not palpable, needle biopsy can be performed under CT guidance. Fine-needle aspiration cytology is rarely used for primary diagnosis but may be used to confirm a recurrence.

2. **Incisional biopsy** involves making an incision over the most protuberant area of the tumor in the direction that the definitive incision for the resection of the tumor would be taking later, if an operation is needed. The incision is deepened through the subcutaneous fat and fascia until the substance of the tumor is reached. It is important to obtain a deep biopsy because a superficial biopsy of the tumor mass can be nondiagnostic.

3. **Excisional biopsy** is reserved for small ($\leq$ 4 cm) tumor that is superficial and the clinical impression is that of benign tumor.

Core needle biopsy is used preferably for the larger tumor masses because most of the time (95%) it provides enough material for definitive histologic evaluation with a minimum of tissue disturbance. If one performs an incisional biopsy, the incision should be carried to the surface of the tumor without raising a flap and, after taking a biopsy, it should be closed in layers so as to avoid hematoma formation or ecchymosis. In some situations a biopsy may not be needed. If the clinical history and physical examination indicate with near certainty that the mass is benign, e.g., a lipoma, one may proceed directly with resection of the mass. In most cases, however, a prior biopsy is advisable.

6. Describe the different types of benign chest wall tumors.

One of the most common benign tumors of the chest wall is a lipoma. **Lipomas** occur in the subcutaneous space, usually between the skin and the investing fascia. Usually they are present for long periods of time and may grow slowly over the years. They should be excised when unsightly, interfering with clothing, causing symptoms, or if there is any concern about malignancy, such as rapid growth of the mass. **Intramuscular lipomas** may occur within the substance of a muscle. They tend to be atypical and require wide excision to avoid local recurrence. **Desmoid** is an intermediate type of lesion that is considered benign, although some regard it as a low-grade fibrosarcoma. It is of fibrous origin, tends to be locally infiltrative, and never metastasizes. About 10% of desmoids affect the chest wall. The treatment of choice for this tumor is wide resection, which provides a high rate of cure. In cases of marginal resection of a desmoid, adjuvant postoperative radiation may be helpful in preventing local recurrence. Benign tumors arising from the ribs are **osteochondroma, chondroma,** and **fibrous dysplasia.** The first two are usually resected due to pain and to ascertain that the entire lesion is benign. Fibrous dysplasia is one of the most common benign lesions of the chest wall, comprising as much as 30% of benign tumors, and should be excised if painful or disfiguring.

7. List the common malignant tumors involving the chest wall.

The most common primary malignant tumors of the chest wall in decreasing order of frequency are chondrosarcoma, fibrosarcoma, multiple myeloma, Ewing's sarcoma, and osteosarcoma. Since multiple myeloma is a disseminated plasma cell neoplasm, the primary approach to its treatment is systemic chemotherapy.

8. Which primary malignant tumors arise from the soft tissues of the chest wall?

The most common types of tumors that may represent a histologic subtype of a soft tissue sarcoma are **liposarcoma** and **malignant fibrous histiocytoma.** Following core needle or incisional biopsy, and after metastatic work-up indicates that there is no extensive metastatic disease, the patient should undergo wide resection with removal of the ribs that are involved or adjacent to the tumor. The prognosis depends on the grade and size of the tumor. Low-grade tumors and those $\leq$ 5 cm in diameter have a better prognosis than high-grade tumors and those that are > 5 cm in diameter. If complete resection (securing a > 2-cm margin around the tumor mass) cannot be obtained, further local therapy in the form of adjuvant radiation is indicated. The role of adjuvant chemotherapy in adults with soft tissue sarcomas is still under clinical investigation.

9. What are the primary malignant tumors arising in the skeletal structures of the chest wall?

Primary malignant tumors arising from the skeletal structures of the chest wall are chondrosarcoma and Ewing's sarcoma. **Chondrosarcoma** requires a wide resection with 4–5-cm margins. Most chondrosarcomas are low-grade and highly curable if adequately resected. **Ewing's sarcoma** is a highly vascular tumor affecting primarily young males. It is the most frequent chest wall tumor in children. Chest wall lesions comprise 6.5% of primary Ewing's sarcoma. These lesions are painful and often associated with generalized malaise, fever, leukocytosis, and an elevated sedimentation rate. Ewing's sarcoma is a radiosensitive tumor, but if the bone can be resected without undue morbidity, such as in a rib lesion, surgical resection is the preferred method of treatment. Chemotherapy is an integral component of the treatment of Ewing's sarcoma.

10. What is the treatment for osteosarcoma?

Osteogenic sarcoma typically occurs during childhood and adolescence. In about 80–90% of cases it affects the long tubular bones. The serum alkaline phosphatase is elevated in 45–50% of patients. Radiographic characteristics, i.e., intramedullary radiodensity, areas of radiolucency, cortical destruction, and extraosseous soft tissue calcification are notable. Following biopsy, the patients undergo 2–3 courses of neoadjuvant chemotherapy followed by resection of the tumor mass. The role of adjuvant chemotherapy in these tumors is of proven effectiveness since surgical treatment alone had a 20% 5-year disease-free survival, whereas a combination of surgery and chemotherapy has a 60% 5-year survival; another 20% of the patients with metastatic lesions can be salvaged with further surgery and chemotherapy for a total 5-year survival of about 80%.

11. What types of primary malignant tumors involve the pleura?

The tumor most frequently involving the pleura is **mesothelioma,** which can be a localized fibrous mesothelioma that is benign, or malignant mesothelioma, which is usually diffuse. The treatment of benign mesothelioma is by simple resection of this mass, while that of malignant mesothelioma should take into consideration the extent of disease and the technical possibility of complete resection. Malignant mesotheliomas restricted to the parietal pleura and diaphragm of one hemithorax should be treated with resection followed by intraoperative photodynamic therapy, intrapleural infusion of chemotherapeutic agents, or systemic chemotherapy. If the visceral pleura is also involved by malignant mesothelioma, as is often the case, pleurectomy of the parietal pleura and pneumonectomy have been practiced by some clinical investigators. However, the cure rate in these cases is very low and new approaches are required to improve survival.

12. Which tumors most commonly metastasize to the chest wall?

Metastatic tumors usually implant themselves through the hematogenous route to the parietal pleura and by extension may involve the other layers of the chest wall. Common sites of primary tumor metastasizing to the chest wall, often through the parietal pleura, are the lung, breast, pancreatic, gastric, colon, genitourinary, and thyroid cancers.

13. What is the treatment of metastatic tumors involving the chest wall?

The treatment of most metastatic tumors is usually nonsurgical because there are other sites of involvement and systemic therapy is preferred. A painful metastatic tumor can be palliated through radiation. In cases of a single metastatic lesion to the chest wall when the primary tumor has been controlled, the chest wall metastasis should be resected. This decision should take into consideration the biologic aggressiveness of the tumor, the disease-free interval between the excision of the primary tumor and the appearance of the metastasis to the chest wall (the longer the better), and the physiologic status of the patient.

14. Is any specific preoperative work-up required before a chest wall resection?

As part of the preoperative evaluation the patient should undergo pulmonary function testing, arterial blood gas analysis, and an assessment of activity. If the sum of these evaluations is a positive value according to the standard thoracic surgery guidelines, the patient can safely undergo the chest wall resection.

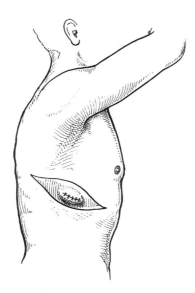

An elliptical incision is carried out around the previous biopsy incision so that the latter will be removed en bloc with the underlying tumor.

15. Describe the technique and incisions used in chest wall resection.

In cases of a previous core or incisional biopsy, an elliptical incision should be performed to encompass the biopsy site. For tumors located in the posterior part of the chest wall near the spine, a longitudinal incision over the center of the protruding mass, parallel to the line of the spinous processes, provides greater exposure. In this case, flaps are developed medially and laterally around the tumor mass, exposing the adjacent soft tissues and ribs for an en bloc resection. In the case of a nearly round tumor involving the lateral chest wall, an elliptical incision over the center of the mass along the direction of the ribs is preferable (see figure above). It is extended well behind and anterior to the tumor mass, flaps are developed, and posteriorly the rib that is certain to be involved is divided and a segment removed so that bimanual palpation through the external aspect of the adipose tissue covering the tumor mass and from the site of the parietal pleura can allow an accurate estimate of the ribs that need to be resected en bloc with the tumor. In the case of a tumor involving the sternum, a longitudinal incision is made from the jugular notch to well below the xiphoid, flaps are developed to beyond the sternal borders on either side, and the ribs are divided at a distance from the sternal border (see figure below). The medial ends of the clavicles are divided with a Gigli saw, the first ribs are divided, superiorly the attachments of the sternocleidomastoid and strap muscles to the sternum are divided making it possible to lift the specimen and separate it from the mediastinal structures. One should be aware of the course of the internal mammary artery as it proceeds from the respective subclavian artery to assume a position behind the medial ends of the ribs, about 0.5 inches from the sternal border starting from below the first costal cartilage and proceeding caudally to divide at the 6th intercostal space into the musculophrenic and superior epigastric arteries.

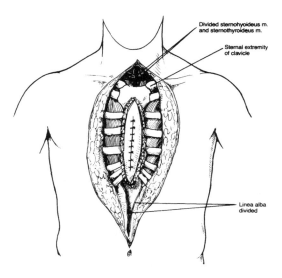

Incision and flap development prior to resection of a sarcoma involving the sternum.

16. Is it necessary to remove the muscles adjacent to the ribs?

The muscles invaded by the tumor or directly adjacent to it should be removed. These muscles can be removed without any significant functional sequelae for the patient. In the posterior chest wall the erector spinae, portions of trapezius and latissimus dorsi, the rhomboid muscles, the levator scapulae, and in the anterolateral chest wall the serratus anterior and pectoralis muscles can be resected en bloc with the tumor mass and the involved ribs and intercostal muscles. If the lung is attached to or involved by the tumor, the respective portion can be wedged out or a formal lobectomy may be performed.

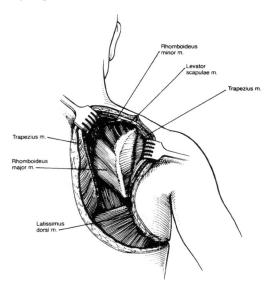

Posterior portion of the incision to expose the upper ribs, which requires division of the muscles around the scapula.

17. Describe the resection of tumors involving the upper ribs.

If there is no involvement of the brachial plexus and vessels, the tumor can be resected. The incision is long and circumscribes the vertebral border of the scapula around its tip to the axillary region, anteriorly over the pectoral muscles to the sternochondral junction. Posteriorly, the trapezius and rhomboid muscles are divided, as well as the latissimus dorsi (see bottom figure on p. 190) as needed, and anteriorly the pectoralis major and minor (see figure below). The serratus anterior is also detached from its origin in the upper ribs. Through this incision, the axillary vessels and brachial plexus are exposed and any connections of the axillary vessels to the chest wall are severed. This exposes the first rib, both anteriorly and posteriorly, which is then divided, and sequentially the other involved ribs are also divided anteriorly and posteriorly, permitting resection of the specimen.

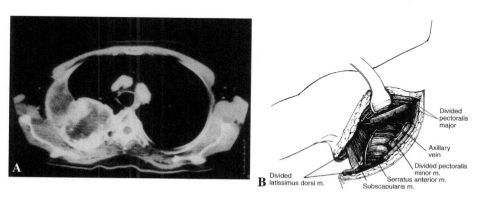

A, Sarcoma involving the upper chest on the right side. *B,* Anterior portion of the incision to expose the upper ribs, dividing the pectoralis major and minor and separating the neurovascular bundle from the chest wall.

18. How is the reconstruction of chest wall defects performed?

Reconstruction is performed by using a mesh such a polypropylene or Gore-Tex. The mesh is sutured to the edge of the defect with nonabsorbable sutures such as Prolene (see figure below). Short-running segments are easier to perform than interrupted sutures. The mesh is folded at the

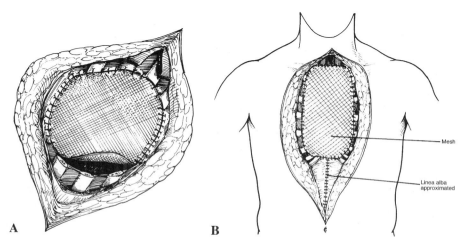

A, A mesh is placed to repair a defect in the lateral chest wall. *B,* A mesh is used to repair the defect after removal of the sternum.

edge for greater strength and the suture is driven between the folded mesh and the surrounding tissue, surrounding fascia or around a rib, as appropriate. As the circumference of the defect is negotiated, the mesh is always held taut and folded continually to accommodate the curvature of this defect so that the center of the mesh remains taut without wrinkles. Prior to placement of the mesh, chest tubes are inserted for drainage of the chest cavity.

19. What can be done surgically for the tumors of the upper chest involving the brachial plexus and vessels?

A tumor of the upper chest wall infiltrating the brachial plexus and axillary vessels is usually associated with swelling of the arm and severe pain along the arm in the distribution of the trunks of the brachial plexus. If there is no detectable metastatic disease present and the likelihood of occult microscopic metastases is low, resection can be performed by doing a forequarter amputation en bloc with resection of the upper chest. In this operation, the incision is modified to obtain a fasciocutaneous deltoid flap: a large flap of skin, subcutaneous tissue, and fascia covering the deltoid muscle is dissected off to the base of the neck in order to provide coverage of any defect in the chest wall. The deltoid flap provides coverage for the upper chest wall and seal for the thoracic cavity. Although this operation is a mutilating one, many patients will accept it if there is a hope of cure and relief of the severe pain caused by the involvement of the brachial plexus and the severe swelling of the arm.

20. How is the chest wall reconstructed following resection of a large part of the overlying skin due to tumor involvement?

Reconstruction of the chest wall with synthetic material is relatively easy if there is overlying skin coverage. Where there is a concomitant skin defect, the situation becomes more complicated. One has to provide a flap to cover the mesh and provide seal for the thoracic cavity. Depending on the location of the defect, flaps that may be used include the latissimus dorsi flap, pectoralis major flap, and the transverse rectus abdominis myocutaneous (TRAM) flap. In some cases, one may borrow a flap from the adjacent arm to cover a defect in the axilla or use a free flap with microvascular anastomosis.

21. What is the morbidity and mortality of chest wall resections?

Chest wall resections are tolerated extremely well, particularly if one does not resect extensive parts of the ipsilateral lung; even resections of several ribs are well tolerated. In the literature, the mortality rate for major chest wall resections involving extensive reconstruction is about 4%.

BIBLIOGRAPHY

1. Anderson BO, Burt ME: Chest wall neoplasms and their management. Ann Thorac Surg 58:1774, 1994.
2. Antman KH, Schiff PB, Pass, HI: Benign and malignant mesothelioma. In DeVita V Jr, Hellman S, Rosenberg SA (eds): Cancer: Principles and Practice of Oncology, 5th ed. Philadelphia, Lippincott-Raven, 1997, pp 1853–1878.
3. Brennan MF, Casper ES, Harrison LB: Soft tissue sarcoma. In DeVita V Jr, Hellman S, Rosenberg SA (eds): Cancer: Principles and Practice of Oncology, 5th ed. Philadelphia, Lippincott-Raven, 1997, pp 1738–1788.
4. Green DM, Tarbell NJ, Shamberger RC: Solid tumors in childhood. In DeVita V Jr, Hellman S, Rosenberg SA (eds): Cancer: Principles and Practice of Oncology, 5th ed. Philadelphia, Lippincott-Raven, 1997, pp 2091–2130.
5. Karakousis CP: Surgery for soft tissue sarcomas. In Bland KI, Karakousis CP, Copeland EM (eds): Atlas of Surgical Oncology. Philadelphia, W.B. Saunders, 1995, pp 283–400.
6. Karakousis CP, Mayordomo J, Zografos GC, Driscoll DL: Desmoid tumors of the trunk and extremity. Cancer 72:1637–1641, 1993.
7. Malawer MM, Link MP, Donaldson SS: Sarcomas of bone. In DeVita V Jr, Hellman S, Rosenberg SA (eds): Cancer: Principles and Practice of Oncology, 5th ed. Philadelphia, Lippincott-Raven, 1997, pp 1789–1852.
8. McCormack P: Chest wall tumors. In Baue AE (ed): Glenn's Thoracic and Cardiovascular Surgery. Norwalk, CT, Appleton & Lange, 1991.

9. Pairolero PC: Chest wall tumors. In Shields T (ed): General Thoracic Surgery, Philadelphia, Lea & Febiger, 1989.

10. Pass HI: Primary and metastatic chest wall tumors. In Roth JA, Ruckdeschel JC, Weisenburger TH (eds): Thoracic Oncology. Philadelphia, W.B. Saunders, 1989.

11. Purut CM: Lesions of the chest wall. In Sabiston Textbook of Surgery, W.B. Saunders, Philadelphia, 1997, pp 1896–1898.

12. Volpe CM, Peterson S, Doerr RJ, Karakousis CP: Forequarter amputation with fasciocutaneous deltoid flap reconstruction for malignant tumors of the upper extremity. Ann Surg Oncol 4:298–302, 1997.

48. CHEST WALL RECONSTRUCTION

Paul G. Ruff IV, M.D.

1. Describe the anatomy of the chest wall.

The chest wall is composed of multiple layers based on a bony framework. The ribs and costal cartilages are hinged upon the vertebral column posteriorly and the sternum anteriorly. They provide a semi-rigid structure that functions to protect the intrathoracic organs and assist in ventilation. The clavicles and scapulae are attached to this framework via the sternoclavicular joint. Intimately associated with the skeletal framework is the neurovascular supply to the chest wall that is derived from the intercostal branches of the aorta, the internal mammary arteries, and branches of the subclavian artery. The neurovascular bundles travel along and just interior to the inferior border of each rib. The muscular layers may be divided into three layers. The innermost layer is the intercostal muscles (internal and external) and the transversus thoracis muscle. These act to stabilize the chest wall during respiration and assist in narrowing the intercostal spaces during inspiration and depressing the rib cage during expiration. The next layer consists of the muscular attachments to the superior and inferior apertures of the chest wall. These include the sternocleidomastoid muscles and the scalenes at the superior aperture, and the rectus abdominis muscles, the internal and external oblique muscles, and the transversus abdominis muscle at the inferior aperture. These muscle groups work to assist inspiration and expiration, respectively. The remaining muscle groups act primarily during movement of the shoulder and arm. These include the pectoralis major, latissimus dorsi, and trapezius. The serratus anterior and the pectoralis minor attach the scapula to the chest wall and assist in elevation of the rib cage.

2. What are the functions of the chest wall?

The chest wall acts as a rigid shell for the protection of the thoracic viscera. As a semi-rigid structure it allows for elevation and depression of the ribs during respiration. The framework acts as a platform for movement of the shoulder and arm. Attached to this platform are the muscles that function in arm, shoulder, and respiratory movements.

3. What are the indications for reconstruction of the chest wall?

Most commonly chest wall reconstruction is necessary in the setting of: (1) trauma, (2) after oncologic resection, (3) infection, (4) radiation wounds, and (5) congenital anomalies.

4. What are the goals of chest wall reconstruction?

Paramount to successful reconstruction is the complete extirpation of the tumor, radiated, or infected tissues. Following this, the priorities are obliteration of intrathoracic dead space, stabilization of the rib cage, adequate soft tissue coverage, and return to function and form.

5. When is skeletal stabilization indicated and what are the options available?

Once more than four ribs or greater than 5 cm of chest wall are removed, these defects must be stabilized. Rigid fixation, autogenous bone grafts, fascial flaps, or large muscle may stabilize the sternum. Various types of prosthetic materials (including Prolene, Gore-Tex or Marlex) may be used to bridge defects in the rib cage. Although these materials provide many options for reconstruction, they also have the disadvantages of producing chronic infection, flaccidity, and dehiscence along the suture line.

6. What flaps are available for chest wall reconstruction?

Certain flaps are more applicable for certain defects. Chest wall defects can be broken down into anterior, lateral, and posterior defects. Anterior reconstruction is commonly achieved using unilateral or bilateral pectoralis major muscle or musculocutaneous flaps, latissimus dorsi muscle or musculocutaneous flaps, rectus abdominis muscle or musculocutaneous flaps, or omentum. Lateral defects are closed with latissimus dorsi or rectus abdominis muscle or musculocutaneous flaps or the omentum. Posterior defects may be treated with trapezius muscle or latissimus dorsi muscle or musculocutaneous flaps. Some cutaneous and fasciocutaneous flaps are used in chest wall reconstruction. These include the breast flap, scapular and parascapular flaps, and the deltopectoral axial pattern flap.

7. What is the blood supply to the pectoralis major muscle?

The pectoralis major is a type V muscle with dual blood supply. The dominant pedicle is the thoracoacromial artery, and the minor segmental blood supply comes from perforators of the internal mammary artery. The muscle may be used as a turn-over flap based on the minor blood supply.

8. What is the blood supply to the latissimus dorsi muscle?

Like the pectoralis major muscle, it is also a type V muscle with respect to blood supply. The dominant pedicle is the thoracoacromial artery and the minor segmental arteries are the lumbar perforators. This muscle may still be advanced based on the serratus anterior branch.

9. How is the rectus abdominis muscle used?

The rectus abdominis is generally used to close anterior midline and anterolateral defects. This is a type III blood supply with dual dominant pedicles: the deep superior epigastric artery and deep inferior epigastric artery. It is usually transposed based on the deep superior epigastric artery. However, it may survive on a large perforator from the eighth intercostal artery. The distal third of the muscle is unreliable in this case. Of note, once the muscle is disinserted, it contracts by approximately 33%.

10. How is the omentum used in chest wall reconstruction?

The omentum may be transposed based on the right or left gastroepiploic artery, and lengthened by unraveling the omental arcade. It is well suited to obliterate intrathoracic dead space or fill defects due to infection or radiation.

11. What congenital defects lead to chest wall reconstruction?

The congenital anomalies that require surgery are sternal clefts, Poland's syndrome, pectus excavatum, and pectus carinatum.

12. What are sternal clefts?

Sternal clefts are rare deformities due to lack or cessation of fusion of the sternum. They leave the essential mediastinal structures unprotected.

13. What is Poland's syndrome?

Poland's syndrome, originally described in 1841, is a congenital anomaly characterized by a partial or completely absent pectoralis major muscle, partial agenesis of the ipsilateral ribs and sternum, brachysyndactyly, mammary aplasia, and hypoplasia or absence of shoulder girdle musculature. The syndrome may present as very mild and minimal findings, or as a severe deformity. In female patients reconstruction must focus on restoration of a symmetric an aesthetically contoured breast mound.

14. What is pectus excavatum and how is it treated?

Also known as funnel chest, this anomaly is characterized by depression of the anterior chest wall usually starting at the sternal angle of Louis caudally to the xiphoid. The incidence of pectus deformities is 1 in 300 live births. In the severe form it can place the patient in respiratory or cardiac discomfort. The commonly employed techniques to correct this deformity are the Ravitch technique and the sternum turnover procedure.

15. What is pectus carinatum and how is it treated?

Pectus carinatum is often referred to as pigeon breast. It is characterized by a protrusion of the anterior chest wall. The reconstruction is similar to that for pectus excavatum.

BIBLIOGRAPHY

1. Arnold PG, Pairolero PC: Chest wall reconstruction: Experience with 100 consecutive patients. Ann Surg 199:725, 1984.
2. Cohen M: Reconstruction of the chest wall. In Cohen M (ed): Mastery of Plastic and Reconstructive Surgery. Boston, Little Brown, 1994, pp 1248–1267.
3. Hester TR, Bostwick J: Poland's syndrome: Correction with latissimus muscle transposition. Plast Reconstr Surg 69:226, 1994.
4. Seyfer A, Graeber G, Wind G (eds): Atlas of Chest Wall Reconstruction. Rockville, MD, Aspen Publications, 1996.
5. Seyfer A: Congenital anomalies of the chest wall. In Cohen M (ed): Mastery of Plastic and Reconstructive Surgery. Boston, Little Brown, 1994, pp 1233–1239.
6. Strauch B, Vasconez L, Hall-Findley E (eds): Axilla and Chest Wall Reconstruction. In Grabb's Encyclopedia of Flaps, Vol. III. Philadelphia, Lippincott-Raven, 1998, pp 1373–1416.

VI. The Diaphragm

49. EMBRYOLOGY AND ANATOMY OF THE DIAPHRAGM

Mark R. Jajkowski, M.D., and Hratch L. Karamanoukian, M.D.

1. When does the diaphragm develop?

The diaphragm develops between the 4th and 8th weeks of gestation.

2. What is the septum transversum?

The septum transversum is a thick plate of mesodermal tissue located between the thoracic cavity and the stalk of the yolk sac.

3. Which portion of the diaphragm is eventually formed by the septum transversum?

Central tendinous portion.

4. Does the septum transversum completely separate the thoracic and abdominal cavities?

No. The septum transversum leaves large posterolateral openings on each side of the foregut, known as the pericardioperitoneal canals.

5. How are the pericardioperitoneal canals obliterated?

During the 5th week of development, the pleuroperitoneal membranes appear. These define the caudal border of the pleural cavities. They extend medially and ventrally from the body wall of the thoracic cavity. By the 7th week they fuse with the septum transversum and the mesentery of the esophagus, thus separating the thoracic and abdominal portions of the coelom.

6. What results from failure of closure of the pericardioperitoneal canal?

Failure of this opening to close results in a posterolateral congenital diaphragmatic hernia (CDH).

7. What is the eponym that refers to the above-described CDH?

Diaphragmatic hernia of Bochdalek.

8. How is the lateral muscular portion of the diaphragm developed?

Myoblasts, which originate in the body wall, invade the pleuroperitoneal membranes and form the lateral muscular portions of the diaphragm.

9. Where are the diaphragmatic crura derived from?

The crura develop from the mesentery of the esophagus.

10. Why is the diaphragm innervated by the phrenic nerves, which are derived from cervical roots 3–5?

The septum transversum initially lies opposite the somites in the 3rd, 4th, and 5th cervical segments at the 4th week of gestation. By the 6th week this structure descends to the level of the thoracic somites. Because of this, innervation of the diaphragm is referred to the ipsilateral shoulder (dermatomes 3–5).

11. What determines the elevated position of the right hemidiaphragm?

It is widely taught that the liver is responsible for the higher position of the right hemidiaphragm. This has been disproved by Reddy et al., who have shown that it is actually the cardiac mass that determines the lower position of the left hemidiaphragm.

BIBLIOGRAPHY

1. Karamanoukian HL, O'Toole SJ, Holm BA, Glick PL: Making the most out of the least: New insights into congenital diaphragmatic hernia. Thorax 52:209–212, 1997.
2. Reddy V, Sharma S, Cobanoglu A: What dictates the position of the diaphragm: The heart or the liver? J Thorac Cardiovasc Surg 108:687–691, 1994.
3. Sadler TW (ed): Langman's Medical Embryology, 7th ed. William & Wilkins, Baltimore, 1995.
4. Schumpelick V, Steinau G, Schluper I, Prescher A: Surgical embryology and anatomy of the diaphragm with surgical applications. Surg Clin North Am 80:213–239, 2000.

50. CONGENITAL DIAPHRAGMATIC HERNIA

Jennifer I. Lin, M.D., and Michael G. Caty, M.D.

1. Describe the embryologic origin of the diaphragm.

The diaphragm develops from the following structures:
1. The transverse septum, which forms the central tendon
2. The pleuroperitoneal membranes, which contribute to the muscular portion of the diaphragm
3. The dorsal and lateral body wall, which also contribute to the muscular portion
4. The mesentery of the esophagus, from which the diaphragmatic crura are formed

2. What is the most common defect in congenital diaphragmatic hernia (CDH)?

Herniation through the foramen of Bochdalek, which occurs in 1:4,000–5,000 live births. This type of hernia occurs in the posterolateral diaphragm and results from lack of fusion between the central tendon and the pleuroperitoneal membrane.

3. What is a foramen of Morgagni hernia?

Herniation through the foramen of Morgagni occurs in the anterior part of the diaphragm, parasternally. It is relatively rare, accounting for <2% of all diaphragmatic hernias, and is almost always asymptomatic.

4. On which side are most CDHs found?

85–90% occur on the left side because the left side of the diaphragm fuses later than the right.

5. What is the pathophysiology of respiratory distress seen with CDH?

The most important cause of respiratory distress is pulmonary hypoplasia. Herniation of abdominal viscera into the thoracic cavity displaces the ipsilateral lung and prevents its normal development. The number and the degree of development of the alveoli are affected, resulting in inadequate gas exchange. The hypoplastic pulmonary vasculature also causes pulmonary hypertension, which results in persistent fetal circulation with a right-to-left shunt through a patent ductus arteriosus, patent foramen ovale, or both.

6. Describe the physical examination findings of an infant with CDH.

The infant is likely to be in severe respiratory distress at birth, requiring resuscitation, mechanical ventilation, and perhaps, extracorporeal membrane oxygenation (ECMO). The abdomen may be scaphoid, and the ipsilateral chest may be prominent from the displaced abdominal viscera. There are decreased breath sounds over the ipsilateral chest, and bowel sounds may be auscultated. The mediastinum may be shifted toward the contralateral side.

7. How is the diagnosis of CDH made?

Usually, CDH is discovered prenatally on routine ultrasound. On a plain chest film, infants with CDH have loops of air-filled bowel in the thoracic cavity. A contrast study, such as a barium swallow or upper GI series, may be necessary if the diagnosis remains uncertain after the plain film.

8. What is the treatment for CDH?

Operative repair. The prognosis for these infants depends more on successful preoperative management than on emergent repair because repair does not appear to provide immediate physiologic benefit.

9. How are infants with CDH managed preoperatively?
- Placement of an orogastric tube to decompress the stomach and bowel
- Mechanical ventilation to decrease acidosis, hypercarbia and hypoxemia
- Hyperventilation to decrease pulmonary artery vasoconstriction
- Vasodilators to decrease pulmonary artery hypertension
- Inotropes to increase systemic pressures and decrease right-to-left shunting
- High-frequency ventilation or ECMO if infant cannot be stabilized with conventional mechanical ventilation

10. What is the prognosis for an infant with CDH?
The overall survival for infants who have CDH and who are symptomatic in the first 12–24 hours of life has been about 50%. Infants with CDH who are asymptomatic during the first day of life have a much better prognosis and tend to have uneventful recoveries after surgical repair. The prognosis for symptomatic infants may be improving because of the use of ECMO.

11. List long-term problems of children with CDH.
- Gastroesophageal reflux
- Chronic lung disease
- Hearing loss
- Pectus excavatum
- Seizures

BIBLIOGRAPHY

1. Karamanoukian HL, Glick PL, Zayek M, et al: Hypoplasia of the lungs due to diaphragmatic hernia or oliohydramnios. Pediatrics 94:1–4, 1994.
2. Karamanoukian HL, O'Toole SJ, Holm BA, Glick PL: Making the most out of the least: New insights into congenital diaphragmatic hernia. Thorax 52:209–212, 1997.
3. Stolar CJH, Dillon PW: Congenital diaphragmatic hernia. In O'Neill JA, Rowe MI, Grosfeld JL,et al (eds): Pediatric Surgery. St. Louis, Mosby-Year Book, 1998.

51. MORGAGNI'S HERNIA AND EVENTRATION OF THE DIAPHRAGM

Mark R. Jajkowski, M.D., and Hratch L. Karamanoukian, M.D.

1. What is Morgagni's hernia?

This is a congenital diaphragmatic hernia located anteromedially or retrosternally between the diaphragmatic attachments to the sternum and the costal cartilages.

2. What percentage of congenital diaphragmatic hernias do Morgagni's hernias represent?

2–3%.

3. How are these hernias usually diagnosed?

In adults, Morgagni's hernias are usually diagnosed incidentally on routine chest x-rays because most cases are asymptomatic. Plain chest radiograph may reveal an enlarged cardiac silhouette or air-fluid levels in the chest.

4. On which side are these hernias usually located?

Ninety percent are right-sided.

5. What is commonly contained within the hernia sac?

In decreasing order of frequency: omentum, colon, stomach, liver, and small intestine.

6. When should surgical repair be undertaken?

In any symptomatic adult as well as in all children.

7. How are they repaired?

These hernias may be repaired by either an abdominal or thoracic approach. More recently laparoscopic or video-assisted thoracic surgery (VATS) repairs have been described.

8. What is diaphragmatic eventration?

This term most commonly describes a congenital or acquired abnormality that results in a weakness and elevation of a portion of the intact diaphragm.

9. What is the cause of acquired diaphragmatic eventrations?

This is caused by unilateral phrenic nerve paralysis as a result of birth trauma, injury during thoracic or cervical operative procedures, tumor invasion, or pleural infection.

10. What is a distinguishing feature of a congenital eventration?

The diaphragm is intact but markedly thin and muscle development is poor or absent.

11. How does an eventration present?

Small eventrations are usually asymptomatic. Infants are more likely to be symptomatic and may present with respiratory insufficiency.

12. How is the diagnosis of eventration made?

Usually by posteroanterior and lateral chest x-ray.

13. How are eventrations treated?

Small asymptomatic eventrations require no treatment. If the patient is symptomatic, operative plication is undertaken through a thoracotomy at the 6th or 7th intercostal space. In infants, a large asymptomatic eventration may also be plicated to prevent further compromise of lung development.

BIBLIOGRAPHY

1. Hussong RL, Landreneau RJ, Cole FH Jr: Diagnosis and repair of Morgagni hernia with video-assisted thoracic surgery. Ann Thorac Surg 63:1474–1475, 1997.
2. La Rosa DV Jr, Esham RH, Morgan SL, Wing SW: Diaphragmatic hernia of Morgagni. South Med J 92:409–411, 1999.
3. Sinclair L, Klein BL: Congenital diaphragmatic hernia—Morgagni type. J Emerg Med 11:163–165, 1993.
4. Weber TR, Tracy TF Jr, Silen ML: The diaphragm. In Bauer AE, et al (eds): Glenn's Thoracic and Cardiovascular Surgery. Stamford, CT, Appleton & Lange, 1996, pp 609–642.

52. DIAPHRAGMATIC TUMORS

Constantine P. Karakousis, M.D., Ph.D.

1. Describe the anatomic structures relevant to the management of diaphragmatic tumors.

The diaphragm on each side is a half-dome layer of musculofibrous tissue between thorax and abdomen. It is convex on its posterosuperior aspect and concave on the anteroinferior surface. It is attached anteriorly to the xiphoid process, the ventral rib ends, and costal cartilages of the 7th to 10th ribs and posteriorly to the 11th and 12th ribs. These attachments are low at the lumbar level posteriorly and laterally, but anteriorly they ascend medially toward the xiphoid level. There are three main apertures: the **aortic aperture** is the lowest and most posterior level with the caudal border of the 12th thoracic vertebra; the **esophageal aperture** at an intermediate level is opposite the 10th thoracic vertebra; and the **vena caval aperture** is at the highest level between the 8th and 9th thoracic vertebrae. The vena caval aperture is centered within the tendinous portion so that its margins are aponeurotic, while the other two apertures are surrounded by muscle fibers of the diaphragm. The aortic aperture anteriorly consists of the median arcuate ligament, which is often poorly defined.

2. Discuss the distribution of the phrenic nerve.

The **phrenic nerve** is the sole motor supply to the diaphragm. The right phrenic nerve comes off the fibrous pericardium covering the right surface of the right atrium and inferior vena cava; it traverses the diaphragm's central tendon either at the caval orifice or just lateral to it. The left phrenic nerve lies between the fibrous pericardium covering the left surface of the left ventricle and mediastinal pleura; it traverses the muscular part of the left hemidiaphragm anterior to the central tendon just lateral to the left cardiac surface on a plane more anterior than that of the right phrenic nerve. The trunk of each nerve then divides into three branches, i.e., an anterior branch, an anterolateral branch, and a short posterior branch, supplying the entire hemidiaphragm on each side. Consideration of the anatomy and distribution of the phrenic nerve makes it clear that a radial incision from the costal margin all the way to the posterior attachment of the diaphragm will denervate the lateral aspect of the diaphragm completely. Therefore, when the diaphragm is incised mainly for the purpose of exposure, it is incised 3–4 cm from its attachment on the costal margin and posterior ribs so that the greatest central portion of the diaphragm will have an intact nerve supply. In the case of tumor involving the diaphragm, the incision should circumscribe the diaphragmatic area of involvement providing an adequate margin around the tumor and disregard the phrenic nerve distribution.

3. What types of tumors involve the diaphragm?

Primary tumors of the diaphragm are rare. More common are extradiaphragmatic tumors that originate in the lung or upper abdominal viscera and involve the diaphragm by direct extension. Metastatic tumors that originate in the thoracic or abdominal cavity may spread to the pleural or peritoneal surface of the diaphragm through exfoliation and migration of cells in each respective cavity or via the lymphatic or hematogenous route.

4. What is the management of the primary tumors of the diaphragm?

Since the diaphragm is composed of a layer of diaphragmatic pleura, the musculotendinous sheet, and a layer of diaphragmatic peritoneum, a tumor that may arise from the diaphragmatic pleura or peritoneum is a **mesothelioma.** There are benign and malignant varieties of mesothelioma. The benign varieties can be cured by resection. Malignant mesothelioma is an aggressive tumor and at the time of diagnosis the tumor has usually disseminated to multiple sites within the cavity where it originated, often with the development of pleural or peritoneal effusion. In the case of surgically manageable localized malignant mesothelioma, resection provides good palliation and often improved survival for the patient. After complete resection of all the gross tumor, intraoperative photodynamic therapy or, later, intracavitary instillation of chemotherapeutic or biologic agents or systemic chemotherapy are options to be considered. In patients with extensive mesothelioma not amenable to surgical resection, systemic chemotherapy may help increase the survival in some cases. Due to the rarity of this tumor, no definitive studies on the choice of chemotherapeutic agents are available. Other primary tumors of the diaphragm may arise from the muscle, tendon, or other soft tissue elements comprising the diaphragm into any of the various soft tissue sarcomas. The treatment for these is surgical resection whenever possible, and the 5-year disease-free survival ranges from 43% to 87%, depending on the grade of the tumor.

5. What is the management of tumors invading the diaphragm by direct contiguity?

Tumors originating in the **ipsilateral lung** and invading the superior aspect of the diaphragm, are often associated with pleural effusion, a sign usually indicative of unresectability. If the biologic aggressiveness of the tumor justifies an extensive procedure, pleuropneumonectomy, i.e., removal of the parietal pleura and the ipsilateral lung, can be performed, providing improved survival in a small percentage of patients. In occasional cases of focal diaphragmatic invasion due to direct spread from an adenocarcinoma of the respective lower lung lobe, the tumor can be completely resected by lobectomy and en bloc resection of the diaphragm. The anticipated survival rates are comparable to those of a T3 resectable tumor (stage IIIa), i.e., 22.4–40% depending on the status of the regional nodes. Tumors invading the peritoneal surface of the diaphragm most commonly are **upper GI tumors,** on the left side originating from the fundus of the stomach and on the right side originating in the liver. Invasion of the diaphragm by adenocarcinomas of the upper GI tract usually signifies a large tumor that often has spread to the regional lymph nodes, decreasing the expected 5-year survival. However, if all macroscopic disease can be encompassed, resection of the ipsilateral involved portion of the hemidiaphragm and the involved viscera is the treatment of choice. The other major category that may involve the peritoneal surface of the diaphragm and its entire thickness is the so-called **retroperitoneal sarcoma** of the upper quadrants of the abdomen, although **sarcomas of the lower chest wall** also may extend directly to the diaphragm, invading initially the pleural surface of the diaphragm. In these cases, if the tumor can be resected completely with adequate margins, the 5-year survival according to the grade of the tumor ranges from a low of 45% for high-grade tumors to a high of 88% for low-grade tumors. Limited involvement of the diaphragm can be dealt with by resecting that portion of the diaphragm en bloc with the adjacent tumor, and this may be possible by either the thoracic or the abdominal approach, depending on the location of the palpable tumor. For large tumors involving the diaphragm extensively, a thoracoabdominal incision is required.

6. Describe the technique of thoracoabdominal incisions for diaphragmatic tumor resection.

The patient is placed in a lateral position and, depending on the location of the bulk of the tumor, one may decide on the starting point of the incision. For tumors that primarily involve the lower thoracic cavity, one may start with a lower thoracic incision, which may be extended to the costal margin. For tumors involving the upper abdomen, such as a retroperitoneal sarcoma, one may be well advised to start with an incision from the midline of the abdomen, midway between the xiphoid and the umbilicus, and extend this incision to the costal margin (see top figure on next page). The peritoneal cavity is entered and a brief exploration is carried out to assess the extent of disease and the presence or absence of any metastases, which may modify the surgical plan. In cases of equal involvement of the space above and below the diaphragm, it is preferable to start with an abdominal incision because it is better tolerated, in order to obtain sufficient information that would either encourage or discourage the completion of the operation. Once a decision is made to proceed with resection of the tumor, the incision is extended into the lowest intercostal space that is deemed appropriate by the assessment of the location of the tumor in the upper quadrant.

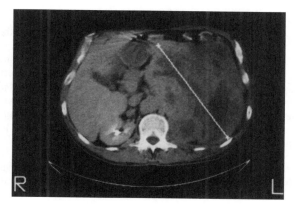

Retroperitoneal sarcoma of the left upper quadrant resected through a left thoracoabdominal incision in combination with a midline incision.

7. Which intercostal space is used?

Usually the 9th or 10th intercostal space is entered for retroperitoneal sarcomas of the upper quadrant of the abdomen. The pleural space is entered and the incision is extended posteriorly enough to permit placement of a self-retaining retractor. The costal margin has to be divided prior to this; it is best to remove a segment of the costal margin of about 1–1.5 cm or so to facilitate exposure. The incision in the diaphragm is extended radially for 3–4 cm and then continued along the periphery of the diaphragm to avoid its denervation. For tumors involving the diaphragm, the incision is dictated by the location of the tumor; it should circumscribe the tumor maintaining a margin of about 2 cm around the entire area of involvement. Retroperitoneal sarcomas involving the diaphragm on the left side often also involve the spleen, tail of the pancreas, the hepatic flexure of the colon, and possibly the greater curvature of the stomach and the left kidney (see figure below). On the right side, a tumor may involve the right lobe of the liver, the right kidney, and the hepatic flexure of the colon.

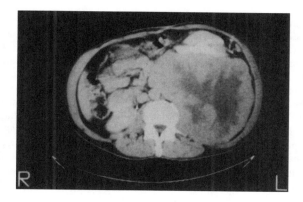

Retroperitoneal sarcoma of the left upper quadrant displacing the left kidney anteriorly, resected through a left thoracoabdominal incision.

8. How does one proceed with the dissection?

Whenever possible, any adjacent organs are dissected from the surface of the tumor in a clean, safe plane in order to better define the extent of the tumor and to free the anterior aspect of the tumor. For large abdominal sarcomas, the thoracoabdominal incision is combined with an upper midline abdominal incision. The main objective remains to dissect the tumor off its posterolateral attachments and mobilize the tumor off its bed. This is important because this plane of dissection is safe and can be carried out with minimal bleeding. This part of the dissection is retroperitoneal, leaving the peritoneum on the surface of the tumor. However, if the tumor infiltrates the tissues posterolaterally, the adjacent layer of the abdominal or lower chest wall may have to be resected en bloc with the tumor mass. The retroperitoneal dissection posterolaterally is carried out through the first plane that appears to be normal and not involved by the tumor. If the colon is attached to the tumor, the involved segment of the colon may be stapled proximally and distally and the mesocolon divided around the area of involvement so that the involved colon and mesocolon may be removed en bloc with the mass.

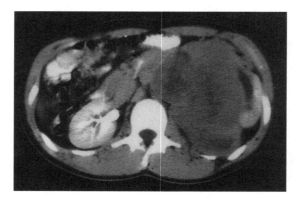

Retroperitoneal sarcoma of the left upper quadrant resected en bloc with the tail of the pancreas, spleen, and left kidney.

9. Are there technical differences between the two quadrants?

On the left side, the lesser sac is entered by dividing the gastrocolic ligament. Any attachments to the curvature of the stomach can be dealt with by stapling across the stomach, allowing the area of involvement to be removed en bloc with the tumor mass. Upon entering the lesser sac, the splenic artery running along the superior border of the pancreas should be identified and ligated (see figure above). The tumor should be mobilized inferiorly, and close to the midline the inferior border of the pancreas should be exposed to allow dissection behind the pancreas from the inferior to the superior border once the tumor mass in the tail of the pancreas has been mobilized. The splenic artery at this level can be ligated and divided. By exposing the posterior aspect of the pancreas, the splenic vein is also ligated and divided. The pancreas can be stapled across or divided between two rows of mattress sutures to control bleeding. In some cases, the kidney is also involved and may have to be mobilized by entering the retroperitoneal space and dissecting it off its bed over the quadratus lumborum muscle. The ipsilateral ureter is ligated and divided, the renal artery posteriorly is ligated and divided, and the renal vein is divided anteriorly between vascular clamps with oversewing of the stumps with a running suture. With the tumor mass that comes very close to or against the aorta, it is important initially to dissect the entire area around the tumor, particularly its posterolateral aspect, and mobilize it off its bed to provide a plane of separation between the tumor mass and the aorta.

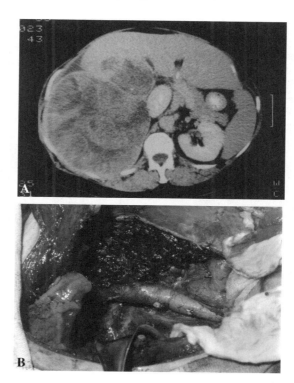

A, Retroperitoneal sarcoma of the right upper quadrant involving the right lobe of the liver and displacing the right kidney medially, resected through a right thoracoabdominal incision. *B,* Operative field after resection of the tumor showing the divided hepatic parenchyma and the inferior vena cava. Part of the right lung is shown on the left.

10. How about the right upper quadrant?

On the right side, the right lobe of the liver may have to be removed en bloc with a retroperitoneal sarcoma in the area involving the diaphragm and the right lobe of the liver (see figure above). After a right thoracoabdominal incision, the diaphragm is incised to free the portion involved by the tumor and leave it on the tumor's surface. The posterolateral attachments of the tumor from the lower chest and upper abdominal wall are divided freeing the tumor posterolaterally and ligating the ureter inferiorly, the renal artery posteriorly, and the renal vein anteriorly in case of renal involvement (see figure on next page). The inferior vena cava has to be exposed clearly by kocherizing the duodenum extensively. If the right lobe of the liver is involved, one has to dissect the hilum after removal of the gallbladder and ligate and divide the right hepatic artery, the right hepatic duct, and the right branch of the portal vein. The right branch of the portal vein is short and should be exposed, placing vascular clamps on it tightly so that it can be divided between the two vascular clamps and the two ends oversewn with a running vascular suture. Superiorly, the confluence of the hepatic veins is exposed and whenever it is easy to distinguish the right hepatic vein, it is ligated and divided. If the stump of the right hepatic vein is short and not easy to dissect out, intrahepatic ligation of the right hepatic vein may be the safest course. After the respective branches in the hepatic hilum have been controlled, it is important to maintain the correct plane as the liver is transected (and thus avoid injuring blood supply to the remaining lobe), which extends anteriorly from the gallbladder fossa to the confluence of the hepatic veins and posteriorly to the right of the inferior vena cava for a right hepatic lobectomy and to the left of the inferior vena cava for a left hepatic lobectomy. Reconstruction of the defect of the right hemidiaphragm or the entire hemidiaphragm is relatively simple, by suturing a mesh to the edge of the diaphragmatic defect.

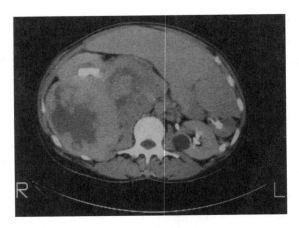

Retroperitoneal sarcoma of the right upper quadrant displacing the right kidney anteriorly, resected through a right thoracoabdominal incision.

11. What should be done in the case of a trunk wall defect with a concomitant defect in the diaphragm?

This situation is more complex. One could start by suturing a piece of mesh to the lower chest wall all the way around the defect to the costal margin, then start with a second piece of mesh suturing it to the diaphragm, starting from the posterior edge of the defect and bringing the mesh all the way to the costal margin where it is sutured to the first mesh. The repair of the defect in the upper abdominal wall is then continued with the first mesh.

12. How about the morbidity and mortality of a thoracoabdominal incision?

There is a widespread but erroneous belief among surgeons that division of the costal margin is associated with high morbidity. This may have been true to some extent in the past due to inadequate methods of postoperative analgesia and a high incidence of postoperative pneumonia in these patients. With the present availability of epidural anesthesia and patient-controlled analgesia, thoracoabdominal incisions are as safe as any other type of incision. This author's experience in the last 5 years involved about 30 cases of retroperitoneal sarcomas of the upper quadrants (all of which had a complete resection), and about as many cases of other tumors; the mortality was zero, the morbidity was very low, and the mean hospital stay was 7.5 days, although many patients were in their 70s or 80s.

13. Does one obtain improved results with the thoracoabdominal incision?

In a collective review, the complete resectability rate of retroperitoneal sarcomas was 53% and the 5-year survival was 33%. In the experience of this author, the resectability rate of retroperitoneal sarcomas is 96% and the 5-year survival rate is 63%. This high rate of complete resectability is accomplished, at least for the upper quadrants of the abdomen, by using the thoracoabdominal incision with the patient in a lateral position and by first mobilizing the tumor off its bed by dividing any posterolateral or anterior attachments, and last dealing with midline structures such as the aorta and inferior vena cava.

BIBLIOGRAPHY

1. Boutin C, Viallat JR, VanZandwijk N, et al: Activity of intrapleural recombinant gamma-interferon in malignant mesothelioma. Cancer 67:2033, 1991.
2. Daly BDT, Mueller JB, Faling LJ, et al: N2 lung cancer outcome in patients with false-negative computed tomographic scans of the chest. J Thorac Cardiovasc Surg 105:904, 1993.

3. Karakousis CP, Gerstenbluth R, Kontzoglou K, Driscoll DL: Retroperitoneal sarcomas and their management. Arch Surg 130:1104–1109, 1995.
4. Karakousis CP, Proimakis C, Walsh DL: Primary soft tissue sarcoma of the extremities in adults. Br J Surg 82:1208–1212, 1995.
5. Karakousis CP, Pourshahmir M: Thoracoabdominal incisions and resection of upper retroperitoneal sarcomas. J Surg Oncol 72:150–155, 1999.
6. Naruke T, Goya T, Tsuchiya R, et al: Prognosis and survival in resected lung carcinoma based on the international staging system for lung cancer. J Thorac Cardiovasc Surg 96:440, 1988.
7. Pass HI, DeLaney TF, Tochner Z, et al: Intrapleural photodynamic therapy: Results of a phase I trial. Ann Surg Oncol 1:28, 1994.
8. Storm FK, Mahvi DM: Diagnosis and management of retroperitoneal soft tissue sarcoma. Ann Surg 214:2–10, 1991.
9. Sugarbaker DJ, Reed MF, Swanson SJ: Mesothelioma. In Sabiston Textbook of Surgery. Philadelphia, W.B. Saunders, 1997, pp 1876–1883.
10. Sugarbaker DJ, Strauss GM, Lynch TJ, et al: Node status has prognostic significance in the multimodality therapy of diffuse, malignant mesothelioma. J Clin Oncol 11:1172, 1993.

53. PACING OF THE DIAPHRAGM

Marco Ricci, M.D., Ph.D, and Raffy L. Karamanoukian, M.D.

1. What is the rationale for pacing of the diaphragm?

To elicit diaphragmatic contractions in patients with diaphragmatic paralysis and intact phrenic nerves.

2. Which patients are candidates for pacing of the diaphragm?

- Patients with **central alveolar hypoventilation** (sleep apnea), in whom there is failure of the respiratory drive mechanisms or upper airway obstruction
- Patients with **spinal cord injuries** (C2–3 or higher)

3. What is central alveolar hypoventilation?

This condition is further divided in two subtypes: **obstructive sleep apnea** and **central sleep apnea.**

- In **obstructive sleep apnea,** the mechanism of respiratory drive is intact, but ventilation is impaired as a result of dysfunction and anatomic closure of the upper airways during sleep. This may be associated with abnormal relaxation of pharyngeal muscles, tumors involving the upper airway, and obesity.
- **Central sleep apnea** is characterized by primary failure of respiratory drive (central) as a result of tumors of the CNS, infections, cerebrovascular accidents, or trauma. These may affect adversely the capacity of the medullary respiratory center to generate respiratory impulses in response to hypoxia and hypercapnia.

4. List the signs of central hypoventilation.

- Somnolence
- Hypercapnia
- Hypoxia
- Pulmonary hypertension with consequent right ventricular dysfunction

5. How can mechanisms of respiratory drive be investigated?

As PCO_2 increases and PO_2 decreases, ventilation should increase. Failure of ventilation to respond adequately to hypercapnia and hypoxia is indicative of central alveolar hypoventilation.

6. How is the respiratory control system organized?

The respiratory control center (involuntary) is located in the medulla oblongata, and its activity is influenced by cortical stimuli (voluntary). From the respiratory control center, where cell bodies of upper motor neurons are located, axons descend to the anterior horns of C3–5, where they synapse with cell bodies of lower motor neurons. Axons of these neurons then form the phrenic nerves, which descend through the mediastinum to innervate the diaphragm.

7. Which patients are not candidates for diaphragm pacing?

Patients with **low** spinal cord injuries (C3–5) because these injuries result in lower motor neuron injury, and phrenic nerve injury.

8. How can phrenic nerve viability be assessed?

Transcutaneous phrenic nerve stimulation in the neck. Phrenic nerve stimulation should elicit diaphragmatic contractions if the nerve is intact.

9. List the components of a pacing apparatus.

- Generator, located outside the body
- Antenna, which is taped to the skin over the area where the receiver is implanted
- Receiver, which resembles the reservoir of a Port-a-cath device and is implanted in a subcutaneous pocket on the anterior chest wall
- Pacing electrode, which is surgically implanted in the mediastinum, adjacent to the phrenic nerve

10. Describe the implantation of the pacing device.

Although implantation of the stimulating electrode can be accomplished through a neck approach, it is most commonly performed through the chest because accessory nerve fibers may join the phrenic nerve in the chest. An anterior small thoracotomy in the third intercostal space is used to access the mediastinum. Once the phrenic nerve is identified, the mediastinal pleura is divided anterior and posterior to the nerve, taking care not to injure the nerve. Then a half-cuff platinum electrode is positioned behind the nerve and secured to the mediastinal pleura. The other end of the electrode is connected to the receiver, which is implanted in the subcutaneous tissue of the anterior chest wall.

11. How is diaphragm pacing performed?

Although the inspiratory duration is usually preset at 1.3 seconds, a respiratory rate of 6–10 breaths/min for bilateral pacing, or 12–14 breaths/min for unilateral pacing is used. Generally, pacing is withheld for the first 2 weeks after implantation because it may cause pleural effusion or bleeding. When pacing is begun, short periods of pacing are usually delivered initially; these are progressively increased over 2–3 weeks, to allow the diaphragm to recover slowly from atrophy. This **conditioning phase** may require longer periods in quadriplegic patients (3–6 months). During pacing, respiratory parameters (tidal volume, minute ventilation, end-tidal CO_2, PaO_2) are carefully monitored. In the presence of inadequate ventilation (diaphragmatic fatigue), diaphragmatic pacing is interrupted temporarily, then resumed.

12. List the complications of diaphragm pacing.

- Nerve injury
- Bleeding
- Infection
- Overpacing
- Underpacing

13. What are the results of pacing of the diaphragm?

Using this technique, complete success in achieving the ventilatory goal can be obtained in approximately 50% of the patients, whereas in the other 50% only a partial benefit is gained, meaning that some other form of ventilatory support is required.

14. List the advantages of pacing of the diaphragm.

- Increased independence from ventilatory support
- Restoration of speech
- Avoidance of sudden death from ventilator malfunction
- Improved survival in quadriplegic patients

BIBLIOGRAPHY

1. Elefteriades JA: Pacing of the diaphragm. In Shields TW (ed): General Thoracic Surgery. Baltimore, Williams & Wilkins, 1994.
2. Elefteriades JA, Hogan JF, Handler A, Loke JA: Long-term follow-up of bilateral pacing of the diaphragm in quadriplegia. N Engl J Med 326:1433, 1992.
3. Glenn WWL: Ventilatory support for pacing of the conditioned diaphragm in quadriplegia. N Engl J Med 310:1150, 1984.

VII. Thoracic Trauma

54. INITIAL MANAGEMENT OF THORACIC TRAUMA

John P. Pryor, M.D., and William J. Flynn, M.D.

1. How does a simple pneumothorax differ from a tension pneumothorax?

A **simple pneumothorax** occurs when the pleural space is violated, either from an opening in the lung parenchyma or from an opening in the chest wall. Air is allowed into the pleural space, equalizing intrapleural pressure with atmospheric pressure. Without a negative intrapleural pressure, effective lung volume is lost in the form of lung collapse. **Tension pneumothorax** occurs when air is forced from a defect in the lung parenchyma and collects in the pleural space under pressure. When the intrathoracic pressure becomes greater than the vena caval or right atrial pressure, flow of blood back into the heart is impeded, decreasing the resultant cardiac output.

2. Describe the clinical syndrome of tension pneumothorax.

The syndrome includes a loss of breath sounds and increased resonance on the side of the collapse, distended jugular veins, and decreased blood pressure. Tracheal deviation occurs more often in pediatric patients who have a more pliable mediastinum but can be seen in the late stages of tension pneumothorax in the adult.

3. What is the treatment for a tension pneumothorax?

Acute treatment of life-threatening tension pneumothorax includes immediate needle decompression with a 14-gauge angiocatheter placed in the second intercostal space at the midclavicular space. This procedure is followed by tube thoracostomy.

4. What is a sucking chest wound?

A large defect in the chest wall that communicates with the pleural space. With inspiration, chest cavity volume increases, intrathoracic pressure decreases, and air gets **sucked** into the pleural space.

5. How is a sucking chest wound managed acutely and definitively?

- **Acute treatment** includes occluding the defect with airtight material such as petroleum jelly (Vaseline) gauze or plastic wrap. One side of the dressing should be left open to allow any air within the chest that is under pressure to be released in expiration, preventing the development of a tension pneumothorax.
- **Definitive treatment** includes debridement and primary closure of the wound. Large wounds with tissue loss can be closed with a synthetic mesh or a tissue flap.

6. What is the concern with a massive or persistent air leak after traumatic pneumothorax?

Large or persistent air leaks may suggest a **major tracheobronchial injury.** Although these injuries are rare, they are usually fatal. If a patient initially survives, he or she is usually found in severe respiratory distress or extremis.

7. Describe the clinical presentation of a major tracheobronchial injury.

The patient is usually found in severe respiratory distress or extremis. Other **collaborating findings** include subcutaneous emphysema, hemoptysis, and pneumomediastinum. **Radiographic signs** include deep subcutaneous air and extraluminal placement of the endotracheal tube evidenced by an abnormally round balloon shadow. The **fallen lung sign** is a pneumothorax that collapses peripherally instead of centrally. This is caused by a major bronchial disruption that forces air centrally, pushing the lung outward.

8. What is the significance of pneumopericardium?

This is a uncommon entity that is usually associated with other major chest injuries. The diagnosis is clearly seen as a radiolucency around the heart on chest radiograph. The causes include pneumothorax, ruptured esophagus, major tracheobronchial injury, or air introduced by a penetrating injury.

9. How is pneumopericardium managed?

Most patients do not have symptoms directly attributed to the air in the pericardial space. In cases of blunt trauma, a diligent search for related injuries should take precedence in management. For patients with isolated penetrating trauma of the anterior chest without associated injuries, many surgeons advocate a subxyphoid pericardial window to rule out the presence of pericardial blood because air in the pericardium alone is not an indication for sternotomy in the asymptomatic patient. There have been several reports of tension pneumopericardium after blunt and penetrating trauma that have been treated successfully with pericardiocentesis and operative pericardiotomy.

10. How is the diagnosis of a ruptured diaphragm made?

Diaphragmatic injuries occur in 1–5% of patients with blunt trauma and 15% of patients with penetrating injury to the lower chest. Blunt ruptures are more commonly diagnosed on the left, in part because of the obturation of the liver in right-sided ruptures. **Radiographic signs** of diaphragm injury include a raised hemidiaphragm, blunted costrophrenic angle, or location of the distal nasogastric tube above the diaphragm. CT scan, diagnostic peritoneal lavage, and MRI all have significant false-negative rates and are not reliable in making the diagnosis. The gold standard for diagnosis is **laparotomy.** Diagnostic thoracoscopy and diagnostic laparoscopy are both highly sensitive in diagnosing even small diaphragmatic injuries and should be considered when diaphragmatic rupture is suspected. All injuries should be diagnosed and treated because missed injuries have a significant rate of becoming symptomatic by herniation of abdominal contents into the chest.

11. What is the treatment for diaphragmatic injuries?

Primary repair with nonabsorbable suture with or without pledgets. Large defects can be closed with a mesh prosthesis.

12. How is the diagnosis of traumatic aortic rupture made?

Traumatic rupture of the aorta (TRA) is a catastrophic injury that is one of the leading causes of immediate death after trauma. Patients who survive this injury require prompt diagnosis and treatment. Any patient who has sustained a high-speed deceleration injury, such as a significant fall or a high-speed motor vehicle accident into a stationary object, should be considered to have a TRA until proved otherwise. Symptoms can be subtle, such as chest and back pain, or absent altogether. Radiographic findings on chest x-ray film that raise the suspicion of TRA include:

- A wide mediastinum (>8 cm on upright film)
- Loss of the aortic knob
- Pleural effusion
- Displacement of the trachea to the right
- Apical pleural cap
- Nasogastric tube deviation to the right.

13. List diagnostic tests that are used to confirm the diagnosis of TRA.

- **Selective aortic angiogram** is sensitive and specific for TRA.

- **Helical CT scan of the thorax** has been shown to be 100% sensitive but only 83% specific in diagnosing TRA.
- **Transesophageal echocardigram** has the advantage that it can be performed in the operating room, while other procedures, such as laporotomy, are being completed.

14. What clinical signs raise the suspicion of esophageal injury?

Chest pain, crepitus, and hematemesis can be subtle or absent. Subcutaneous air, pneumomediastinum, or pneumothorax may be the only early signs.

15. How is esophageal injury diagnosed?

Diagnosis is best made by meglumine diatrizoate **(Gastrografin) swallow** or by **endoscopy**. Each of these has an approximately 10% false-negative rate, and many surgeons perform both in cases that have a high index of suspicion for injury. Rigid esophagoscopy is believed by some to be superior in visualizing proximal injuries, but it has a high risk of iatrogenic injury when performed by inexperienced clinicians. Blunt ruptures almost always occur at the cervical level or at the gastroesophageal junction. Penetrating injuries often have associated vascular or organ injury that may delay diagnosis.

16. What is traumatic asphyxia?

A clinical syndrome of increased venous pressure and backflow to the upper torso after a crush injury to the chest. The appearance is dramatic with marked edema and cyanosis of the head and neck. Subconjunctival hemorrhages may also be present. Cerebral edema from venous hypertension is the major sequel of the syndrome. Patients with traumatic asphyxia may also have significant underlying chest, abdomen, and neck injuries. Treatment is guided toward airway control, diagnosis of related injuries, and management of the cerebral edema.

17. Define Beck's triad.

Beck's triad comprises (1) hypotension, (2) jugular venous distention, and (3) muffled heart sounds. It is frequently quoted as evidence for pericardial tamponade. Heart sounds are not able to be assessed as muffled in a busy trauma department. Tamponade is frequently associated with mental status changes, which along with hypotension and jugular venous distention forms a useful triad. Additional aids in diagnosis include an elevated central venous pressure, equalization of right-sided and left-sided heart pressures, and variation of systolic pressure during inspiration (pulsus paradoxus).

18. Discuss the role of bedside ultrasound in diagnosing pericardial tamponade.

Modern trauma care includes ultrasonographic visualization of the pericardial space as part of the **focused assessment sonography for trauma (FAST) exam.** Pericardial fluid can be diagnosed by experienced surgical ultrasonographers with 100% sensitivity and 96.9% specificity. Ultrasound examinations of the pericardium should be done at least twice early in the course to rule out an evolving fluid collection.

- Clinically unstable patients with a **positive study** can proceed directly to median sternotomy.
- **Equivocal studies** can be confirmed by traditional subxiphoid pericardial window in the operating room.
- In patients with a **negative** study, many surgeons perform a collaborating study, such as a pericardial window, or admit the patient for observation.
- Penetrating injuries to the pericardium can be missed by ultrasound when pericardial blood decompresses into the pleural space

19. What is the hemodynamic consequence of air embolus?

As little as 0.5–1 mL of air in the coronary circulation can cause cardiac arrest. Air embolism in patients with penetrating or blunt trauma is usually a result of a bronchopulmonary fistula. Typically, even in the presence of a communication between the airway and a pulmonary vein, the pressure gradient favors blood to enter the airway, instead of air entering the veins. With significant pulmonary vein hypotension or with increased airway pressure from positive-pressure ventilation, the gradient reverses, and air enters the pulmonary vasculature. The clinical picture is one of cardiac and CNS collapse in patients with significant chest trauma, usually after the initiation of positive-pressure ventilation.

20. How is the diagnosis of air embolus made?

- A high index of suspicion must be kept in mind with penetrating chest injuries.
- Air bubbles within small vessels can sometimes be seen on funduscopic examination of the retina.
- Transthoracic echocardiography and transesophageal echocardiography may show air bubbles in the chambers.
- Air can be seen on direct inspection of the coronary vessels.
- Air aspirated from the ventricle or aorta is diagnostic of embolism.

21. What is the treatment for air embolus?

Position the patient in the left lateral decubitus position. If possible, avoid positive-pressure ventilation. Definitive treatment includes occluding the source of embolism and evacuating air from the ventricle. Hyperbaric oxygen may benefit patients with CNS air embolism.

22. What is blunt cardiac injury (BCI)?

Injuries to the heart include chamber rupture, valvular rupture, pump failure, and cardiac contusion. Anatomically, BCI refers to blunt injury to the myocardium without rupture or valvular injury. Most cases of BCI are asymptomatic and have no clinical sequelae. In a small percentage of severe contusions, complications can occur, including:

- Ventricular arrhythmias (41%)
- Supraventricular arrhythmias (36%)
- Bradycardia (7%)
- Hypotension (7%)

Patients with normal admission electrocardiograms (ECGs) and cardiac enzymes rarely developed complications.

23. How is BCI diagnosed?

The presumptive diagnosis is made when there are clinical indicators of myocardial damage after trauma. Many studies have been able to show some correlation between abnormal admission ECGs, **creatinine kinase(CK)-MB fraction,** and **troponin I levels** with cardiac complications after trauma. Troponin-I has been shown to be more specific than CK-MB for cardiac muscle injury in the context of blunt trauma. The use of troponin I requires two samples, one at the time of admission and one 12 hours later. **Echocardiogram** may aid in the diagnosis of related ruptures, pericardial effusions, valvular injuries, or mural thrombi.

24. What is the treatment for BCI?

Treatment of severe cases is aimed at supporting hemodynamics with fluid resuscitations, invasive cardiac monitoring, and inotropes. Routine antiarrhythmics are not recommended.

25. What is the principal risk of forming emergent thoracotomy for trauma?

Inadvertent needle stick and cut injuries to the health professionals from patients at high risk for transmittable blood-borne diseases.

CONTROVERSY

26. Discuss the indications for emergent thoracotomy for trauma.

The survivability of an emergent thoracotomy for trauma is generally <1%. The specific situation in which the outcome is improved is in patients who have penetrating injuries of the chest who arrive in extremis but with vital signs. Many surgeons perform emergent thoracotomy as a last effort for salvage in patients with blunt trauma who arrive with signs of life or in patients with penetrating injuries who had signs of life within 5 minutes of arrival at the hospital. Signs of life are defined as spontaneous movements, spontaneous respirations, a pulse, or cardiac electric activity.

BIBLIOGRAPHY

1. Adams JE 3rd, Davila-Roman VG, Bessey PQ, et al: Improved detection of cardiac contusion with cardiac troponin I. Am Heart J 131:308–312, 1996.
2. Allen GS, Coates NE: Pulmonary contusion: A collective review. Am Surg 62:895–900, 1996.
3. Asensio JA, Stewart BM, Murray J, et al: Penetrating cardiac injuries. Surg Clin North Am 76:685–722, 1996.
4. Demetriades D, Asensio JA, Velmahos G, Thal E: Complex problems in penetrating neck trauma. Surg Clin North Am 76:661–683, 1996.
5. Fabian TC, Davis KA, Gavant ML, et al: Prospective study of blunt aortic injury: Helical CT is diagnostic and antihypertensive therapy reduces rupture. Ann Surg 227:666–677, 1998.
6. Gammie JS, Shah AS, Hattler BG, et al: Traumatic aortic rupture: Diagnosis and management. Ann Thorac Surg 66:1295–1300, 1998.
7. Hill SL, Edmisten T, Holtzman G, Wright A: The occult pneumothorax: An increasing diagnostic entity in trauma. Am Surg 62:895–900, 1996.
8. Ho AM, Ling E: Systemic air embolism after lung trauma. Anesthesiology 90:564–575, 1996.
9. Meye DM, Jessen ME, Wait MA, Estrera AS: Early evacuation of traumatic retained hemothoraces using thorascopy: A prospective randomized trial. Ann Thorac Surg 64:1396–1400, 1997.
10. Moon RM, Luchette FA, Gibson SW, et al: Prospective, randomized comparison between epidural versus parenteral opioid analgesia in thoracic trauma. Ann Surg 229:684–692, 1999.
11. Powell MA, McMahon D, Peitzman AB: Thoracic injury. In Peitzman AB, Rhoades M, Schwab CW, Yearly DM (eds): The Trauma Manual. Philadelphia, Lippincott-Raven, 1998, pp 199–225.
12. Reber PU, Schmied B, Seiler CA, et al: Missed diaphragmatic injuries and their long term sequelae. J Trauma 44:183–188, 1998.
13. Richardson JD, Miller FB, Carrillo EH, Spain DA: Complex thoracic injuries. Surg Clin North Am 76:725–748, 1996.
14. Roszycki GS, Feliciano DV, Ochsner MG, et al: The role of ultrasound in patients with possible penetrating cardiac wounds: A prospective multicenter study. J Trauma 46:543–552, 1999.
15. Voggenreiter G, Neudeck F, Aufmkolk M, et al: Operative chest wall stabilization in flail chest—outcomes of patients with and without pulmonary contusion. J Am Col Surg 187:130–133, 1998.
16. Wisner DH: Trauma to the chest. In Sabiston DC, Spencer FC (eds): Surgery of the Chest, 6th ed. Philadelphia, W.B. Saunders, 1995, pp 456–493.

55. INDICATIONS FOR THORACOTOMY IN TRAUMA

Paula Michele Flummerfelt, M.D.

1. Is it true that most patients sustaining serious thoracic trauma will require operative intervention?

No. Outside of minor surgical procedures, such as tracheostomy, pericardiocentesis, chest tube placement, and suturing of chest wall lacerations, formal thoracotomy is required in only 12–15% of patients.

2. Is thoracotomy indicated after penetrating or blunt truncal trauma when the patient is exsanguinating or has pericardial tamponade?

Yes. These conditions are not conducive to successful resuscitation by external cardiac massage and urgent thoracotomy is indicated.

3. What is the survival of patients with truncal trauma who have had external cardiac massage for >5 minutes and then have thoracotomy?

Patients are resuscitated at a rate 30%, but the overall survival is around 5–8%.

4. Regarding the previously mentioned group of patients, name the group of patients with the highest survival rates.

Patients with penetrating wounds to the heart.

5. What is the survival rate of patients who are lifeless at the scene?

0.

6. What is the survival rate of patients who are lifeless on arrival to the emergency department but showed signs of life in the field?

30% with immediate thoracotomy.

7. Which has a better prognosis—stab wounds or gunshot wounds?

Stab wounds. Multiple chamber injury, coronary artery injury, and significant associated injuries worsen the prognosis.

8. What is the mortality rate after emergency department thoracotomy for cardiac arrest after blunt trauma?

> 98%.

9. Name the condition associated with the classic triad of muffled heart sounds, narrow pulse pressure, and elevated central venous pressure.

Pericardial tamponade.

10. Is pericardiocentesis the best treatment of pericardial tamponade?

No. Currently, it is used as a temporary procedure only. **Subxiphoid pericardiotomy** should be done if there are adequate facilities for thoracotomy. Pericardiocentesis has its greatest value as a diagnostic tool in the patient who actually does not have any intrapericardial injury.

11. Name a clinical situation in which a large air leak is seen in the underwater seal of the Pleur-evac.

In the presence of a wide open tracheal or proximal bronchial tear.

12. List three injuries that are associated with pneumomediastinum.
   1. Tracheal tear
   2. Bronchial tear
   3. Esophageal injury

13. For continuing hemothorax (after initial egress of blood), is there a strict criteria set for thoracotomy?
   No. A minimum rate needs to be set by the surgeon, and if the hourly rate exceeds that minimum rate per hour, thoracotomy should be performed.

14. Is a bullet traversing the mediastinum an indication for thoracotomy?
   Yes, even if the patient does not have an air leak, continued hemothorax, or pericardial tamponade.

15. What incision is made for thoracotomy in the patient with a bullet traversing the mediastinum?
   Usually a bilateral anterolateral thoracotomy with or without a transsternal extension.

16. Describe the treatment for right-sided air embolism.
   Conservative treatment by aspiration through a Swan-Ganz catheter or central venous pressure catheter usually is effective.

17. Describe the treatment for left-sided air embolism.
   Thoracotomy, involving cross-clamping the aorta, removing the source (by cross-clamping the pulmonary hilum), and aspiration of air from the left ventricle and ascending aorta concomitantly before cardiac resuscitation.

18. List some chronic conditions that also require thoracotomy.
   - Unevacuated clotted hemothorax
   - Fibrothorax
   - Chronic diaphragmatic hernia
   - Late valvular insufficiency from blunt or penetrating trauma
   - Chronic false aneurysms
   - Chronic nonclosing thoracic duct fistula
   - Chronic empyema
   - Infected intrapulmonary hematoma
   - Missed tracheobronchial injury
   - Traumatic arteriovenous fistula

19. Does the mere removal of a bullet require thoracotomy?
   When specific organ injuries are also present, they may warrant thoracotomy.

20. Can one expect spontaneous healing from a hemothorax that was <1000 mL initially, then < 50 mL/hour for 8–12 hours?
   Yes; thoracotomy is not indicated.

21. List the structures for which the right posterolateral thoracotomy incision is useful in visualization.
   - Trachea
   - Proximal esophagus
   - Right atrium
   - Left atrium
   - Superior vena cava
   - Inferior vena cava
   - Azygos vein

22. List the acute indications for thoracotomy in trauma.
- Cardiac tamponade
- Acute deterioration after penetrating trauma
- Vascular injury at the thoracic outlet
- Massive air leak from the chest tube
- Tracheal or bronchial injury
- Esophageal injury
- Evidence of a great vessel injury
- Massive or continuing hemothorax
- Penetrating wound that traverses the mediastinum

BIBLIOGRAPHY

1. Mattox KL: Indications for thoracotomy: Decision to operate. Surg Clin North Am 69:47–59, 1989.

56. DEFINITIVE MANAGEMENT OF THORACIC TRAUMA

John P. Pryor, M.D., and William J. Flynn, M.D.

1. What is flail chest?

A segment of chest wall that moves independently from the rest of the chest as a result of multiple ribs being fractured in at least two places. This flail segment does not expand with the intact chest and is seen moving in what appears to be the opposite direction. This paradoxical movement hinders proper ventilation and causes severe pain. A flail segment does not show paradoxical motion in patients that are being ventilated with positive pressure because all parts of the chest are being expanded outward together.

2. How is flail chest managed?

Management is directed at **pulmonary support** and **pain relief.** Many patients with significant flail should receive positive-pressure ventilation. Pain relief is best delivered by thoracic epidural or patient-controlled anesthesia (PCA). Open fixation of the segment has been shown to decrease significantly the ventilatory support time and allow for earlier extubation.

3. Some traumatic pneumothoraces are not evident on chest radiograph but seen on abdominal CT scan. Do all of these occult pneumothoraces need thoracostomy?

No. Most pneumothoraces that are not diagnosed on chest radiograph but are seen only on abdominal CT scan are small (< 5%). Most of these patients neither develop symptoms nor expand the pneumothorax and can be observed without a chest tube. A second chest radiograph is required to document that the pneumothorax has not expanded. Most surgeons continue to place a thoracostomy tube in patients who receive positive-pressure ventilation to eliminate the risk of forced expansion of an air leak and a subsequent tension pneumothorax.

4. Discuss the acute and definitive management of a traumatic bronchopulmonary disruption.

Most tracheobronchial injuries occur within 2.5 cm of the carina. The right bronchus is more often injured than the left. Patients are usually in severe distress, and **endotracheal intubation** should be attempted emergently. **Fiberoptic bronchoscopy** is the most direct way to diagnose an injury to the upper airway. An **armed bronchoscope** has an endotracheal tube in place over the scope, ready to be placed into position as the bronchoscope is advanced past the injury. This is especially helpful if single-lung ventilation is needed to bypass a major primary bronchial injury in the opposite bronchus. Surgical exposure to the trachea is through a collar-type neck incision, with extension through a sternotomy if needed. The carina and right bronchus are best approached through a right anterolateral thoracotomy. Repair of the injury is possible with interrupted 3–0 absorbable suture. Care should be taken to avoid excessive dissection because the tracheal blood supply is segmental.

5. Do all hemothoraces need to be drained?

Yes. Untreated or retained hemothorax occurs in 5–30% of patients with thoracic trauma. These undrained collections place the patient at a high risk to develop subsequent empyema, fibrothorax, lung entrapment, and impaired pulmonary function.

6. What is the management for persistent hemothorax after thoracostomy?

1. Primary attempts at drainage should include a large (38–42F), well placed thoracostomy tube. A second tube may be placed if the first drains the cavity inadequately.

2. If a fluid collection persists, operative drainage should be considered. Many surgeons

prefer using video-assisted thoracoscopic surgery to evacuate clots from the thorax in the first few days after injury.

3. After 4–7 days, thoracoscopy becomes difficult secondary to the fibrous adhesions in the chest cavity and a limited open thoracotomy is often necessary.

7. Discuss the appropriate management of pulmonary contusion.

There are varying degrees of pulmonary contusion from a mild self-limiting problem to respiratory collapse. The primary objective is to **secure the airway** and **relieve any pneumothorax or hemothorax.** Endotracheal intubation and positive-pressure ventilation are required if there is significant tachypnea, respiratory acidosis, or hypoxemia. Pain control is important to allow full ventilatory capacity. This may include local infiltration of associated rib fractures (rib block), a thoracic epidural, or PCA. Positive end-expiratory pressure should be added to the ventilation scheme to keep alveoli recruited. Patients should be maintained as close to euvolemic as possible. Fluids needed for adequate resuscitation should not be withheld because of a pulmonary contusion. Fluid resuscitation with hypertonic saline may have some benefit in patients with concomitant pulmonary contusion by improving hemodynamics without causing pulmonary edema. Diuretics may have some direct benefits of reducing pulmonary capillary pressures but should be used only with extreme caution to avoid hypovolemia and hypotension.

8. What is the general treatment of multiple rib fractures without flail?

Treatment is aimed at **pain relief** and **treatment of the underlying pulmonary injury.** After adequate treatment of pneumothoraces and hemothoraces, management of pain relief becomes paramount because inadequate pain relief of chest wall injury leads to splinting, atelectasis, inadequate ventilation, decreased mobilization of secretions and ultimately decreased pulmonary function, and increased risk of pulmonary infection. Pain relief of significant chest wall trauma can be provided by:

- Standard opioid injections
- PCA
- Intrapleural opioid injection
- Regional block by intercostal injection

Continuous epidural infusion of morphine and bupivacaine has been shown to be superior to PCA in decreasing chest wall pain and improving pulmonary function in randomized prospective studies and should be considered the treatment of choice for pain relief in patients with significant chest wall trauma.

9. Describe the surgical options for controlling pulmonary parenchymal bleeding and air leak.

Bleeding and massive air leaks are the two most common reasons for emergent thoracotomy for trauma. When the chest is entered, the source of the bleeding or leak is usually found early, but repair is difficult secondary to ongoing bleeding. Maneuvers for controlling hemorrhage include:

- Manual compression of the lung parenchyma
- Cross-clamping the pulmonary hilum with a Satinsky vascular clamp
- Applying a large Roummel tourniquet to the hilar structures

If time allows, the inferior pulmonary ligament can be taken down sharply and the lung twisted 180° around the hilum, compressing the vessels and controlling blood loss and air leaks. For deep parenchymal injuries, exposure of the injury facilitates repair. This can be accomplished with a **tractotomy,** a method to open the lung parenchyma over a deep injury. One of the blades of a GIA 75 stapler is placed into the wound, and the other is connected with the blade on the outside of the lung surface. When fired, a tract is made that exposes the base of the injury, allowing repair.

10. Do all penetrating injuries to the neck need to be explored?

No. Patients with active bleeding, loss of an airway, expanding hematomas, a bruit, or shock need immediate exploration to control hemorrhage and treat major injuries to the aerodigestive tract. For patients with minimal or no symptoms, nonoperative techniques can be used.

11. What nonoperative techniques are used for evaluating patients with penetrating neck injuries?
- Angiography
- Bronchoscopy
- Upper endoscopy

Angiography is most helpful with suspected vascular wounds in zone III (above the angle of the mandible) and zone I (below the cricothyroid cartilage) of the neck. In these areas, preoperative angiography aids in planning surgical approaches to injured vessels. **Upper endoscopy** and **barium swallow** can used to rule out injuries to the cervical esophagus and pharynx with about equal sensitivity.

12. Describe the order of maneuvers during an emergent thoracotomy for trauma.
1. Time is not wasted preparing a sterile field.
2. The left chest is opened at the fourth interspace in an anterolateral manner, with extension as posterior as possible. Division of the third and fourth rib posteriorly aids in exposure.
3. Blood present in the left chest is evacuated, and any exsanguinating wounds to the lung are controlled.
4. The pericardium is then opened sharply to relieve any tamponade.
5. The heart is herniated out of the pericardium to perform closed compression.
6. The right pleural space should be opened to look for hemorrhage and to relieve any possible tension pneumothorax.
7. The coronary vessels are inspected for air emboli, and the apex of the left ventricle is aspirated for air.
8. If these maneuvers fail to regain adequate pulses, the descending aorta may be clamped in an effort to increase circulation to the heart, lung, and brain. Proper placement of the aortic clamp requires sharp incision of the parietal pleura overlying the distal descending aorta and blunt finger dissection around the aorta. A large vascular clamp is then used to occlude flow in the aorta.
9. If these measures fail, the resuscitation is ended.

13. What are the indications for thoracotomy in patients with blunt or penetrating trauma?
- Severe blood loss
- Massive air leak
- Retained hemothorax
- Suspected air embolism

14. What is the approach for thoracotomy in patients with severe blood loss?
More than 1500 mL of blood out of the chest tube after thoracostomy raises the suspicion of a major vascular injury and should prompt emergent thoracotomy. Any amount of blood that is evacuated and causes a drop in the systolic blood pressure by >10 mm Hg should be considered significant. If the decision is made to go to the operating room, the chest tube Pleurevac should be converted to a cell-saver unit so that blood can be recycled. The acceptable amount of blood drainage over time is controversial but is generally concerning when a rate of 200 mL an hour is sustained over 2–3 hours.

15. Discuss the appropriate surgical approach to injuries to the right and left proximal subclavian arteries.
If the patient is hemodynamically stable, an aortogram with selective views of the great vessels is extremely helpful in planning the operative repair. Often, the patient's status does not allow for preoperative angiographic diagnosis, and empiric decisions need to be made about the exposure. The arch of the aorta, innominate artery, proximal right subclavian artery, and proximal

right common carotid artery can all be easily accessed through a median sternotomy with a right neck extension. The proximal left common carotid and proximal left subclavian artery can be exposed through a left posterolateral thoracotomy. The left mid and distal subclavian can be exposed by a left supraclavicular incision. Both distal common carotids can be accessed by neck incisions along the sternocleidomastoid muscle. A combination of these incisions is sometimes required to obtain control of vessels and to complete repairs. Generally, repair of large vessels can be accomplished with either dacron or polytetrafluoroethylene graft. Smaller vessels, including the subclavian vessels, can be repaired with saphenous vein graft.

16. What is the Sauerbruch maneuver?

Sauerbruch in 1907 described a maneuver for occluding inflow to the heart to allow the surgeon to repair a cardiac wound. The third finger is placed into the transverse sinus of the pericardium as the fourth and fifth fingers are placed in the posterior pericardium, compressing the vena cava and pulmonary veins. The first and second fingers are free to help hold the heart stable.

17. Describe the strategy for repairing cardiac wounds.

The standard approach to most cardiac wounds is by a **median sternotomy.**

1. If an emergent left thoracotomy was performed, extension across the sternum (**clam-shell**) facilitates exposure.

2. The pericardium is opened, and the heart is inspected anteriorly and posteriorly.

3. Simple lacerations of the chambers can be closed with interrupted 3–0 or 2–0 Prolene with pledgets. Lacerations near coronary vessels can be closed by passing the sutures under the artery to avoid ligation.

4. Distal coronary artery injuries can be ligated, whereas proximal injuries should be formally bypassed.

5. Injuries to the atria or vena cava may be repaired with the aid of a side-occluding Satinsky clamp.

6. Inflow can be controlled by clamping the inferior and superior vena cavae, but ischemia and cardiac arrest usually occur after 3 minutes of total inflow arrest.

7. Repair of septal and valvular injuries can usually be delayed until the patient is hemodynamically stable. In cases of acute heart failure resulting from septal or valvular injury, repair during cardiopulmonary bypass may be necessary.

18. Describe the management of esophageal wounds.

Treatment consists of debridement of the injury, primary closure, reinforcement of the closure, and adequate drainage. Exposure to the cervical esophagus is by a lateral neck incision. Most of the upper and mid esophagus is best approached through a right thoracotomy. A left thoracotomy allows adequate exposure of the lower esophagus and hiatus. Primary closure can be performed with two layers of absorbable material; the closure should be reinforced with a flap of diaphragm, pleura, or intercostal muscle. Drainage is accomplished with Jackson-Pratt drains in the neck or large chest tubes if the repair is in the thorax. In cases of extensive tissue loss or delayed diagnosis with significant mediastinitis, a lateral cervical esophagostomy may be needed to divert the injury. A gastrostomy is also constructed for distal diversion. The need for diversion is rare, and diversion should not be used routinely for injuries to the esophagus.

CONTROVERSIES

19. Are there any maneuvers to stabilize a patient with traumatic rupture of the aorta until definitive management is possible?

Most surgeons agree that prompt surgical management of the injury should take place after diagnosis. If surgery is delayed, there may be benefit to reducing the shearing forces in the vessel by administering β-blockers. At least one prospective study reported a 0% rupture rate for delayed repair of traumatic rupture of the aorta with the use of β-blockers with and without nitroprusside, keeping the systolic pressure around 100 mm Hg. β-blockade should be used with extreme caution in patients with significant hypotension and shock.

20. Discuss the surgical options for repair of traumatic rupture of the aorta.

Repair of a traumatic aortic laceration is usually accomplished by replacement with a straight dacron interposition graft. The patient is positioned in the right lateral decubitus position, and a double-lumen endotracheal tube is placed. Exposure is best through a generous left posterolateral thoracotomy. The current controversy is how to manage distal flow during the repair because interruption of flow can cause spinal cord ischemia. The **clamp and sew** technique does not use any type of shunt during the repair. The aorta is clamped between the left carotid and left subclavian artery, the left subclavian artery is clamped and the distal aorta is clamped. The graft is then sewn in as fast as possible. This method has a the highest risk of distal ischemia and can cause permanent paraplegia. The **Gott shunt** is a 9-mm heparin-bonded tube that is placed from the ascending aorta or left ventricular apex to the descending aorta or femoral artery. This is a passive shunt that has been shown to decrease the rate of paraplegia. An active shunt that uses a pump can be placed from the left atrium to the femoral artery and has been shown to have the lowest risk of paraplegia. Generally, in all types of repairs, keeping the clamp time to <30 minutes significantly decreases the rate of paraplegia.

21. Do emergent cricothyroidotomies performed for trauma need to be converted to tracheostomies?

Probably not. Emergency cricothyroidotomy is truly a life-saving maneuver that should be performed without regard to potential complications. After successful resuscitation, there has been a controversy about whether the airway should be converted to a formal tracheostomy. The damage of a cricothyroidotomy is done mostly at the time of insertion. Complications such as thyroid cartilage fracture, cricothyroid fracture, and subglottic stenosis are not relieved by tracheostomy.

BIBLIOGRAPHY

1. Adams JE 3rd, Davila-Roman VG, Bessey PQ, et al: Improved detection of cardiac contusion with cardiac troponin I. Am Heart J 131:308–312, 1996.
2. Allen GS, Coates NE: Pulmonary contusion: A collective review. Am Surg 62:895–900, 1996.
3. Asensio JA, Stewart BM, Murray J, et al: Penetrating cardiac injuries. Surg Clin North Am 76:685–722, 1996.
4. DeLaurier GA, Hawkins ML, Treat RC: Mansberger AR. Acute airway management: Role of cricothyroidotomy. Am Surg 56:112–115, 1990.
5. Demetriades D, Asensio JA, Velmahos G, Thal E: Complex problems in penetrating neck trauma. Surg Clin North Am 76:661–683, 1996.
6. Fabian TC, Davis KA, Gavant ML, et al: Prospective study of blunt aortic injury: Helical CT is diagnostic and antihypertensive therapy reduces rupture. Ann Surg 227:666–677, 1998.
7. Gammie JS, Shah AS, Hattler BG, et al: Traumatic aortic rupture: Diagnosis and management. Ann Thorac Surg 66:1295–1300, 1998.
8. Hawkins ML, Shapirom MB, Cue JL, Wiggins SS: Emergency cricothyroidotomy: A reassessment. Am-Sur. 61(1):52–5, 1995.
9. Hill SL, Edmisten T, Holtzman G, Wright A: The occult pneumothorax: An increasing diagnostic entity in trauma. Am Surg 62:895–900, 1996.
10. Ho AM, Ling E: Systemic air embolism after lung trauma. Anesthesiology 90:564–575, 1996.
11. Meye DM, Jessen ME, Wait MA, Estrera AS: Early evacuation of traumatic retained hemothoraces using thorascopy: A prospective randomized trial. Ann Thorac Surg 64:1396–1400, 1997.
12. Moon RM, Luchette FA, Gibson SW, et al: Prospective, randomized comparison between epidural versus parenteral opioid analgesia in thoracic trauma. Ann Surg 229:684–692, 1999.
13. Powell MA, McMahon D, Peitzman AB. Thoracic injury. In Peitzman AB, Rhoades M, Schwab CW, Yearly DM (eds): The Trauma Manual. Philadelphia, Lippincott-Raven, 1998, pp 199–225.
14. Reber PU, Schmied B, Seiler CA, et al: Missed diaphragmatic injuries and their long-term sequelae. J Trauma 44:183–188, 1998.

15. Richardson JD, Miller FB, Carrillo EH, Spain DA: Complex thoracic injuries. Surg Clin North Am 76:725–748, 1996.
16. Roszycki GS, Feliciano DV, Ochsner MG, et al: The role of ultrasound in patients with possible penetrating cardiac wounds: A prospective multicenter study. J Trauma 46:543–552, 1999.
17 Voggenreiter G, Neudeck F, Aufmkolk M, et al: Operative chest wall stabilization in flail chest—outcomes of patients with and without pulmonary contusion. J Am Col Surg 187:130–138, 1998.
18. Wisner DH: Trauma to the chest. In Sabiston DC, Spencer FC (eds): Surgery of the Chest, 6th ed. Philadelphia, W.B. Saunders, 1995, pp 456–493.

57. LARYNGEAL TRAUMA

Jennifer Wingate, M.D.

1. What are the mechanisms of laryngeal injury?
Internal injury
- Inhalation—chemical vapors, steam, smoke
- Chemical—caustic ingestion
- Iatrogenic—intubation or extubation trauma
- Foreign bodies

2. What is the incidence of laryngeal trauma?
External injury

Blunt or penetrating trauma to the larynx (rare).

The incidence in major centers has been reported as 1 to 15,000–30,000 trauma victims, with blunt laryngeal injury accounting for <1% of all blunt trauma injuries. Although blunt injuries used to prevail, increasingly **penetrating injuries** are becoming more common in the United States. This is due to the fact that improved motor vehicle safety—use of seat belts, air bags, and decreased speed limits—has decreased the number of motor vehicle–related injuries, whereas there has been an increasing number of personal assaults involving gunshots and knife injuries.

3. How are injuries caused by external laryngeal trauma classified?
A description of the mechanism of injury, site and extent of injury, and structures involved helps define the severity of the injury.

Severity of Laryngeal Trauma

	SYMPTOMS	SIGNS	MANAGEMENT
Group 1	Minor airway symptoms	Minor hematomas Small lacerations No detectable fractures	Observation Humidified air Head of bed elevation
Group 2	Airway compromise	Edema/hematoma Minor mucosal disruption No cartilage exposure	Tracheostomy Direct laryngoscopy Esophagoscopy
Group 3	Airway compromise	Massive edema Mucosal tears Exposed cartilage Vocal cord immobility	Tracheostomy Direct laryngoscopy Esophagoscopy Exploration/repair No stent necessary
Group 4	Airway compromise	Massive edema Mucosal tears Exposed cartilage Vocal cord immobility	Tracheostomy Direct laryngoscopy Esophagoscopy Exploration/repair Stent required

Modified from Schaefer SD: Primary management of laryngeal trauma. Ann Otol Rhinol Laryngol 91:399–402, 1982.

4. Describe the important initial steps in evaluating a patient with laryngeal injury.
- Before treatment can begin, one first has to **identify the injuries.** External laryngeal trauma is not a common occurrence, and because even minor trauma can lead to life-threatening consequences, the astute physician must have a high index of suspicion to identify and manage properly an acute laryngeal injury.
- As with other patients that present to the emergency department, a thorough history and physical examination are essential, being mindful of the **ABCs** (airway, breathing, circulation) of trauma care.

- **Concomitant injuries** to the cervical spine and chest, including vascular and soft tissue structures, must be considered and precautions taken to prevent further injury while identifying or excluding these injuries.

5. List the most common signs and symptoms of laryngeal injury.
- Hoarseness
- Dysphagia
- Odynophagia
- Mid-neck tenderness
- Subcutaneous emphysema
- Hemoptysis
- Difficulty breathing

6. Do the signs of symptoms of laryngeal injury correlate with the severity of the injury?
With the exception of **airway obstruction on initial presentation,** the other signs and symptoms have not been shown to correlate with the severity of injury. For example, a patient who initially presents with only minimal hoarseness may subsequently develop airway compromise a few hours later due to increasing edema.

7. Discuss the diagnostic modalities that are most useful in identifying laryngeal injury.
Flexible fiberoptic laryngoscopy (FFL).

In addition to better patient tolerance and less gagging and coughing, which may compromise the airway further, with FFL, the examination is performed easily on gurney bound patients. In patients whose airway is stable on presentation, evaluation by FFL is considered a routine and integral portion of the physical examination. Improved visualization of the larynx by FFL allows identification of abnormalities and the extent of injury, including soft tissue edema, hematomas, mucosal tears, vocal fold paresis or paralysis, arytenoid dislocation, presence of exposed cartilage, and other structural irregularities. Recognition of endolaryngeal abnormalities helps dictate further management (i.e., the need for CT scanning, conservative vs. surgical treatment).

CT

The use of CT three-dimensional viewing has significantly aided the identification of suspected laryngeal injury as well as elucidating the extent of known injuries (to determine whether patients require operative intervention or conservative therapy). Patients who would not benefit from CT are those who have obvious fractures or large endolaryngeal lacerations necessitating open exploration, a history of minimal trauma, or laryngeal tenderness or subcutaneous emphysema, and a normal FFL examination. All others should undergo CT scanning to evaluate the laryngeal framework for occult fractures, dislocated cartilages, and endolaryngeal soft tissue not visualized on the FFL examination.

8. What other injuries are associated with laryngeal trauma?
- Pharynx and esophagus
- Vascular structures
- Closed head injury
- Spinal injury
- Chest injury
- Facial fractures

9. How are associated esophageal injuries evaluated?
Esophageal injuries are infrequently seen with blunt trauma as opposed to penetrating laryngeal trauma. **Rigid esophagoscopy** is the preferred method for evaluation and can be performed after the airway is secured. Barium swallow is an effective means for evaluating the integrity of the esophagus but is less sensitive than rigid esophagoscopy.

10. How should the airway be managed initially in acute laryngeal trauma?

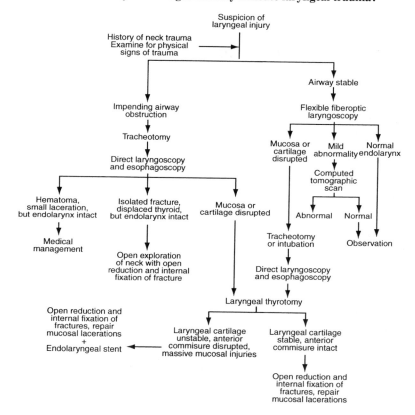

Management protocol for the acutely injured larynx. (From Schaefer SD: Acute management of extreme laryngeal trauma: A 27-year experience. Arch Otolaryngol 118:603, 1992, with permission.)

11. List the indications for surgical management.
Not including the surgical airway:
- Large endolaryngeal mucosal lacerations
- Displaced arytenoids
- Lacerations involving the anterior commissure or free margin of the vocal fold
- Displaced or comminuted fractures of the laryngeal skeleton
- Exposed cartilage

12. List the indications for nonoperative management.
- Endolaryngeal edema
- Hematomas
- Minor mucosal disruptions without exposed cartilage and not involving the anterior commissure
- Single nondisplaced paramedian fracture of the thyroid cartilage

13. What is nonoperative management for laryngeal trauma?
- Head of bed elevation
- Monitored observation for at least 24 hours
- Humidification of inspired air or oxygen

- Antibiotic and antireflux therapy for mucosal injuries
- Steroids (effective only if they can be given within hours after injury)

14. When is stenting the airway employed?
- Massive endolaryngeal lacerations with or without mucosal grafts to prevent adhesions and stenosis
- Multiple cartilage fractures in which open reduction/internal fixation is not feasible
- Avulsion injury that precludes restoration of the anterior commissure

15. What is the function of the laryngeal stent?
- To splint the laryngeal skeleton
- To maintain the lumen of the airway
- To serve as a keel to maintain the scaphoid shape of the anterior commissure

16. List the main goals of management in laryngeal trauma.
- Maintain an airway
- Restore the voice to the preinjury state
- Prevent aspiration

17. How critical is the timing of management?
Optimal results are best achieved by **early recognition and management.** When surgery is required, the timeliness of intervention (within **24–48 hours** of injury) has been shown to improve outcomes with regard to voice, airway, and deglutition.

18. List the major complications of external laryngeal trauma.
- Possibility of tracheostomy for initial airway stability
- Permanent tracheostomy
- Hoarseness
- Dysphagia

19. Explain the rationale for performing tracheostomy initially as management for airway stabilization.
The best and appropriate management for airway stabilization is **tracheostomy** performed under local anesthesia. This applies to patients with severe injuries and airway embarrassment as well as patients with only minor intraluminal injuries (lacerations or hematomas), who require intubation for other reasons. The rationale for avoiding endotracheal intubation in patients with minor endolaryngeal abnormalities is based on the possibility of aggravating preexisting injuries, leading to more severe injury; creating a false passage; or producing airway compromise in a previously stable airway. Others argue that intubation can be accomplished safely if the patient has minor intraluminal injury, it is performed by a skilled physician, and when there is no suspicion of possible laryngotracheal disruption. Cricothyrotomy has a high risk of exacerbating laryngeal injuries and is contraindicated in the event of laryngotracheal separation.

20. How does pediatric laryngeal trauma differ from that in adults?
- **Diagnosis is more difficult.**
  Laryngotracheal trauma is rare in children.
  Pediatricians are not familiar with this type of injury.
  Caregivers are often distracted by the severity of concomitant injuries.
- **Laryngeal injuries tend to be less severe as well as less common** than in adults:
  Pediatric patients are less likely to be involved in assaults and high-impact activities.
  The immature larynx is anatomically positioned higher in the neck, receiving greater protection from the mandible; pediatric cartilage is more pliable and mobile and more resistant to fracture.

- **Extensive laryngeal injuries tend to have more long-term sequelae** with regard to airway, voice, and deglutition than in adults with similar injuries treated in a similar fashion.
- **Airway embarrassment can occur with only a minor reduction in airway diameter** because of the overall smaller size of the laryngotracheal inlet and smaller pulmonary reserve. Adults can tolerate 50% narrowing of the airway without signs of respiratory distress.
- **CT scanning limitations in children** secondary to the delay in ossification of the thyroid cartilage make interpretation more difficult.
- **Children have a greater predisposition for soft tissue injury** (hematoma and edema) because the submucosal tissues of the larynx are attached loosely to the underlying perichondrium.

21. What is the treatment approach for laryngeal trauma in children?

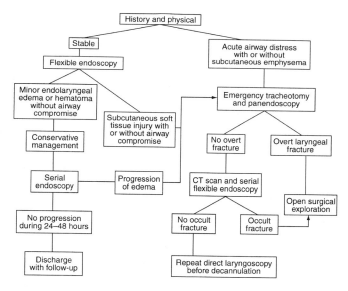

Treatment algorithm for blunt laryngotracheal trauma in children. (From Gold SM: Blunt laryngotracheal trauma in children, Arch Otol Head Neck Surg 123:86, 1997, with permission.)

BIBLIOGRAPHY

1. Ganzel TM, Mumford LA: Diagnosis and management of acute laryngeal trauma. Am Surg 55:303–306, 1989.
2. Gold SM, Gerber ME, Shott SR, et al: Blunt laryngotracheal trauma in children. Arch Otolaryngol Head Neck Surg 123:83–87, 1997.
3. Jewett BS, Shockley WW, Rutledge R: External laryngeal trauma: Analysis of 392 patients. Arch Otolaryngol Head Neck Surg 125:877–880, 1999.
4. Kadish H, Schunk J, Woodward GA: Blunt pediatric laryngotracheal trauma: Case reports and review of the literature. Am J Emerg Med 12:207–211, 1994.
5. Merritt RM, Bent JP, Porubsky ES: Acute laryngeal trauma in the pediatric patient. Ann Otol Rhinol Laryngol 107:104–106, 1998.
6. O'Keeffe LJ, Maw AR: The dangers of minor blunt laryngeal trauma. J Laryngol Otol 106:372–373, 1992.
7. Schaefer SD: Laryngeal and esophageal trauma. In Cummings CW (ed): Otolaryngology Head and Neck Surgery, 3rd ed. St. Louis, Mosby-Year Book, 1998, pp 2001–2012.

8. Schaefer SD: The acute management of external laryngeal trauma: A 27-year experience. Arch Otolaryngol Head Neck Surg 118:598–604, 1992.
9. Schaefer SD: The treatment of acute external laryngeal injuries: State of the art. Arch Otolaryngol Head Neck Surg 117:35–39, 1991.
10. Schaefer SD: Use of CT scanning in the management of the acutely injured larynx. Otolaryngol Clin North Am 24:31–36, 1991.
11. Schaefer SD: Primary management of laryngeal trauma. Ann Otol Rhinol Laryngol 91:399–402, 1982.
12. Schockley WW: Laryngeal trauma. In Shockley WW (ed): The Neck. St. Louis, Mosby-Year Book, 1994, pp. 189–208.
13. Stack BC, Ridley MB: Arytenoid subluxation from blunt laryngeal trauma. Am J Otolaryngol 15:68–73, 1994.
14. Trone TH, Schaefer SD, Carder HM: Blunt and penetrating laryngeal trauma: A 13-year review. Otolaryngol Head Neck Surg 88:257–261, 1980.
15. Yen PT, Lee HY, Tsai MH, et al: Clinical analysis of external laryngeal trauma. J Laryngol Otol 108:221–225, 1994.

58. PENETRATING NECK TRAUMA

Mohammad H. Eslami, M.D., and John J. Ricotta, M.D.

1. What is the most common cause of penetrating neck trauma in the U.S.?
Iatrogenic injury to the cervical vasculature or esophagus.

2. What anatomic landmarks are used to help with the management of the neck trauma?
Neck is divided into three anatomic zones: (1) **zone I** is the space between the sternal notch and the cricoid cartilage. This area includes thoracic outlet vasculature, proximal carotid and vertebral arteries, apex of the lung, trachea, esophagus, thoracic duct, and major cervical trunks; (2) **zone II** encompasses the area between the cricoid cartilage and the angle of the jaw. It includes the common carotid arteries, proximal portion of the internal and external carotid arteries, vertebral arteries, jugular veins, esophagus, trachea, and larynx; and (3) **zone III** is the area between the angle of the jaw and the base of the skull and includes pharynx, vertebral arteries, branches of external carotid arteries, and distal internal carotid arteries. Common to all three zones is the spinal cord.

3. How should one approach trauma to the neck?
Neck injuries can be fatal as they may involve many vital organs and large vessels. Nonetheless, one should approach these patients similar to any other trauma patients, following the guidelines of the Advanced Trauma Life Support. Quickly access and secure the airway (chin thrust, oxygen mask, intubation, chest tubes, surgical airway), proceed with blood pressure and circulation control (large-bore IVs, initial fluid bolus, control life-threatening bleeding [never blindly apply clamps, control by manual compression]). Then move on to quick evaluation of neurologic deficits ("mini" neurologic exam with cervical spine mobilization). Every injured patient needs to be completely disrobed. Evaluate the entrance and exit wounds and record your findings. Never explore penetrating neck wounds in the emergency room. Then proceed with a complete secondary exam, obtain appropriate laboratory tests, and radiographic studies.

4. Which penetrating neck wounds warrant exploration?
This is an area of controversy. The old dictum was to explore any patient with suspected penetration of the platysma. This resulted in great number of false-negative explorations. Current recommendation is to perform exploration in the following situations:

- Hemodynamically unstable patient;
- High-velocity injuries or transaxial gunshot wounds;
- Expanding hematoma (uncontrolled vascular injuries, compromised airway);
- Air bubbling in the wound (tracheoesophageal injuries);
- Worsening of lateralized neurologic deficit (carotid/vertebral injuries).

5. If none of the above criteria are met, how is the patient managed?
In patients with penetrating neck trauma but without any signs and symptoms of organ injury (e.g., expanding hematoma, active bleeding, air in the wound or crepitus, saliva or food particles in the wound, or lateralizing neurologic deficit), treatment depends on the site of injury. Observation may be combined with angiography, esophagoscopy, or rigid bronchoscopy. Contrast studies of the esophagus and occasionally trachea may be indicated to identify and localize lesions. The degree to which patients are invasively evaluated depends on the level of suspicion that the injury is present. In general, observation alone is adequate for zone II injuries, while diagnostic studies are indicated in zones I and III, where the risk of occult injury is higher.

6. What is the current recommendation for the management of the penetrating neck injury in zone I?

In a hemodynamically stable patient, further studies should be done to evaluate the areodigestive organs and aortic arch, including aortic arch and great vessel angiogram, tracheobronchoscopy, esophagogram, and/or esophagoscopy. If these studies are negative, patient can be observed. Injuries of the esophagus are treated by drainage with or without diversion. Injuries to pharynx and hypopharynx are mainly treated conservatively. Tracheal injuries may be treated by intubation with or without tracheostomy. Vascular injuries may be treated by exploration or, in some instances, endovascular repair. Surgical exploration may require cervical, thoracic, or combined incision for adequate access.

7. What is the current recommendation for the management of the penetrating neck injury in zone II?

Similar to all trauma patients, an unstable patient suffering from penetrating neck trauma should undergo prompt surgical exploration. Stable patients with no signs or symptoms of injury to any of the neck organs can be observed with no further studies. In stable patients with any signs or symptoms of vascular or tracheoesophageal injuries, other tests are needed in order to proceed with either exploration or careful observation. These tests include angiography, esophagography (with or without esophagoscopy), and bronchoscopy. Even without the presence of the hard signs and symptoms, if high clinical suspicion remains, one should obtain these tests to rule out any organ injury. There is currently great interest in the use of duplex ultrasound in the diagnosis of zone II carotid injury.

8. What is the current recommendation for the management of the penetrating neck injury in zone III?

Similar to the injuries in zone I, unstable patients should undergo exploration while stable patients require further studies regardless of signs or symptoms. These include a complete oropharyngeal exam, laryngoscopy, and four-vessel angiogram. If exploration is imminent and if the patient's condition allows it, an emergent angiogram should be considered before exploration since exposure and repair of vascular injuries in zone III can be both difficult and hazardous.

9. How do you expose and control the vascular injuries in zone I?

The most important principle in the management of any vascular trauma is proximal and distal control before repairing the injured vessel. Vascular injuries in zone I are managed through different incisions depending on the location of injury. Common carotid and vertebral arteries can be approached through the standard incision anterior to sternocleidomastoid muscle (SCM). The right and left subclavian arteries (SCAs) can be exposed through a supraclavicular incision. However, when the hematoma extends to the clavicle or there is evidence of intrathoracic injury, exposure of intrathoracic proximal carotid may be required. For both carotids and right subclavian vessels this is done through a sternal split, which may be partial or, more often, total. The left SCA is controlled through a left anterolateral fourth interspace thoracotomy. A "trap door" incision can be used on either side, although it is more morbid than other approaches. Recently, endovascular control and possibly repair of these vessels have been reported using endovascular covered stents and balloon catheters. This can be done via a femoral or retrograde brachial approach. A combined open/endovascular approach with proximal balloon control may avoid thoracotomy in selected patients.

10. How do you expose and control the vascular injuries in zone II?

Zone II carotid artery and jugular vein injuries can be approached by a standard anterior SCM incision. Vertebral artery anatomy makes the exposure of this vessel difficult. Only a very short segment of the proximal distal artery is outside the bony vertebral canal. After a short course, the vertebral artery enters the bony transverse process at the level of C6. Ongoing bleeding from vertebral artery in a stable patient should be managed angiographically whenever possible. Even with proximal control, back bleeding through the basilar artery remains problematic. Ideally, such incisions are packed and the patient is taken to the angiography suite for distal and proximal balloon occlusion. As is the case with hypogastric arteries, proximal ligation should be avoided since it complicates later angiographic embolization.

11. How do you expose and control the vascular injuries in zone III?

To gain control of distal internal carotid artery (ICA), an anterior SCM incision is used. If this is not adequate, additional exposure of the distal ICA can be managed by performing the following maneuvers: (1) posterolateral approach; approaching the high ICA from behind the SCM; (2) division of the digastric muscle; (3) division of the ansa hypoglossal nerve and/or the occipital artery; (4) mandibular subluxation; and (5) detachment of the SCM from the mastoid process. In stable patients who have undergone angiographic evaluation, distal arterial injuries may be controlled by angiographic embolization.

12. When do you ligate the carotid arteries?

Injury to the carotid arteries were managed by ligation prior to WWII when it was noted that selective repair led to improved outcome. Ligation of the common or internal carotid arteries in the presence of a competent circle of Willis can be done with expectation of preserved cerebral perfusion. However, a competent arch of Willis is absent in 20% of the population. Also, proximal ligation combined with perioperative hypotension may lead to infarction. Therefore, carotid arteries should be repaired whenever feasible.

Patients with focal acute injuries that can be repaired should be revascularized even in the face of coma. Patients whose injuries are subacute, cannot be repaired within 60–120 minutes of injury, or who have evidence of significant brain infarction on CT scan should have their arteries ligated. Reperfusion in these cases may exacerbate the deficit through hemorrhage or edema. In addition, patients with thrombus extending up to the carotid siphon (as evidenced by no back bleeding after thrombectomy) should have distal ligation, as the chance of reversing their situation is limited.

Patients with minimal or no neurologic deficit and a thrombosed ICA present a particular clinical challenge. They often have a carotid dissection, which is in the acute phase best managed by anticoagulation and close follow-up.

13. Are there maneuvers that can help you decide with certainty in the OR that ligation of carotid artery would cause minimal neurologic morbidity?

There are operative findings that can help guide that determination, but none are absolute. Vigorous back bleeding from the ECA or ICA stumps and stump pressure above 50 mmHg have been used as indicators of adequate collateral flow to support ligation.

14. How is artery repair accomplished?

Repair is only applicable to the carotid artery injury, whereas vertebral artery injuries have to be either embolized or ligated. Carotid artery injury is repaired after debridement of devitalized edges of the injured site. In the case of complete transection of the vessel, after debridement of the edges, the two ends can be sutured in an end-to-end fashion if there is minimal tension on both ends. Up to 2 cm of the common carotid artery can be removed without significant difficulty in the repair of the artery. However, extensive mobilization is time-consuming and should be avoided. If devitalized segments are further than 2 cm apart, the repair is best done by a vein interposition graft. Tangential injury to the carotid artery can be repaired by use of autogenous vein patch. Synthetic patch is discouraged except in unique selected cases. If necessary, ECA can be managed by ligation. An intact ECA should not be sacrificed to facilitate primary anastomosis. Shunts are used liberally once the lesion is defined and thrombus removed. This allows an unhurried repair with prograde perfusion.

15. How do you manage the jugular vein injury?

Venous injuries are the most common injuries encountered in a patient with penetrating neck trauma. If the injury to the vein is complex or the patient is unstable, the vein can be ligated to reduce the operative time. Simpler injuries or injuries in a stable patient can be repaired by patch venography. Note that injury to either the internal or external jugular vein can cause air embolus. Positive-pressure ventilation will help avoid this complication.

16. What are the signs of esophageal injury?
Most clinical presentations of esophageal injuries are occult, but patients may present with cervical pain, fever, dysphagia of their saliva, crepitus, and hematemesis.

17. What is the most common cause of esophageal injury in the U.S.?
Iatrogenic instrumentation.

18. What are some of the signs that may be seen on a routine chest x-ray?
Chest x-ray may show no abnormalities. Nonetheless, common findings include pneumothorax, pneumopericardium, presence of retropharyngeal air, exaggeration of cardiac silhouette, and pleural effusion.

19. How do you diagnose a suspected esophageal injury?
The best available studies are esophagoscopy and esophagogram. Both are sensitive and specific, but combined procedures yield sensitivity and specificity of close to 100%. Esophagogram should be performed first, followed by esophagoscopy. Esophagoscopy is ordered if esophagogram is negative and there is still high clinical suspicion of esophageal injury.

20. What is the most common site of esophageal injury?
The cervical esophagus near the upper sphincter.

21. What is the most significant prognosticator of morbidity and mortality with esophageal injury?
Time to diagnosis. Different studies have shown that early diagnosis is the most significant factor associated with good outcome. It has been shown that mortality in the patients diagnosed after 24 hours is significantly higher than in those who were diagnosed less than 24 hours from the injury.

22. How do you manage an early diagnosed cervical esophageal injury?
After debridement of devitalized tissue and irrigation, primary repair in a two-layer fashion is the recommended technique. Drains are placed and oral feeding is initiated after a normal barium swallow that shows no leak on postoperative days 5–7. If the primary repair is not possible, the treatment may require esophageal resection with gastric pull-up. In unstable patients or in the presence of significant devitalized tissue, drainage of mediastinum, creation of cervical esophagostomy (a controlled fistula), and institution of total parenteral nutrition (TPN) in anticipation of delayed repair may be prudent.

23. What is the best incision to expose the cervical esophagus?
An incision in front of the left sternocleidomastoid muscle. Lateral mobilization of the carotid sheath and anteromedial traction of the trachea exposes the cervical esophagus.

24. What organ is commonly injured during this exposure or with left-sided cervical esophageal injury?
Thoracic duct. This is diagnosed by the high concentration of triglycerides in the drainage.

25. How do you manage injury to the thoracic duct?
Small thoracic duct injuries that manifest with drainage from the wound several days after injury can be managed conservatively. Keeping the patient on NPO, TPN, and closed-suction drainage closes the small injuries. If the drainage slows, patient can be advanced slowly. If the drainage cannot be controlled conservatively, it requires ligation of the thoracic duct by thoracotomy. Large injuries diagnosed during the initial neck exploration should be treated by primary ligation of the site of injury.

26. How do you manage penetrating hypopharyngeal wounds?

Conservatively, by keeping the patient NPO with a nasogastric tube for 7 days along with IV antibiotics.

27. What are some of the signs and symptoms of laryngotracheal injuries?

Difficulty breathing and speaking, stridor, air bubbling in the neck wound, cervical tenderness, and subcutaneous emphysema.

28. How would you manage patients with laryngotracheal injuries?

Airway control is the critical first step. This can be managed by surgical cricothyrotomy, insertion of an endotracheal tube at the site of injury (such as a hole created by a bullet), followed by prompt exploration in the operating room.

29. How do you diagnose tracheal injury?

By laryngoscopy and bronchoscopy. Recall that tracheal injuries are often associated with other injuries and evaluation of the esophagus is of particular significance.

30. How do you repair the cervical tracheal injury?

Tracheal injuries can be repaired primarily in an interrupted fashion using polyglycolic sutures. The most significant technical consideration is adequate mobilization of the trachea to achieve a tension-free repair.

31. Bonus question: A patient with penetrating neck trauma requiring exploration for active bleeding presents to the emergency room. In the OR, you find a thyroid injury with active bleeding. How do you manage this?

Thyroid injuries are uncommon and can be managed by simple suture ligation of the bleeding site of manual compression of the gland.

BIBLIOGRAPHY

1. Apffelstaedt JP, Muller R: Results of mandatory exploration of penetrating neck trauma. World J Surg 18:917–920, 1994.
2. Ballard JL, McIntyre WB: Cervicothoracic vascular injuries. In Rutherford RR (ed): Vascular Surgery, 5th ed. Philadelphia, W.B. Saunders, 2000, pp 893–902.
3. Britt LD, Peyser MB: Penetrating and blunt neck trauma. In Mattox KL, Feliciano DV, Moore EE (eds): Trauma, 4th ed. New York, McGraw-Hill, 2000, pp 437–451.
4. Bufkin BL, Miller JI Jr, Mansour KA: Esophageal perforation: Emphasis on management. Ann Thorac Surg 61:1447–1451, 1996.
5. Cohen ES, Cohen ES, Breaux CW, et al: Penetrating neck injuries: Experience with selective exploration. South Med J 80:26, 1987.
6. Chagnon FP, Mulder DS: Laryngotracheal trauma. Chest Surg Clin North Am 6:733–748, 1996.
7. Cohn HE, Hubbard A, Patton G: Management of esophageal injuries. Ann Thorac Surg 48:309, 1989.
8. Demetriades D, Asensio JA, Velmahos G, Thal E: Complex problems in penetrating neck trauma. Surg Clin North Am 76:661–683, 1996.
9. Demetriades D, Charalambides D, Lakhoo M: Physical examination and selective conservative management in patients with penetrating injuries of the neck. Br J Surg 80:1534–1536, 1993.
10. Mathison DJ, Grillo H: Laryngotracheal trauma. Ann Thorac Surg 43:254, 1987.
11. Menawat SS, Dennis JW, Laneve LM, Frykberg ER: Are arteriograms necessary in penetrating zone II neck injuries? J Vasc Surg 16:397, 1992.
12. Perry MO: Injuries of carotid and vertebral arteries. In Borgord FS, Wilson SE, Perry MO (eds): Vascular Injuries in Surgical Practice. East Norwalk, CT, Appleton & Lange, 1991, pp 95–105.
13. Wisner DH: Cervical vascular injury. In Trunkey DD, Lewis FR Jr (eds): Current Therapy of Trauma, 4th ed. St. Louis, Mosby, 1999, pp 190–197.
14. Yugueros P, Sarmiento JM, Garcia AF, Ferrada R: Conservative management of penetrating hypopharyngeal wounds. J Trauma 40:267, 1996.

59. INJURY TO THE THORACIC GREAT VESSELS

Mohammad H. Eslami, M.D., and John J. Ricotta, M.D.

1. Name the thoracic great vessels.

Thoracic aorta, brachiocephalic branches of aorta, the superior and inferior vena cava, and innominate and azygos veins.

2. How do you approach a patient with a suspected injury to the thoracic great vessels?

Thoracic great vessel injury (TGVI) can have devastating consequences, including death at the scene of an accident. Nonetheless, the trauma patient should be approached by following the ABC of trauma care, as dictated by Advanced Trauma Life Support (ATLS). First secure the airway (chin thrust, oxygen mask, intubation, chest tubes, and surgical airway). In patients with chest injury attention should be paid to pneumothorax, especially tension pneumothorax. This can be evaluated by insertion of a large-bore needle followed by a chest tube. Then proceed with blood pressure and circulation control (large-bore IVs in the lower and upper extremities, initial fluid bolus, control of life-threatening hemorrhage). The possibility of cardiac injury with pericardial tamponade should always be considered with chest trauma. Then perform a quick evaluation of neurologic deficits ("mini" neurologic exam with cervical spine mobilization). The exposure is of utmost importance and every injured patient should be disrobed completely. Evaluate the entrance and exit wounds and record your findings. Never explore the penetrating neck wounds during the initial evaluation. Following the initial assessment, proceed with a complete secondary exam and obtain appropriate laboratory tests and radiographic studies.

3. How is pericardial tamponade evaluated?

Possibility of cardiac injury with chest trauma should always be suspected. These patients present with hypotension, distended neck veins, and muffled heart sounds. Pericardiocentesis followed by a pericardial exploration may be life-saving in these cases.

4. What injury mechanisms may lead to TGVI?

Certain types of accidents are more prone to causing TGVI. These include severe deceleration injuries, such as fall from more than 20 feet (3 floors), motor vehicle accidents involving a crushed steering wheel or pedestrian hit by a car, transmediastinal gunshot wounds, any gunshot or stabbing wounds to the neck zone I or thorax (insertion of a central lines using internal jugular or subclavian vein), and crush injuries.

5. What physical exam findings may point to TGVI?

- First or second rib fracture
- Scapular fracture
- Bruising over the anterior chest
- Unstable sternum
- Thoracic outlet hematoma
- Unequal peripheral pulses or blood pressures
- Focal neurologic deficits (hemiparesis, paraplegia)

6. What is the single most important initial screening tool for the diagnosis of TGVI?

An anteroposterior chest x-ray.

7. What are the signs that point to TGVI on chest x-ray?

- Abnormal thoracic contour/size
- "Widened" mediastinum
- Opacification of aortopulmonary window
- Depression of left main stem bronchus
- Tracheal shift to the right
- Deviation of NGT to the right
- Widening of the right paratracheal stripe
- Presence of an apical cap
- Widening of paraspinal line
- Hemothorax

8. What is the best modality to accurately diagnose TGVI?

The current gold standard for the diagnosis of TGVI is digital subtraction angiography. There is a great deal of interest in spiral CT scanning as several studies have shown promising results, but at the present time they are still experimental. Transesophageal echocardiography (TEE) is used in some centers for diagnosis of TGVI. Each of these modalities has its advocates, and they may be combined to increase diagnostic sensitivity.

9. What is the most important initial step in the management of TGVI?

Expeditious diagnosis. Many of these injuries documented by angiogram may require operation. Prior to operation, the patients must be judiciously resuscitated to maintain a systolic blood pressure of 70–90 mmHg. Restoration of normal blood pressure is contraindicated, as aggressive hydration may exacerbate the bleeding. When indicated, blood pressure and heart rate should be controlled with beta-blockers and afterload-reducing agents. Failure to control the blood pressure and overzealous fluid resuscitation on the way to the operating room can be fatal.

10. Discuss the role of emergency room thoracotomy in the management of TGVI.

Emergency room thoracotomy is a significantly morbid procedure with a low salvage rate. It is contraindicated in patients with no EKG signs of cardiac activity. In one series, without any signs of life at the accident scene, the overall survival following emergency room thoracotomy was 2%. The patients who survived sustained significant neurologic deficits. When there was evidence of cardiac activity at the scene, the overall survival rate was 13%. In cases of blunt trauma, survival was only 3% regardless of cardiac condition. The survival rates in the pediatric population are even lower. Nonetheless, there are selected cases in which this procedure is indicated and should be considered, such as post-injury cardiac arrest (secondary to tamponade), persistent severe post-injury hypotension due to ongoing bleeding, in patients with penetrating trauma who present with signs of life, and occasionally to resuscitate patients with profound abdominal bleeding.

11. Is surgery always necessary in the setting of TGVI?

The vast majority of patients with acute TGVI will require surgery. In selected group of patients with severe multitrauma injuries, surgery may be delayed by using heart rate and blood pressure control and afterload-reducing agents while the patient's condition is stabilized. In some stable patients with radiographic evidence of intimal flaps but no disruption of aorta, close observation with ICU monitoring with heart rate and blood pressure control may be appropriate.

12. What are the indications for surgery in a patient with TGVI?

- Initial blood loss > 1500 ml from the chest tube or ongoing bleeding (> 200 ml/hr for 2 hours)
- Pericardial tamponade or hemopericardium
- Expanding hematoma at the thoracic outlet
- Exsanguinating bleeding from a supraclavicular wound
- Radiographic evidence of acute TGVI
- Radiographic evidence of changes in the known chronic thoracic great vessel condition

Recently, successful endovascular repair of some TGVIs with covered stents has been reported.

13. What are the three key principles in approaching TGVI?

TGVI should be approached with the objectives of **proximal and distal control** followed by **restoration of vascular continuity** whenever possible.

14. How do you expose the injury?

If the site of injury is unknown, the incisions that provide the best exposure are anterolateral thoracotomy on the left and median sternotomy on the right. If the site of the injury is known, different type of incisions are possible. For the exposure of proximal common carotid, vertebral arteries, and jugular vein, the incision depends on the side of the injury (the types and locations of incisions are discussed in Chapter 58). Median sternotomy is used for exposure of pulmonary artery, ascending aorta, transverse aortic arch, innominate artery, intrathoracic vena cava, and right subclavian artery or vein. Left thoracotomy is useful for exposure of the left subclavian artery or vein and the descending thoracic aorta. Repair of the ascending aorta, aortic arch, and innominate artery may require cardiopulmonary bypass (CPB) or vascular shunts for the repair of the injury (see also Chapter 58).

15. What is the initial management of suspected air embolism?

Venous injury and penetrating lung trauma may cause air embolism. This devastating complication is very difficult to diagnose because the key presenting signs, cardiac arrest and seizure, are nonspecific and may have many causes in patients with TGVI. Nonetheless, if the diagnosis is suspected or made, air embolism is initially managed by placing the patient in Trendelenburg position with the right side up, thus allowing the air to be trapped in the right ventricle. Removal of air requires CPB.

16. What are some other complications that may accompany TGVI?

Bullet embolus, thoracic duct injury (see Chapter 58), tracheal injuries, and esophageal injuries.

17. Bonus question: You are called to the ICU to insert a chest tube in an acutely hypotensive patient with right chest hemothorax. You notice a temporary dual-chamber dialysis catheter that was placed 20 days previously. After inserting the chest tube, you immediately encounter 3 L of dark blood. What do you think happened?

Although traumatic chest tube insertion may lead to hemothorax, the most likely cause of bleeding is erosion of the superior vena cava by the old dialysis catheter. Patient needs to be taken to the OR. Placement of subclavian catheters also may acutely lead to rupture of subclavian vessels that may result in cardiac tamponade, cardiac arrest, and death.

BIBLIOGRAPHY

1. Biffl WL, Moore EE, Harken AH: Emergency department thoracotomy. In Mattox KL, Feliciano DV, Moore EE (eds): Trauma, 4th ed. New York, McGraw-Hill, 2000, pp 245–260.
2. Feliciano DV, Mattox KL, Graham JM, et al: Major complications of percutaneous subclavian catheters. Am J Surg 138:969, 1979.
3. Gammie JS, Shah AS, Hattler BG, et al: Traumatic aortic rupture: Diagnosis and management. Ann Thorac Surg 66:1295–1300, 1998.
4. Mansour MA, Moore EE, Moore FA, Read RR: Exigent post injury thoracotomy; analysis of blunt vs. penetrating trauma. Surg Gynecol Obstet 175:97–101, 1992.
5. Mattox KL, et al: Injury to the thoracic great vessel. In Mattox KL, Feliciano DV, Moore EE (eds): Trauma, 4th ed. New York, McGraw-Hill, 2000, pp 559–580.
6. Mattox KL, Wall MJ Jr: Newer diagnostic measures and emergency management. Chest Surg Clin North Am 7:213–226, 1997.
7. Ohki T, Veith FJ, Marin ML, et al: Endovascular approaches of traumatic arterial lesions. Semin Vasc Surg 10:272–285, 1997.
8. Rousseau H, Soula P, Perreault P, et al: Delayed treatment of traumatic rupture of the thoracic aorta with endoluminal covered stent. Circulation 99:498–504, 1999.

60. ESOPHAGEAL TRAUMA

Burke Thompson, M.D.

1. In the evaluation of penetrating neck injury, how is the neck anatomically divided?
- **Zone I** extends from the clavicle to the cricoid cartilage.
- **Zone II** extends from the cricoid cartilage to the angle of the mandible.
- **Zone III** extends from the angle of the mandible to the base of the skull.

2. How common is esophageal injury in patients with penetrating neck trauma?
Uncommon. It occurs in 7–9% of patients with penetrating injuries to the neck. It is one of the most commonly missed injuries in this patient population, however.

3. How can the esophagus be injured by blunt trauma?
Injury occurs as the esophagus is compressed between the trachea and the vertebral column. This injury may go undetected initially and present with fistulization 4–5 days after the injury. Most often, the perforation forms in a contusion along the anterior wall.

4. What are the findings seen with penetrating injury to the esophagus?

HISTORY	PHYSICAL EXAMINATION	CHEST RADIOGRAPH
Dysphagia	Subcutaneous emphysema	Pneumothorax
Odynophagia	Neck tenderness	Pneumomediastinum
Hematemesis	Air escaping from wound	Hydrothorax

5. How is an esophageal injury identified?
Rigid esophagoscopy and **esophagography** may identify a lesion; if negative, however, these studies do not rule out injury completely. **Surgical exploration,** when needed, requires meticulous inspection. Advancing a nasogastric tube to the level of suspected injury and instilling saline may be helpful. Air may be instilled if the surgical field is flooded. The instillation of methylene blue may also be useful.

6. Describe the surgical repair of penetrating injuries to the esophagus.
Early perforations are treated with primary repair. This is done in two layers. The mucosa is approximated with fine absorbable sutures, and the muscularis is repaired with fine nonabsorbable sutures. A closed drainage system, esophageal tube, and gastrostomy tube should always be used.

Late perforations are treated with cervical esophagostomy, distal esophageal ligation, and gastrostomy in addition to the primary repair.

7. What is the most important factor affecting outcome in patients with penetrating esophageal injuries?
Delay in diagnosis and delay in surgical repair can raise the mortality associated with this injury from 2% to nearly 100%.

8. How should the esophagus be evaluated after corrosive ingestion?
- As in all cases of trauma, the airway must be secured first.
- Esophagoscopy should be done promptly to evaluate the extent of injury. It is critical that the scope be advanced only to the proximal extent of the injury to avoid perforation.
- The distal extent of the injury should be evaluated radiographically at a later date.

9. Discuss the indications for emergency surgery after corrosive ingestion.

Laparotomy is warranted if there is free air in the abdomen, interstitial air in the wall of the stomach, or radiologic confirmation of perforation. The abdomen should also be explored if a nasogastric tube was placed in a patient found to have extensive esophageal injury. Thoracotomy is warranted if there is pneumothorax, pneumomediastinum, pleural effusion, or signs and symptoms of mediastinitis.

10. List the late sequelae of ingestion of corrosive substances.
- Stricture
- Gastroesophageal reflux
- Cancer
- Tracheoesophageal fistula

11. How are strictures that form after caustic esophageal burns treated?

Dilatation is standard. This may need to be done repeatedly and is often performed in a retrograde manner by a gastrostomy. Refractory strictures require esophagectomy or bypass.

12. What is the prognosis of patients who develop esophageal cancer after ingestion injury?

Malignant degeneration must be suspected in patients with strictures who experience a change in symptoms. When they do develop, these cancers have a better prognosis than sporadic epidermoid cancers. Resection is often curative if detection is early.

13. A patient complains of chest pain and fever after esophagoscopy. How should this be evaluated initially?

A **water-soluble contrast study** should be done first. If no perforation is seen, the study should be repeated with barium. Repeat esophagoscopy should be avoided because the risk of extending a perforation.

BIBLIOGRAPHY

1. Adolfo A, Kaledzi Y, Parsa M, Freeman H: Penetrating neck wounds: Mandatory versus selective exploration. Ann Surg 202:563, 1985.
2. Deziel D: Rush University Review of Surgery, 3rd ed. Philadelphia, W.B. Saunders, 2000.
3. Greenfield LI, Mulholland M, Oldham KT, et al: Surgery—Scientific Principles and Practice, 2nd ed. Philadelphia, Lippincott-Raven, 1997.
4. Jones R, Terrell J, Salyer K: Penetrating wounds of the neck: An analysis of 274 cases. J Trauma 7:228, 1967.
5. Schwartz SI, Shires GT, Spencer FC: Principles of Surgery, 7th ed. New York, McGraw-Hill, 1999.
6. Weigelt J, Thal E, et al. Diagnosis of penetrating cervical esophageal injuries. Am J Surg 154:619, 1987.
7. Winter RP, Weigelt JA: Cervical esophageal trauma: Incidence and cause of esophageal fistulas. Arch Surg 125:849, 1990.

61. TRAUMATIC DIAPHRAGMATIC HERNIA

Mark R. Jajkowski, M.D., and William J. Flynn, M.D.

1. On which side do most diaphragmatic ruptures occur after blunt trauma?

80–90% occur in the left hemidiaphragm. This is thought to be due to protection of the right hemidiaphragm from the liver, which may act to buffer direct force on the right side. Also, some authors believe that the left hemidiaphragm may be congenitally weaker.

2. What is the mortality associated with diaphragmatic injury?

0–41% (average, 15%). The mortality is generally due to associated injuries, which are common with injury to the diaphragm. In general, blunt trauma has a higher associated mortality (27–41%) than penetrating trauma (5%).

3. What is the incidence of diaphragmatic rupture in blunt trauma?

Injury to the diaphragm occurs with approximately 1–3% of blunt traumas. The incidence is higher with penetrating trauma (approximately 15%). Because of the difficulty in diagnosing these injuries, the actual incidence may be higher than reported.

4. What is the rate of associated injury secondary to blunt trauma?

90%; these injuries may cover the spectrum of intraabdominal, intrathoracic, intracranial, or extremity injuries.

5. Where is the defect usually located after blunt trauma?

Posteriorly on the left hemidiaphragm. The defect is usually a large (10–15 cm) radial tear.

6. When should an injury to the diaphragm from penetrating trauma be suspected?

When the entrance wound lies between the level of the nipples and the costal margin. In this situation, combined thoracic and abdominal injuries must be suspected because of the excursion of the diaphragm during inspiration and expiration.

7. List the most common intra-abdominal viscera to herniate through a defect in the diaphragm.

In decreasing order of frequency:
- Stomach
- Spleen
- Colon
- Small intestine
- Liver

8. What are some of the early signs and symptoms of diaphragmatic herniation?

Blunt trauma generally produces no external signs pathognomonic of diaphragmatic injury, and many patients are asymptomatic, making diagnosis difficult. Some patients may present with **respiratory insufficiency** or **cardiac compromise** resulting from shift of the mediastinum to the contralateral side. One may appreciate a decrease in breath sounds, the presence of bowel sounds, or a decrease in the mobility of the affected thorax. If a diagnostic peritoneal lavage was performed, drainage of the lavage fluid from a chest tube would indicate injury to the diaphragm on that side.

9. What signs on chest radiograph would suggest a diaphragmatic herniation?

An initial chest radiograph is interpreted as normal in half of the cases of diaphragmatic herniation. Some signs that may suggest such an injury include:
- Finding of the nasogastric tube above the diaphragm in the left thorax

- An elevated hemidiaphragm
- An obscured diaphragm shadow
- A blunted costophrenic angle
- Air-fluid level or hollow viscus in the thorax

10. How are most of diaphragmatic injuries diagnosed?

Most of these injuries are unsuspected preoperatively and are found at laparotomy or thoracotomy performed for associated injuries. For this reason, both hemidiaphragms should be inspected thoroughly during operation for either blunt or penetrating trauma. Laparoscopy and thoracoscopy are becoming more widely used as diagnostic modalities in trauma. They may prove useful in the setting of penetrating trauma.

11. When recognized in the acute phase, how is a diaphragm injury managed?

A laparotomy is performed, and exploration for associated injuries is undertaken. After reduction of the herniated viscera, the defect may be closed primarily with interrupted nonabsorbable, monofilament suture. As familiarity is gained with laparoscopic techniques, these injuries may eventually be repaired with these minimally invasive means.

12. If a patient undergoes a thoracotomy for an acute thoracic injury and a diaphragmatic herniation is discovered, how is this best managed?

Although this injury may be managed through a thoracotomy, reduction of the herniated viscera is performed most easily through a separate laparotomy incision. This also allows for thorough examination of the abdominal cavity for identification and management of associated injuries.

13. What can be done if massive destruction of the diaphragm is encountered?

Immediate reconstruction may be undertaken by detaching the hemidiaphragm from its abdominal wall attachments. The diaphragm is then resutured to an area superior to the wound. This procedure effectively converts this to an abdominal wall defect, which may then be managed with local wound care with eventual split-thickness skin grafting or myocutaneous flap closure. Alternatively the defect may be repaired with a nonabsorbable synthetic mesh prosthetic. This must be done with caution if contamination of the wound is present because of the increased risk of infection of the prosthetic.

14. What late complications may occur if a diaphragmatic hernia is undiagnosed?

Obstruction, strangulation, or perforation of intra-abdominal viscera that are incarcerated in the defect.

15. What is the risk of intestinal obstruction and strangulation associated with an undiagnosed diaphragmatic hernia?

80% within 3–5 years (average, 4.6 years).

16. What organs are most commonly involved with intestinal obstruction and strangulation?

- Colon
- Stomach
- Omentum
- Small bowel

17. How is repair of a chronic diaphragmatic hernia managed?

An undiagnosed diaphragm injury continues to enlarge with subsequent increases in visceral herniation. This eventually leads to symptoms of cardiopulmonary compromise or intestinal obstruction. Several months to years after the initial injury, repair is more difficult because of muscle atrophy and dense adhesions. Repair is performed through a thoracotomy or laparotomy depending on the relevant anatomy and surgeon preference. If the tissue is viable and in good condition, this may be repaired primarily as described earlier if it can be done in a tension-free manner. If repair cannot be accomplished without tension, a synthetic mesh prosthetic may be used to reinforce the repair.

BIBLIOGRAPHY

1. Asenio JA, Demetriades D, Rodriguez A: Injury to the diaphragm. In Feliciano DV, Moore EE, Mattox KL (eds): Trauma. Stamford, CT, Appleton & Lange, 1996, pp 461–485.
2. Fildes JJ: Traumatic diaphragmatic hernia. In Nyhus LM, Condon RE (eds): Hernia. Philadelphia, J.B. Lippincott, 1995, pp 567–574.
3. Symbas PN, Vlasis SE, Hatcher C Jr: Blunt and penetrating diaphragmatic injuries with and without herniation of organs into the chest. Ann Thorac Surg 42:158–162, 1986.
4. VanTrigt P: Diaphragm and diaphragmatic pacing. In Sabiston DC, Spencer FC (eds): Surgery of the Chest, 6th ed. Philadelphia, W.B. Saunders, 1995, pp 1081–1099.
5. Weber TR, Tracy TF Jr, Silen ML: The diaphragm. In Baue AE, et al (eds): Glenn's Thoracic and Cardiovascular Surgery. Stamford,CT, Appleton & Lange, 1996, pp 609–642.

62. PENETRATING THORACIC INJURY

Harry W. Donias, M.D., and Raffy L. Karamanoukian, M.D.

1. What is the goal of treatment in the patient sustaining penetrating thoracic trauma?

To restore a survivable physiology. The current approach to seriously injured trauma patients includes three stages:

1. Temporary management of critical injuries with control of bleeding and contamination
2. Physiologic restoration and optimization in the SICU
3. Planned reoperation for definitive treatment

In penetrating thoracic trauma, this approach needs to be modified. Although the philosophy of terminating the operation before exceeding the patient's physiologic limits is similar, vascular structures of the chest, such as the great vessels, heart, and lung, require definitive repair at the initial operation, resulting in less emphasis on reoperation and more emphasis on simpler and quicker but definitive procedures.

2. List clinical variables that indicate the need for an abbreviated procedure.

- Number of injuries
- Initial systolic blood pressure
- Intraoperative estimated blood loss
- Number of units transfused
- Anticipation of hypothermia, acidosis, or coagulopathy (which may result in an irreversible physiologic insult to the patient)

3. Which incision should be used for surgical treatment of penetrating thoracic injuries?

- The standard empiric incision for a patient in extremis is the **left anterolateral thoracotomy.** It is used principally for resuscitation and for cross-clamping the aorta, while anterior repairs are performed. By keeping the patient supine, this position increases venous return; creates less hypotension; decreases the chance of getting blood into the dependent lung; and provides better exposure of the heart, great vessels, and descending aorta. This incision may be extended across the sternum to a bilateral anterolateral thoracotomy for extensive bilateral injuries, including traversal of the mediastinum by a missile.
- A **median sternotomy** may be performed for anterior stab wounds and for thoracic outlet great vessel injuries. Injuries to the trachea may also be approached through this incision.
- A **book** or **trapdoor incision** is used primarily for injuries of the intrathoracic left subclavian artery.
- The **posterior incision** is used for injuries to the descending thoracic aorta, the esophagus, the diaphragm, posterior aspects of the lung, right and left main stem bronchi, and trachea in the area of the carina.

4. What is the goal of emergent resuscitative thoracotomy (ERT)?

To attempt resuscitation of the patient in extremis. ERT consists of opening the pericardium for release of pericardial tamponade, cross-clamping the descending thoracic aorta, and open cardiac massage. Depending on the initial findings, direct repair of cardiac injuries, vascular control of great vessel injuries, or hilar cross-clamping for control of hemorrhage and air embolism can be life-saving maneuvers performed in the emergency department.

5. What is the outcome of ERT?

Patients with penetrating cardiac wounds, especially stab wounds, have proved to be the greatest beneficiaries of ERT, with an overall survival rate of about 10%. If no signs of life are present on arrival to the emergency department, the survival rate drops to 1.4%. The survival for patients with noncardiac penetrating injuries who undergo ERT is 25% if they are hypotensive with signs of life on presentation to the emergency department. This rate drops to 8% if they have no detectable blood pressure but a cardiac rhythm on admission and 3% for those presenting without signs of life. Chances for survival for all patients with blunt trauma who undergo ERT are universally dismal. Even if vital signs are present on admission, survival is extremely rare.

6. After ERT, how is an identified cardiac wound managed?

Once a cardiac wound is visualized, digital control with pressure is attempted. After release of the pericardial tamponade, the patient usually improves and can be transported while the wound is controlled digitally to the operating room for definitive repair. Attempts at repair of the heart in the emergency setting should be avoided. If sutures are not carefully placed and pledgeted, they can tear through the myocardium, enlarge the traumatic defect, and convert a salvageable wound into one that cannot be repaired. Only in the patient who is exsanguinating through a wound that cannot be controlled with digital pressure should further attempts at control be made. Further control may be achieved with sutures, staples, Foley catheters, or inflow occlusion (Sauerbruch grip). Skin staples have been shown to be quicker, to pose less risk of needle-stick injury to the trauma team, and to be of equal mechanical strength as sutures.

7. Penetrating cardiac injuries most commonly affect what structure?

The right ventricle because it is anteriorly located and more vulnerable.

8. How are cardiac injuries immediately adjacent to a coronary artery repaired?

The defect should be repaired without damaging or occluding the coronary circulation. Horizontal mattress sutures should be placed under the coronary artery and the knots tied at a distance from the artery.

9. Discuss the role of surgeon-performed ultrasound in penetrating thoracic trauma.

In patients with a precordial or transthoracic penetrating wound with a suspicion of cardiac injury, a sensitive and rapidly available diagnostic modality is essential. Surgeon-performed cardiac ultrasound has been described with a mean examination time of 0.8 minute with a 98–100% accuracy rate for detecting pericardial blood. With aid of real-time imaging, the time interval from diagnosis to operation is markedly reduced, which enables the surgeon to make earlier decisions regarding patient management. 100% sensitivities and specificities have been described.

10. Are false-positive or false-negative results possible with surgeon-performed ultrasound?

A massive hemothorax may surround the pericardium and produce a false-positive result, or the hemopericardium may decompress into the thoracic cavity, yielding a false-negative result.

11. What does hemopericardium look like on ultrasound?

Blood or fluid is visualized as an anechoic or echolucent dark area. In contrast, structures with higher density, such as pericardium, appear echogenic or bright. In the normal heart, the epicardium and parietal layers of the pericardium show as a single echogenic line. When blood accumulates between the pericardial layers, each layer is visualized as a distinct echogenic line with an echolucent zone (blood) between them, consistent with hemopericardium.

12. Should subxiphoid pericardiotomy be used to diagnose traumatic pericardial effusion?

No. Although subxiphoid pericardial window performed in the emergency department or operating room has been shown to be sensitive and highly specific, it is invasive and time-consuming (30–40 minutes). The small incision used is beneficial only if no injury to the heart is present. If a cardiac injury is present, this small incision results in extensive blood loss during the time that a median sternotomy or anterolateral thoracotomy is performed to expose the injury. If a cardiac wound is suspected, the incision of choice is one that allows repair.

13. What is pulmonary tractotomy?

A simple, easily accomplished procedure aimed at obtaining control of lung parenchymal injuries in the trauma patient that eliminates the need for formal lung resection. It is indicated for through-and-through lung injuries that do not involve hilar vessels or airways. The wound tract is opened by dividing the overlying bridge of tissue with a linear cutter stapler or with a knife between vascular clamps. The exposed tract is carefully inspected to ensure no major vascular or bronchial injury is present that would require repair or resection. The tractotomy is a diagnostic as well as therapeutic maneuver. Bleeding points and air leaks are selectively ligated with figure-of-eight sutures. If the lung tissue was divided between vascular clamps, it is oversewn beneath the clamps with a continuous suture. The tractotomy is left open, and the chest is closed in the standard manner. Pulmonary tractotomy is contraindicated in hilar injuries and in injuries that can be treated by simple pneumonorrhaphy.

14. How is air embolism associated with penetrating thoracic trauma?

Air embolus occurs when air moves from the airway into the pulmonary venous system through a traumatic fistula. With penetrating injuries of the lung, especially when entrance and exit sites have been oversewn and marked Valsalva maneuver by the patient (coughing or straining) or positive-pressure ventilation >60 mm Hg occurs, systemic air emboli can be created from bronchioloalveolar-to-pulmonary venous fistula. The air embolus can cause mortality or major morbidity if delivered to critical arteries, such as those in the cerebral or coronary circulation. Manifestations of this condition include seizure activity, confusion, and cardiac arrest. In a patient with penetrating chest trauma, air embolus should be suspected if there is evidence of a stroke or cardiac failure shortly after initiation of positive-pressure ventilation.

15. How is air embolism treated?

Once recognized, immediate thoracotomy and cross-clamping of the hilum to control the bronchopulmonary fistula is required. The heart should be exposed, and the left atrium, left ventricle, and root of the aorta should be vented with needles. After the air has been vented, the bronchopulmonary fistula should be repaired, or the affected area of lung should be resected to prevent further embolization. Success in reversing this process is rare.

16. What findings are suggestive of tracheobronchial injury?

- Pneumothorax
- Pneumomediastinum
- Atelectasis
- Subcutaneous emphysema
- Unusually large and persistent air leak
- Need for a second (or third) chest tube
- Incomplete expansion of pneumothorax despite functioning chest tubes
- Inability to keep lung expanded
- Refractory and recurrent lobar or whole-lung atelectasis
- Chest radiograph showing a pneumothorax with downward displacement of the lung hilum

17. Should prophylactic antibiotics be used in patients receiving a chest tube for trauma?

Yes. 2–25% of patients who undergo tube thoracostomy for treatment of thoracic injuries develop infectious complications. The most common infectious complications associated with tube thoracostomy are empyema and pneumonia. Contaminating bacteria are potentially introduced into the pleural space by damaged bronchial airways or external contamination from a penetrating missile, improper chest tube placement, presence of necrotic parenchymal tissue, foreign bodies, and retained hemothorax. The most commonly isolated pathogen is *Staphylococcus aureus,* and the recommended prophylactic antibiotic is a first-generation cephalosporin, such as cefazolin.

18. How is hemothorax in a trauma patient with stable vital signs treated?

Tube thoracostomy and monitoring of chest tube output and vital signs.

19. What are the indications for thoracotomy in trauma patients with a hemothorax and stable vital signs?

The amount of chest tube drainage is >1500 mL with initial tube thoracostomy or >200 mL/h for 3 consecutive hours. The hemodynamic status and physiologic state of the patient must be strongly considered with any decision to perform thoracotomy.

20. Can autotransfusion be performed in the trauma patient with hemothorax?

Yes. Blood evacuated from a tube thoracostomy can be collected in a suction device and mixed with citrate anticoagulant. This blood can be reinfused 4 hours after time of collection.

21. What complications are seen with autotransfusion in the trauma patient with hemothorax?

Complications usually arise after the infusion of >1500 mL of salvaged blood and are typically associated with the excessive use of anticoagulant or the administration of activated products of coagulation and fibrinolysis that are present in the collected blood.

22. Is there a role for video-assisted thoracic surgery (VATS) in penetrating thoracic trauma?

VATS can be used safely in hemodynamically stable patients with no cardiovascular or great vessel injury, sparing many patients the pain and morbidity associated with thoracotomy. Emergency VATS has the potential to remove the uncertainty and the waiting period before definitive treatment by allowing direct inspection of intrathoracic organs and the chest wall.

23. List indications for VATS in the stable trauma patient.

- Suspected diaphragmatic injury
- Continued bleeding after tube thoracostomy
- Clotted hemothorax unresponsive to tube thoracostomy

24. What is the thoracoabdominal region?

That area of the body that contains portions of both the thoracic and the abdominal cavities. The upper limits of the abdomen are bounded by the diaphragm, which in full expiration elevates to the level of the nipples anteriorly and the tips of the scapula posteriorly. These correspond to the levels of the fourth and sixth intercostal spaces. Because the thoracic cavity extends inferiorly to the costal margins, many intra-abdominal organs are within the region of the lower chest. Although all penetrating injuries should be suspected of involving both cavities, this is especially important for penetrating injuries in the thoracoabdominal region.

25. Which patients with penetrating thoracic injury should undergo laparoscopy?

All patients with **penetrating left thoracoabdominal trauma** without indications for an open procedure should undergo laparoscopy to exclude occult injuries to the diaphragm. Physical and radiographic changes are nonspecific or absent in patients with diaphragmatic injuries form penetrating trauma. The overall incidence of diaphragmatic injuries with penetrating left thoracoabdominal trauma is 42%. Frequently, patients with previous penetrating injuries present with delayed diaphragmatic hernias. These may appear hours to years after the injury with potentially fatal complications. The rate of mortality of patients presenting late after diaphragmatic injury is 25%, as compared with 3% when diagnosed early. For these reasons, laparoscopy is recommended. Laparoscopy has the added advantage of allowing visualization of the abdominal viscera. Perforation of the diaphragm may be repaired with laparoscopic technique in the absence of other associated injuries. If there is concern about intra-abdominal visceral injuries or bleeding from solid organs, a celiotomy should still be performed to ensure that no injuries are missed.

26. What is bullet embolism?

Bullet embolism is unique to penetrating trauma. Rarely a bullet or bullet fragment enters the venous circulation through an iliac vein, inferior vena cava, or another large vein. Once in the venous system, the bullet can pass through the right side of the heart and into the pericardial vasculature. If embolization of an intact bullet occurs, the bullet should be removed because of the danger of erosion of the pulmonary vasculature and potential pulmonary infarct. The bullet is removed with isolation of the affected portion of the pulmonary artery, arteriotomy, and removal of the bullet. Sometimes bullet fragments can be left in place.

BIBLIOGRAPHY

1. Asensio JA, Berne JD, Demetriades D, et al: One hundred five penetrating cardiac injuries: A 2-year prospective evaluation. J Trauma 44:1073–1082, 1998.
2. Bartek JP, Grasch A, Hazelrigg SR: Thoracoscopic retrieval of foreign bodies after penetrating chest trauma. Ann Thorac Surg 63:1783–1784, 1997.
3. Branney SW, Moore EE, Feldhaus KM, Wolfe RE: Critical analysis of two decades of experience with postinjury emergency department thoracotomy in a regional trauma center. J Trauma 45:87–95, 1998.
4. Brown SE, Gomez GA, Jacobson LE, et al: Penetrating chest trauma: Should indications for emergency room thoracotomy be limited? Am Surg 62:530–534, 1996.
5. Gonzalez RP, Holevar MR: Role of prophylactic antibiotics for tube thoracostomy in chest trauma. Am Surg 64:617–621, 1998.
6. Liu D, Liu H, Lin PJ, Chang C: Video-assisted thoracic surgery in treatment of chest trauma. J Trauma 42:670–674, 1997.
7. Mattox KL, Wall M Jr: Thoracic trauma. In Baue AE (ed): Glenn's Thoracic and Cardiovascular Surgery, 6th ed. Stamford, CT, Appleton & Lange, 1996, pp 91–115.
8. Mayrose J, Jehle DV, Moscati R, et al: Comparison of staples versus sutures in the repair of penetrating cardiac wounds. J Trauma 46:441–444, 1998.
9. Murray JA, Berne J, Ascensio JA: Penetrating thoracoabdominal trauma. Emerg Med Clin North Am 16:107–128, 1998.
10. Rozycki GS, Feliciano DV, Ochsner MG, et al: The role of ultrasound in patients with possible penetrating cardiac wounds: A prospective multicenter study. J Trauma 46:543–551, 1999.
11. Thourani VH, Feliciano DV, Symbas PN, et al: Penetrating cardiac trauma at an urban trauma center: A 22-year perspective. Am Surg 65:811–818, 1999.
12. Velmahos GC, Degiannis E, Souter I, et al: Outcome of a strict policy on emergency department thoracotomies. Arch Surg 130:774–777, 1995.
13. Wall MJ, Soltero E: Damage control for thoracic injuries. Surg Clin North Am 77:863–879, 1997.
14. Wall MJ, Villavicencio RT, Millerce III, et al: Pulmonary tractotomy as an abbreviated thoracotomy technique. J Trauma 45:1015–1023, 1998.
15. Wisner DH: Trauma to the chest. In Sabiston DC, Spencer FC (eds): Surgery of the Chest, 6th ed. Philadelphia, W.B. Saunders, 1995, pp 456–493.

63. TRAUMATIC CHYLOTHORAX

Hratch L. Karamanoukian, M.D., Jeffrey Visco, M.D.,
and Raffy L. Karamanoukian, M.D.

1. What is chylothorax?

Chylothorax is the presence of lymphatic fluid in the pleural cavity resulting from a leak of the thoracic duct or one of its tributaries.

2. What are the general categories for the etiology of chylothorax?

Chylothorax can be congenital in origin, traumatic resulting from operative procedures and blunt or penetrating trauma, or from nontraumatic causes (neoplasms).

3. What are the causes of chylothorax following neck surgery?

Excision of lymph nodes and radical neck dissection.

4. What are the causes of chylothorax after thoracic surgery?

Ligation of patent ductus arteriosus (PDA), excision of coarctation of the aorta, esophagectomy, resection of aortic aneurysm, and resection of mediastinal tumor.

5. What are the serious complication of esophagogastrectomy?

Anastomotic leakage, impaired gastric emptying, respiratory failure requiring prolonged ventilation, and chylothorax are the most significant complications of esophagogastrectomy. Early recognition of chylothorax is important because of the large amounts of protein and fluid that may be lost if this drainage is allowed to continue. If this fistula persists for more than a week following esophagogastrectomy, the duct must be ligated surgically in order to allow prompt recovery of the already malnourished patient.

6. What is the latent period for development of chylothorax after thoracic duct injury?

The latency period is 3–7 days between the time of injury of the thoracic duct or one of its tributaries and the development of chylothorax.

7. In which part of the chest is the thoracic duct more apt to be damaged?

In the upper left part of the chest. This happens after mobilization of the aortic arch, left subclavian artery, or the esophagus.

8. Does damage of the thoracic duct above T5 more commonly cause right- or left-sided chylothorax?

The thoracic duct originates in the cisterna chyli (midline at L2) and ascends through the diaphragm just to the right of the aorta (at T10–T12) and crosses over to the left behind the aortic arch (T5–T6). It empties near the angle of union of the subclavian and internal jugular veins. Damage to the thoracic duct below T5 or T6 more commonly results in right-sided chylothorax. Damage of the thoracic duct above T5 or T6 more commonly causes left-sided chylothorax.

9. What is the most common cause of nonpenetrating injury to the thoracic duct?

Sudden hyperextension of the spine. In such cases, the duct ruptures just above the level of the diaphragm. Penetrating trauma from a gunshot or stab wound can also cause injury to the thoracic duct.

10. What are some conservative measures to help treat chylothorax?

In addition to adequate drainage of the chest by tube thoracostomy, central hyperalimentation and an NPO order are helpful. The thoracic duct will close spontaneously in more than 50%

of cases using this approach. If drainage continues for more than 14 days despite conservative therapy, surgical intervention is recommended to prevent nutritional, metabolic, and immune deficiencies.

11. What is the operative approach for chylothorax?

Although the thoracic duct can be approached from the right or left chest, ligation just above the diaphragm through a right posterolateral thoracotomy is favored. If the thoracic duct is found, direct ligation is curative using nonabsorbable sutures. In most cases, however, mass ligation of tissue between the aorta and the azygos vein over the vertebral body just above the diaphragm is performed. Care should be taken not to injure the esophagus or aorta during this procedure.

BIBLIOGRAPHY

1. Miller JI Jr: Anatomy of the thoracic duct and chylothorax. In Shields TW, LoCicero J III, Ponn RB (eds): General Thoracic Surgery, 5th ed. Philadelphia, Lippincott Williams & Wilkins, 2000.
2. Karamanoukian HL, Bergsland J, Karamanoukian RL: ABSITE Combat Manual, 2nd ed. New York, Magalhaes Scientific Press, 2000.
3. Karamanoukian RL, Karamanoukian HL: Surgery 101: Basic Science Review, Vol. 2. New York, Magalhaes Scientific Press, 1999.

VIII. Minimally Invasive Thoracic Surgery

64. THORACOSCOPY: TROCAR PLACEMENT

Marco Ricci, M.D., Ph.D., and Hratch L. Karamanoukian, M.D.

1. What type of lesion in the chest is amenable to video-assisted resection?

With recent advances in video technology and endoscopic instrumentation, a wide variety of diseases are amenable to thoracoscopic resection. These include, among others, mediastinal masses, mediastinal lymph nodes and cysts, and pleural and pulmonary lesions. Each type requires careful planning and optimal placement of multiple trocars through the chest wall in order to obtain adequate visualization. Simply stated, posterior lesions are generally better visualized using trocars placed through the anterior chest wall, which allow to direct the video camera and the thoracoscopic instruments posteriorly. Conversely, lesions located anteriorly may be better exposed by inserting the trocars through the posterior chest wall.

2. Why is trocar placement important in thoracoscopic surgery?

Proper positioning of the thoracoscopic instruments through the chest wall is of paramount importance to obtain adequate visualization. In contrast to conventional thoracic surgery, trocars should be placed at a certain distance from the area where the lesion or surgical target is located in order to have adequate space to maneuver the instruments. Similarly, thoracoscopic instruments should not enter the chest too close to each other, as this would also impair visualization and surgical manipulation.

3. What is the triangulation technique?

In thoracoscopic surgery, trocar placement is commonly undertaken according to the triangulation technique, which entails the use of three incisions for port placement. The first incision is located 2 cm below the tip of the scapula, and represents the apex of the hypothetical triangle. A second and a third port are then placed anteriorly and posteriorly (see figure below), at the base of the triangle. While most of the thoracoscopic procedures can be performed by using three trocars, more complex operations often require placement of additional ports. When using only three trocars, one is used for the video camera (frequently the one at the apex of the triangle), whereas the other two are used for other instruments such as graspers, endoscissors, or endostaplers.

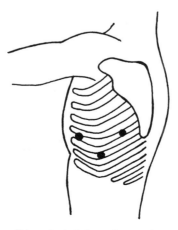

Triangular technique of trocar placement.

4. Is single-lung ventilation required for video-assisted thoracoscopic surgery (VATS)?

Single-lung ventilation is a prerequisite for all thoracoscopic procedures, either on the mediastinum, pleura, or pulmonary parenchyma. This is necessary in order to have sufficient space within the pleural cavity in order to maneuver the thoracoscopic instruments. As a result, patients with extensive pleural adhesions or those who for various reasons do not tolerate single-lung ventilation are not candidates for VATS.

5. What is important when inserting the first trocar?

As stated previously, patients with extensive pleural adhesions are not candidates for VATS. Great care should be taken when inserting the first trocar, as this would reveal the presence of unexpected adhesions. A technique similar to that used for inserting a thoracostomy tube is used. As the parietal pleura is entered bluntly, digital exploration of the incision is undertaken to ensure that the lung has been collapsed and adhesions are not present.

6. Where are the trocars placed for posterior mediastinal masses?

While a trocar is placed at the midaxillary line on the 5th or 6th intercostal space, two additional trocars are placed at the anterior axillary line above (4th intercostal space) and below (6th or 7th intercostal space) the first trocar. Great care should be taken in avoiding placement of the instruments too anteriorly, as visualization may be impaired by the lung, particularly if complete collapse has not been accomplished. If the lung needs to be retracted away from the operating field, an additional trocar may be necessary.

7. Where are the trocars placed for anterior mediastinal masses?

As for posterior mediastinal masses, the first trocar is routinely placed at the midaxillary line through the 5th intercostal space. Additional trocars are placed at the midaxillary line on the 3rd intercostal space, and at the posterior axillary line on the 4th intercostal space. If the trocars are placed too posteriorly, an incompletely collapsed lung may impair visualization.

8. Can thymectomy be performed through the left chest?

Although thymectomy can be performed from either right or left chest, it is ordinarily performed through the right chest. However, in the presence of thymic lesion growing toward the left pleural cavity, a thoracoscopic approach through the left chest may be preferable.

BIBLIOGRAPHY

1. Landreneau RJ, Mack MJ, Hazelrigg SR, et al: Video-assisted thoracic surgery: Basic technical concepts and intercostal approach strategies. Ann Thorac Surg 54:800, 1992.

65. DIAGNOSTIC THORACOSCOPY

Marco Ricci, M.D., Ph.D, and Hratch L. Karamanoukian, M.D.

1. Who are candidates for diagnostic thoracoscopy?
Patients with:
- Undetermined pleural disease
- Interstitial or neoplastic lung disease
- Mediastinal adenopathy of unknown origin
- Mediastinal tumors

2. Discuss the contraindications to diagnostic thoracoscopy.
Because one-lung ventilation and lung collapse are required to perform diagnostic thoracoscopy, **inability to tolerate one-lung ventilation** represents a contraindication for thoracoscopy. A **history of previous thoracotomy and history of severe pleural and pulmonary infectious disease** are generally considered contraindications to diagnostic thoracoscopy, because these patients are likely to have extensive pleural adhesions that may preclude lung collapse and visualization of the intrathoracic structures. Occasionally, thoracoscopy in these patients may be attempted because pleural adhesions can be divided thoracoscopically. In this setting, conversion to an open thoracotomy is carried out when adequate visualization cannot be accomplished.

3. How is diagnostic thoracoscopy performed?
1. Single-lung ventilation to obtain lung collapse and proper visualization is accomplished by placing a left-sided double-lumen endobronchial tube. Alternatively a single-lumen endotracheal tube with bronchial blocker may be used.

2. As in laparoscopy, intrathoracic visualization is obtained by using a camera connected to a monitor (video-assisted thoracoscopic surgery).

3. In contrast to laparoscopy, insufflation of CO_2 is not necessary because the rigid chest wall provides space to maneuver inside the chest once the lung is collapsed. Chest wall rigidity may adversely affect visualization and ability to operate using thoracoscopic instruments so that correct positioning of the operating trocars is important.

4. The thoracoscope is usually inserted through a small incision at the sixth or seventh intercostal space on the midaxillary line, although this may vary depending on the location of the intrathoracic targets.

5. One or two additional small incisions to insert thoracoscopic instruments are necessary and are usually placed anterior and posterior to the one used for the camera. Because of the rigidity of the chest wall, proper placement of the incisions is essential to reach targets with the proper **angle of attack.**

4. Discuss the role of diagnostic thoracoscopy in the management of pleural disease.
Work-up of pleural effusion of unknown cause is usually begun with thoracentesis. Diagnostic thoracoscopy plays little role in the diagnosis of transudative effusions because these are commonly related to dysfunction of other organs (liver, kidneys, heart). The role of thoracoscopy as a diagnostic modality in the management of effusions resulting from pneumonia or tuberculosis is limited.

Diagnostic thoracoscopy is especially useful when investigating malignant effusions. This technique allows for the visualization of intrathoracic organs and pleural malignancies, such as mesotheliomas. The extension of the tumor and involvement of intrathoracic structures can be defined accurately, and thoracoscopically directed pleural biopsies can be performed in areas where the disease is present. The accuracy of this technique in obtaining diagnostic pleural biopsy specimens is extremely high, in contrast to blind percutaneous biopsies, which are often negative in the presence of pleural malignancies (as a result of the localized nature of most of these tumors).

5. Discuss the role of diagnostic thoracoscopy in the management of parenchymal and interstitial lung disease.

In many instances, obtaining the exact diagnosis in the presence of acute or chronic interstitial lung disease may be problematic because the yield of other diagnostic procedures, such as sputum analysis, bronchoalveolar lavage, and bronchoscopy with transbronchial biopsy, is low. Diagnostic thoracoscopy allows for direct visualization of the involved lung in its entirety as well as other intrathoracic structures. Performance of thoracoscopically guided lung biopsies may be accomplished easily using endo-staplers. Biopsies can be performed in areas of lung parenchyma where the disease is most prominent, in contrast to conventional open-lung biopsy, in which visualization and access to the lung are limited by the small thoracic incision. Evaluation of the mediastinum, mediastinal nodes, and pleural surface can be undertaken easily; these structures cannot be exposed sufficiently by conventional minithoracotomy and open-lung biopsy. The main disadvantage of diagnostic thoracoscopy is represented by the fact that patients who do not tolerate single-lung ventilation are not candidates for this procedure and require open-lung biopsy.

6. Discuss the role of thoracoscopy in the diagnosis of mediastinal masses.

Diagnostic thoracoscopy can be used in the setting of unresectable mediastinal tumors of unknown cause as an alternative to modified mediastinoscopy (retrosternal) or mediastinotomy (Chamberlain procedure). When the mediastinal mass is thought to be resectable based on preoperative diagnostic tests (i.e., CT scan of the chest), it should probably be resected, and the role of diagnostic thoracoscopy is limited.

Diagnostic thoracoscopy may be employed in the management of mediastinal lymphadenopathy when a primary lymphoma of the mediastinum is suspected to obtain adequate biopsy tissue. It may be used in patients with mediastinal adenopathy secondary to lung cancer, in combination with or as an alternative to cervical mediastinoscopy. In contrast to mediastinoscopy, aortopulmonary nodes and nodes of the pulmonary hilum can be approached easily. The location and extension of the primary tumor can be accurately defined as well as the involvement of mediastinal structures or chest wall.

7. What is the role of thoracoscopy in the diagnosis of pulmonary nodules?

In the presence of a solitary pulmonary nodule, lung cancer has to be ruled out. In these patients, thoracoscopy and wedge biopsy may be employed as an alternative to CT-guided needle biopsy, with an accuracy approximating 100%.

BIBLIOGRAPHY

1. Gaensler EA, Carrington CB: Open biopsy for chronic diffuse infiltrative lung disease: Clinical, roentgenographic and physiological correlations in 502 patients. Ann Thorac Surg 30:411–426, 1990.
2. Hucker J, Bhatnager NK, Al-Jilaihawi AN, Forrester-Wood CP: Thoracoscopy in the diagnosis and management of recurrent pleural effusions. Ann Thorac Surg 52:1145–1147, 1991.
3. Landreneau RJ, Hazelrigg SR, Mack MJ, et al: Thoracoscopic mediastinal lymph node sampling: Useful for mediastinal lymph node stations inaccessible by cervical mediastinotomy. J Thorac Cardiovasc Surg 106:554–558, 1993.
4. Landreneau RJ, Mack MJ, Hazelrigg SR, et al: Video-assisted thoracic surgery: Basic technical concepts and intercostal approach strategies. Ann Thorac Surg 54:800–807, 1992.
5. Mack MJ, Shennib H, Landreneau RJ, Hazelrigg SR: Techniques for localization of pulmonary nodules for thoracoscopic resection. J Thorac Cardiovasc Surg 106:550–553, 1993.
6. Menzies R, Charbonneau M: Thoracoscopy for the diagnosis of pleural disease. Ann Intern Med 114:271–276, 1991.

66. VIDEO-ASSISTED THORACOSCOPIC PLEURODESIS

Mark R. Jajkowski, M.D., and Hratch L. Karamanoukian, M.D.

1. What is pleurodesis?

The purposeful irritation of the pleural surface. The irritation may be produced by chemical or mechanical means. This produces an inflammatory pleuritis that promotes adherence of the visceral pleura to the parietal pleura. The adherence of the pleurae obliterates the pleural space.

2. Why is pleurodesis performed?

- The presence of a malignant pleural effusion
- Persistent or recurrent spontaneous pneumothorax

3. What is the most common cause of spontaneous pneumothorax?

Rupture of small blebs in the lung.

4. List the goals of treatment of spontaneous pneumothorax.

- Reexpansion of the lung
- Obliteration of the blebs
- Permanent pleurodesis to prevent recurrence

5. What is the most effective agent used for chemical pleurodesis?

Talc; the success rate when it is used for malignant pleural effusion is reported to be >90%. The usual dose is 5 g of talc mixed into 50 mL of saline. This slurry is instilled into the thorax through a tube thoracostomy.

6. Discuss the traditional treatment for spontaneous pneumothorax.

A **tube thoracostomy** is placed for reexpansion of the lung. With chest tube drainage alone, the recurrence rate is 20–50%. Because of the high recurrence rate, a slurry of talc or tetracycline may be instilled through the chest tube to create a **chemical pleurodesis.** With continued persistence of the pneumothorax or recurrent disease, a **thoracotomy** is performed. Resection of blebs is performed along with **mechanical pleurodesis.**

7. How has the development of thoracoscopy or viseo-assisted thoracoscopic surgery (VATS) changed the management of malignant pleural effusions and spontaneous pneumothorax?

VATS has brought a minimally invasive therapy to the treatment of these conditions. With VATS, the need for thoracotomy is decreased.

8. What different modalities have been described for performing VATS pleurodesis?

Essentially any modality used for pleurodesis during thoracotomy may be employed during a VATS procedure. These include the various methods of chemical and mechanical pleurodesis and pleurectomy. Additionally treatment with Nd:YAG laser via thoracoscopy has been described. Not only is one able to perform pleurodesis with the laser, but also blebs <2 cm in size may be resected successfully with low-power laser pulses.

9. List the advantages of VATS pleurodesis over tube thoracostomy chemical pleurodesis.

- VATS permits the same treatment that is possible with open thoracotomy.
- One is able to visualize the entire thoracic cavity, and because of this, bleb resection is possible along with the ability to biopsy any suspicious lesions that may be encountered.
- Recovery is faster with comparable results when compared with thoracotomy.

10. List the disadvantages of VATS over tube thoracostomy.
- Morbidity and mortality associated with general anesthesia
- Increased cost

11. Is talc pleurodesis through a tube thoracostomy more effective than when done by VATS?

Several studies have not shown VATS talc insufflation to be superior to installation of talc slurry through a tube thoracostomy. When a more invasive procedure is required in complicated cases, VATS has many advantages over thoracotomy with comparable results.

BIBLIOGRAPHY

1. Cohen RG, et al: Talc pleurodesis: Talc slurry versus thoracoscopic talc insufflation in a porcine model. Ann Thorac Surg 62:1000–1004, 1996.
2. Colt HG, et al: A comparison of thoracoscopic talc insufflation, slurry, and mechanical abrasion pleurodesis. Chest 111:442–448, 1997.
3. Danby CA, et al: Video-assisted talc pleurodesis for malignant pleural effusions utilizing local anesthesia and IV sedation. Chest 113:739–742, 1998.
4. Torre M, et al: Nd:YAG laser pleurodesis via thoracoscopy. Chest 106:338–341, 1994.
5. Yim APC, et al: Thoracoscopic talc insufflation versus talc slurry for symptomatic malignant pleural effusion. Ann Thorac Surg 62:1655–1658, 1996.

67. VIDEO-ASSISTED THORACOSCOPIC STAGING OF LUNG CANCER

Marco Ricci, M.D., Ph.D., and Hratch L. Karamanoukian, M.D.

1. What is the role of thoracoscopic staging in lung cancer?

Video-assisted thoracoscopy (VAT) has been introduced as an adjunctive procedure in the management of lung cancer patients. This technique may be employed in combination with conventional techniques of preoperative staging, such as chest radiograph, CT scan, and mediastinoscopy.

2. Discuss the limitations of conventional staging techniques.

Lung cancer staging routinely employs CT scanning of the chest and bronchoscopy. Although the strategy of using mediastinoscopy in all patients with lung cancer who are potential operative candidates has been advocated by some, this procedure is most often used selectively, when mediastinal lymphatic involvement is suspected based on preoperative CT scan (mediastinal nodes >10 mm) findings. These techniques used in combination usually offer valid information regarding the extension of the primary tumor and the presence or absence of lymph node metastases or distant metastases. In a few patients, they may fail to detect specific characteristics of the neoplastic disease, such as involvement of the parietal pleura, spread of the tumor across the interlobar fissure, and unsuspected lymph node metastases in the mediastinum.

3. What is the role of VAT in detecting invasion of the parietal pleura?

Data from the literature have shown that CT scan or chest radiograph may fail to detect tumor invasion of the parietal pleura, especially if its occurrence is not accompanied by pleural effusion. When VAT is employed, 4–5% of patients with lung cancer who would otherwise be candidates for pulmonary resection are found to have unsuspected tumor dissemination on the parietal pleura. Because these patients do not benefit from pulmonary resection, the potential morbidity and mortality of an exploratory thoracotomy are avoided.

4. What is the role of VAT in detecting tumor spread across the interlobar fissure?

VAT may give precise information regarding tumor spread across a fissure into the adjacent lobe, which is often difficult to detect on CT scan. Preoperative definition of tumor extension may alter the operative strategy substantially (i.e., pneumonectomy instead of lobectomy). Precise knowledge of tumor extension may be especially important in patients with borderline pulmonary function tests, in whom the extent of pulmonary resection is limited by poor functional respiratory parameters.

5. What is the role of VAT in investigating mediastinal lymph node involvement?

Although conventional cervical mediastinoscopy remains the most commonly employed method of assessing involvement of mediastinal nodes, this technique does not allow access to several groups of mediastinal nodes, such as those located at the aortopulmonary window, perihilar nodes, posterior mediastinal nodes along the inferior pulmonary vein, and posterior subcarinal nodes. Data from the literature have shown that false-negative results after mediastinoscopy occur in 10–33% of patients. VAT may be employed in combination with mediastinoscopy to improve the accuracy of mediastinal staging.

6. Discuss the advantages of VAT over the Chamberlain procedure.

Mediastinomy (Chamberlain procedure) has been employed to assess metastic involvement of anterior mediastinal and aortopulmonary nodes. These nodes frequently may be involved in the setting of lung cancer arising from the left upper lobe and cannot be reached during cervical mediastinoscopy. VAT can be used as an alternative to the Chamberlain procedure to biopsy these nodes. VAT also allows for visualization of the primary tumor and evaluation of other lymphatic stations.

9. How does VAT relate to new multi-modality approaches?

As knowledge of various types of lung cancer increases, new modalities of treatment are tested. Neoadjuvant chemotherapy, with or without radiation therapy, has been introduced in an attempt to improve outcomes of patients with locally advanced non–small cell lung cancer (N2 and T3 disease). The use of VAT as an adjunct to conventional staging procedures may help in identifying patients with locally advanced lung cancer who may benefit from a multimodality approach (i.e., N2 disease undetected by mediastinoscopy).

BIBLIOGRAPHY

1. Miller JD, Goronstein LA, Patterson GA: Staging: The key to rational management of lung cancer. Ann Thorac Surg 53:170–178, 1992.
2. Wain JC: Video-assisted thoracoscopy and the staging of lung cancer. Ann Thorac Surg 56:776–778, 1993.
3. Yashar J, Weitberg AB, Glicksman AS: Preoperative chemotherapy and radiation therapy for stage IIIa carcinoma of the lung. Ann Thorac Surg 53:445–448, 1992.

68. VIDEO-ASSISTED LOBECTOMY

Paul C. Kerr, D.O.

1. What are the current indications for video-assisted lobectomy of the lung?

The current role of video-assisted lobectomy in malignant disease of the lung is under investigation. There is general agreement that the tumor should be small (< 5 cm) and well localized. Patients with stage I lung cancer are optimal candidates for this procedure. Benign disease of the lung requiring lobectomy can be managed effectively using video-assisted thoracic surgery (VATS) techniques. Benign indications for lobectomy using VATS include giant bullae (e.g., involving the entire upper lobe), pulmonary sequestration, and bronchiectasis.

2. What are the contraindications to VATS lobectomy?

Current contraindications to VATS lobectomy include any nodal disease (N1, N2, N3) chest wall involvement, endobronchial tumors, and patients requiring neoadjuvant therapy. These conditions may preclude a standard thoracotomy if nodal involvement is present. As such, they may preclude a less invasive approach, such as VATS lobectomy, because of the inability to perform a complete tumor resection; VATS lobectomy may also be unsafe or technically impossible because of dense adhesions or central location of the tumor.

3. How is the specimen removed following VATS lobectomy?

There are case reports of recurrence of tumor in the thoracoscopic incisions before the routine use of specimen bags. Placing the resected lobe in a specimen bag prior to removal prevents seeding of tumor cells in the port incisions.

4. Are there any complications specific for VATS compared to standard thoracotomy and lobectomy?

No. Prolonged air leak, pneumonia, respiratory failure, and bronchial stump leak are not unique to VATS lobectomy. No current reports have shown an increase in the incidence of these postoperative complications after VATS lobectomy for either benign or malignant disease. They can occur after any operation on the lung, regardless of the approach.

5. What are the advantages of video-assisted lobectomy over thoracotomy?

In the two randomized prospective studies that compared VATS lobectomy to standard lobectomy using thoracotomy, the only statistically significant difference between the two groups was the degree of postoperative pain. Not surprisingly, there was less postoperative pain following VATS lobectomy.

BIBLIOGRAPHY

1. Kirby TJ, Mach MJ, Landreneau RJ, et al: Lobectomy: Video-assisted surgery versus muscle sparing thoracotomy: A randomized trial. J Thorac Cardiovasc Surg 109:997–1000, 1995.
2. Kirby T, Rice T: Thoracoscopic lobectomy. Ann Thorac Surg 56:784–786, 1993.
3. Lewis RJ, Caccavale RJ: VATS lobectomy. Semin Thorac Cardiovasc Surg (in press).
4. McKenna RJ: VATS lobectomy with mediastinal lymph node dissection. Chest Surg Clinic North Am 4:223–232, 1995.

69. VIDEO-ASSISTED THORACOSCOPY FOR TUMORS OF THE MEDIASTINUM

Paula Michele Flummerfelt, M.D.

1. Is video-assisted thoracoscopic surgery (VATS) an accepted diagnostic and treatment alternative for selective mediastinal tumors?

No. Although we have been acquiring knowledge and improving skill, the utility of VATS for mediastinal tumors is still under investigation. Only retrospective multicenter case reviews are available for review with their attendant limitations.

2. In general, is it usually easier to perform VATS for a benign tumor rather than a malignant one?

Yes.

3. Should VATS be considered for all thin-walled mediastinal cysts?

Yes, because they can be decompressed and delivered through a small port. Portions of the cyst wall can be left behind if in contact with vital structures. (Cysts may recur in the future, so one needs to try to obliterate the mucosa to prevent the risk of recurrence.)

4. Is VATS recommended as first-line treatment for malignant tumors?

No. More time is needed to determine whether resection of malignant tumors results in findings similar to those of open resection.

5. Concerning the technical aspects of removing benign mediastinal cysts with VATS, should aspiration be attempted at the onset?

Yes. Aspiration makes grasping of the cyst easier and expedites resection and removal.

6. When is thoracoscopic biopsy appropriate?

When resection is inappropriate or not possible. Thoracoscopy is an operation and should be undertaken only after less invasive tests prove nondiagnostic.

7. What are the principles of thoracoscopic surgery for the posterior mediastinum?
- The sites for trocar placement are selected in the anterior chest somewhat away from the mass.
- Lower mediastinal posterior masses should be approached through upper anterior trocar sites, and upper posterior mediastinal masses should be approached by low anterior trocar sites.

8. Is carbon dioxide insufflation required for thoracoscopy?

No.

9. Why are specimen bags especially helpful in removing specimens through the thoracoscope?

When removing specimens through small incisions, this may cause malignant or infected material to be spilled into the pleural space. A surgical glove can be used as well as Endobag and a Pleatman sac.

10. List the indications for thoracoscopic surgery in the anterior mediastinum.
- Resection of a benign cyst
- Simple thymectomy in early myasthenia gravis
- Diagnostic procedures (e.g., rule out lymphoma or other unknown tumor)

11. Do current data support resection of malignant anterior mediastinal masses?
No; this awaits further study.

12. Name the anesthetic mode for VATS resection of anterior mediastinal masses.
A double-lumen tube is used, split-lung ventilation, with continuous positive airway pressure on the inflated lung if hypoxemia is a problem.

13. Describe the patient positioning and placement of the ports for resection of a left-sided mass of the anterior mediastinum.
- The patient is placed in a 45° off-center position with a small roll under the side to be approached.
- The placement of the ports is as follows:
  Medial port is in the fourth intercostal space, 2–3 cm lateral to the internal mammary artery
  Camera port is in the fifth or sixth intercostal space off the midclavicular line
  Lateral port is in the fourth or fifth intercostal space

BIBLIOGRAPHY

1. Demmy T, et al: Multicenter VATS experience with mediastinal tumors. Ann Thorac Surg 66:187–192, 1998.
2. Hazelrugg S, et al: Thoracoscopic resection of mediastinal cysts. Ann Thorac Surg 56:659–660, 1993.
3. Naunheim KS: Video thoracoscopy for masses of the posterior mediastinum. Ann Thorac Surg 56:657–658, 1993.
4. Rovariaro G: Videothoracoscopic excision of mediastinal masses: Indications and technique. Ann Thorac Surg 56:1679–1684, 1994.
5. Sugarbaker, D: Thoracoscopy in the management of anterior mediastinal masses. Ann Thorac Surg 56:653–656, 1993.

70. VIDEO-ASSISTED DECORTICATION OF THE LUNG

Mohammad Pourshahmir, M.D., and Sung Yoon, M.D.

1. Describe the classification of empyema.

According to the American Thoracic Society, there are three different stages of empyema:

1. **Exudative empyema** (stage I) consists of thin fluid with a low cellular content and low viscosity. The underlying lung readily re-expands.

2. **Fibrinopurulent empyema** (stage II) is characterized by abundant polymorphonuclear (PMN) cells and by deposition of fibrin on the visceral and parietal surfaces of the pleura. This is the transitional phase between acute and chronic empyema. There is an increasing tendency towards loculation that is accompanied by initial fixation of the lung.

3. **Organizing or chronic empyema** (stage III) is characterized by thick exudate. In this stage 75–80% of the fluid consists of sediment. This stage begins about 6 weeks after the onset of illness. The wall of the empyema organizes by ingrowth of capillaries and fibroblasts and the lung will not expand by simple evacuation of the cavity.

2. Describe the algorithm for treatment of empyema.

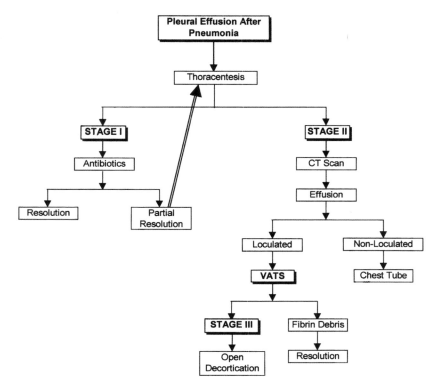

Strategic algorithm for treatment of empyema. CT, computed tomography; VATS, video-assisted thoracic surgery.

3. What are the indications for surgical intervention?

Stage I empyema is treated with intravenous antibiotics and placement of large-bore tube thoracostomy. Stage II or fibrinopurulent empyemas are characterized by the presence of increased leukocytes and the deposition of intrapleural fibrin leading to the development of loculations and fibrinous pleural peel, which can limit lung expansion. Stage II disease usually cannot be treated with tube thoracostomy alone and requires surgical intervention either via video-assisted thoracic surgery (VATS) or open thoracotomy. Stage III empyemas are usually treated with decortication through an open surgical approach.

4. What is the main principle of surgical intervention for empyema?

Early decortication results in better infection control and restoration of lost lung function.

5. What are the advantages of video-assisted decortication?

- Accurate inspection of the entire pleural cavity
- Direct visualization of all surgical maneuvers at the time of operation
- Shorter postoperative hospital stay compared to open thoracotomy
- Decreased amount of pain
- Shorter duration of postoperative chest tube drainage compared to open thoracotomy
- Better cosmesis

6. What are the contraindications to video-assisted decortication?

According to Striffeler and colleagues at the University of Bern, Switzerland, the exclusion criteria for video-assisted decortication consist of clinical evidence of stage III empyema, including evidence of thickened visceral peel or shrunken hemithorax, as well as any suspicion of lung abscess or malignancy.

7. Describe the surgical technique for video-assisted decortication.

Double-lumen endotracheal intubation is obtained and the patient is placed in the lateral position and unilaterally ventilated. The first port is placed one interspace below the angle of the scapula. The rigid camera is introduced through this port. The second port is made more anteriorly and inferiorly. The exact placement depends on the location of the loculations and adhesions. A blunt-ended metal sucker is then used to aspirate the pus and fibrinous septae in the pleural cavity. The space is then irrigated with normal saline and a large-bore chest tube is inserted under direct visualization in the dependent portion of the affected hemithorax.

BIBLIOGRAPHY

1. Angelllilo Mackinlay T, Lyons G, Chimnodeguy D, et al: VATS debridement versus thoracotomy in the treatment of loculated postpneumonia empyema. Ann Thorac Surg 61:1626–630, 1996.
2. Kaiser D, Ennker C, Hartz C: Video-assisted thoracoscopic surgery: Indications, results, complications, and contraindications. Thorac Cardiovasc Surg 41:330–334, 1993.
3. Lawrence D, Ohri S, Moxon R, et al: Thoracoscopic debridement of empyema thoracis. Ann Thorac Surg 64:1448–1450, 1997.
4. Linder A, Friedel G, Toomes H: Prerequisites, indications, and techniques of video-assisted thoracoscopic surgery. Thorac Cardiovasc Surg 41:140–146, 1993.
5. Pearson FG, Deslauriers J, Ginsberg RJ, et al (eds): Thoracic Surgery. New York, Churchill Livingstone, 1995, pp 549–553.
6. Sabiston D: Textbook of Surgery: The Biological Basis of Modern Surgical Practice, 15th ed. Philadelphia, W.B. Saunders, 1997, p 1835.
7. Striffeler H, Gugger M, Hof V, et al: Video-assisted thoracoscopic surgery for fibrinopurulent pleural empyema in 67 patients. Ann Thorac Surg 65:319–323, 1998.

71. VIDEO-ASSISTED ANTIREFLUX SURGERY

Harry W. Donias, M.D., and Hratch L. Karamanoukian, M.D.

1. Discuss the advantages of video-assisted antireflux surgery.

In the early 1990s, many reports showed that video-assisted antireflux surgery could be accomplished reliably and safely in most patients; the immediate results were comparable to (and in some instances better than) those obtained with traditional open techniques, hospital stay was shorter than with open techniques, and total expenses associated with the operation were lower. Today, patients treated with video-assisted antireflux surgery benefit from the superb exposure afforded by the use of modern optics, cameras, and high-resolution monitors. Easier identification of structures in the field decreases the incidence of intraoperative complications and allows for a more accurate construction of an effective antireflux barrier. Less manipulation of intraabdominal organs, small incisions, no need for traumatic retraction, and a dry field all result in a faster recovery.

2. Describe the primary indications for antireflux surgery.

Objective evidence of gastroesophageal reflux disease (GERD) plus:

1. Persistent GERD symptoms or development of complications not responding to medical therapy (failure to resolve symptoms or heal esophagitis after 12 weeks of acid suppression with proton-pump inhibitors and prokinetics, alteration in dietary habits, weight loss, and sleeping with head of bed elevated).

2. GERD symptoms interfering with lifestyle, despite medical therapy.

3. Paraesophageal hernia with GERD.

4. Need for continuous drug treatment in a patient desiring discontinuation of medical therapy (young age, financial burden, noncompliance, or lifestyle choice).

3. What are other indications for antireflux surgery?

Complications of GERD:

- Continued esophagitis
- Esophageal stricture
- Recurrent aspiration or pneumonia
- Barrett's esophagus

4. What is a fear of long-term medical management of GERD?

Chronic suppression of normal gastric acid secretion coupled with unchecked bile acid effects on the gastric and esophageal mucosa may be primary contributors to the rising incidence of adenocarcinoma of the distal esophagus and gastric carcinoma seen today.

5. List the absolute contraindications to laparoscopic antireflux surgery (LARS).

- Inability to tolerate a general anesthetic or laparoscopy
- Uncorrectable coagulopathy
- Severe chronic obstructive pulmonary disease
- Pregnancy

6. Discuss relative contraindications to LARS.

Previous upper abdominal surgery, particularly around the diaphragm or esophageal hiatus, renders LARS more difficult. In morbidly obese patients access to the abdominal cavity is not a problem, but the omentum and gastrosplenic ligament may be bulky and difficult to retract adequately, and fatty infiltration of the left lateral segment of the liver may make exposure of the esophageal hiatus impossible. Significant esophageal shortening (>5 cm) when coupled with esophageal stricture and poor peristalsis may be better treated with esophagectomy. Large hiatal hernias, especially paraesophageal hernias, may be difficult to repair and should be avoided until the surgeon has gained significant experience with this operation.

7. What tests are used in the preoperative evaluation of patients for LARS?

- **Upper GI endoscopy** with biopsy specimens of suspicious lesions should be performed. Esophagitis should be described and graded with a standardized tool, such as the Savary-Miller score. Hiatal hernia and esophageal length can be assessed as well as ulceration, stricture, or Barrett's esophagus.
- **Esophageal manometry** should be performed to assess esophageal body and lower esophageal sphincter function. Esophageal dysmotility (diminished contraction amplitude, diminished peristalsis) should be recognized and treated with partial fundoplication. Patients with aperistalsis may have achalasia and require a different therapy.
- **24-hour ambulatory pH monitoring** is the **gold standard** in defining and quantifying reflux. This test requires prolonged cessation of proton-pump inhibitors and an indwelling nasoesophageal tube in an outpatient setting, which is time-consuming, uncomfortable, and relatively expensive. For these reasons, most use 24-hour pH monitoring selectively if prior studies are inconclusive.
- **Barium swallow** is used selectively to assess anatomic reasons for dysphagia, such as stricture, ring, or web. It also gives the surgeon an idea about the size of the hiatal hernia and length of the esophagus confirms endoscopy results from an outside institution.
- Other tests, such as **esophageal transit, gastric emptying, video esophagram, esophageal endosonography,** and **CT scan** are used only occasionally to establish the diagnosis further or evaluate the anatomy of the region.

8. List the technical principles that are common to all fundoplications.

1. Dissect away from the esophagus to avoid injury to the esophageal wall.
2. All dissection must be performed under direct vision.
3. The fundus, rather than any other part of the stomach, must be plicated around the esophagus, rather than around the proximal stomach, and must be fixed to the esophagus to remain in place permanently.
4. There must not be tension present at the completion of the fundoplication, either axially (tending to pull the repair up through the hiatus into the mediastinum) or rotationally (pulling the fundus counterclockwise back to the left, creating a twist of the lower esophagus).
5. The esophagus must never be grasped directly or manipulated with the tip of a pointed instrument.
6. A total fundoplication always should measure 2 cm in length in its anterior aspect. It is always longer posteriorly. Partial fundoplications (anterior or posterior) are usually 1.5 to 2 times the length of a total fundoplication.
7. The diaphragmatic hiatus must be secured gently around the esophagus above the fundoplication. The esophagus, at the hiatus, must easily accommodate a 54–60F dilator.

9. Describe the typical port placement for LARS.

Most surgeons perform LARS from between the patient's legs, either on a split leg table or with the patient in the lithotomy position. Five trocar ports are used. Additional ports may be added to assist in retraction or suturing the gastric wrap. A 45° laparoscope is placed 15 cm below the xiphoid and to the left of midline. A liver retractor is placed 15 cm from the xiphoid just below the right costal margin. The surgeon operates with the left hand through a trocar 7 cm from the xiphoid under the right costal margin, which is angled through the falciform ligament; for the right hand, a trocar is placed 10 cm from the xiphoid under the left costal margin. A final trocar is placed 20 cm from the xiphoid under the left costal margin to retract the stomach and esophagus.

10. What are the borders of the retroesophageal triangle?

The **posterior surface of the esophagus** anteriorly, the **left crus** superiorly and posteriorly, and the **posterior gastric cardia** inferiorly (note that only the right crus surrounds the esophageal hiatus, and its left leg is incorrectly but customarily called the **left crus**). Each border should be identified clearly during the retroesophageal dissection. Generally, dissection performed outside of this border results in serious complications. Dissection performed too far superiorly results in penetration of the pleura, resulting in a simple or tension pneumothorax. Dissection performed too far anteriorly results in esophageal perforation and too far inferiorly results in gastric perforation. Posteriorly the dissection is relatively safe.

11. List the measures that are taken to ensure proper placement of the fundoplication.
   1. The stomach posterior to the esophagus is pulled anterior and cephalad until the angle of His is identified.
   2. The anterior aspect of the greater curvature is grasped and elevated in cephalad direction. These two portions of the upper stomach are lifted, and using a to-and-from motion (the **shoeshine maneuver**), any redundancy in the fundic wrap is removed.
   3. The stomach is brought together anteriorly to ensure that adequate length is available to wrap the esophagus without tension.

12. Discuss the main concern of performing a laparoscopic Rosetti-Nissen fundoplication.
   This procedure is associated with a higher rate of early and persistent dysphagia than either laparoscopic **floppy** Nissen or Toupet fundoplication. When the anterior wall of the stomach is used for fundoplication rather than the true fundus, only half of the tissue available for creating the nipple valve at the gastroesophageal junction is used. The redundancy of tissue available in the posterior gastric wall is wasted, lessening the likelihood that a tension-free fundoplication will be created. When the fundus remains tethered to the spleen, by not dividing the short gastric vessels, tension on the Rosetti-Nissen fundoplication results from elasticity in the stomach and gastrosplenic attachments. This tension occasionally causes the fundoplication and distal esophagus to twist counterclockwise when surgical traction and the dilator are removed, resulting in a narrow **spiral** gastroesophageal valve. This valve deformity may cause obstruction to bolus food passage, but because there is no stricture, it may be refractory to dilation. The manometric finding of incomplete lower esophageal sphincter relaxation is associated with this deformity. Another anatomic trap of the Rosetti-Nissen fundoplication is the potential for creating a two-compartment (**bilobed**) stomach, which requires reoperation to correct.

13. List complications seen with LARS.

Intraoperative	Postoperative
• Viscous perforation	• Dysphagia
• Bleeding	• Early satiety
• Pneumothorax	• Gas bloat syndrome
• Subcutaneous or mediastinal emphysema	• Inability to belch/vomit
	• Nausea
	• Hyperflatulence
	• Diarrhea
	• Recurrent GERD symptoms

14. What is the most frequent site of bleeding during LARS?
   The undersurface of the left lobe of the liver, as a result of retractor injury or inadequate control of epiphrenic vessels, frequently a phrenic arterial branch lying adjacent to the left crus of the diaphragm. Dissection of phrenogastric attachments close to the stomach generally avoids injuring this vessel.

15. Where else does bleeding occur in association with LARS?
   At division of the short gastric vessels.

16. What is the most common fundoplication-associated complication after LARS?

Transhiatal migration of the fundoplication into the mediastinum, most frequently because of postoperative vomiting. This has led many surgeons to administer intravenous ondansetron at the completion of the case and every 6 hours thereafter until postoperative nausea subsides. Obesity and increased intraabdominal pressure also is associated with the transdiaphragmatic migration. It has been described after heavy weight-lifting or motor vehicle accidents. Patients with Barrett's esophagus may be more prone to the development of this complication.

17. Discuss complications that can arise from dividing the hepatic branch of the vagus nerve.

The gastrohepatic ligament is divided to gain access to the gastroesophageal junction early in the operation. The gastrohepatic ligament usually is divided with cautery above the hepatic branch of the vagus nerve, revealing the caudate lobe posteriorly and the lateral aspect of the right crus of the diaphragm medially. If necessary, the hepatic branch of the vagus nerve may be divided to provide further exposure, and some surgeons divide it routinely. Division carries the risk of increasing cholelithiasis and damage to a replaced left hepatic artery, arising from the left gastric artery, which is present in 25% of patients. Division of a replaced left hepatic artery could result in necrosis of the liver.

18. What steps must be taken if the pleura is inadvertently lacerated?

The surgeon must communicate with the anesthetist that this event has occurred. Assuming that the lung parenchyma is not damaged, the carbon dioxide pneumothorax generally poses no serious complications to the patient and is absorbed quickly at the end of the case. The anesthetist can increase the airway pressure, while the surgeon can slightly decrease the insufflator pressure limit, and adequate ventilation and perfusion can be maintained. Pneumothorax occurs in 1–5% of LARS. Chest tube placement almost never is required because of the rapid reabsorption of carbon dioxide. Postoperative chest radiographs, initially routine, are now reserved for patients who have difficulties in the recovery room.

19. What is the probable cause of hyperflatulence seen after LARS?

This is most likely related to the body's homeostatic attempts to mitigate the effects of acid reflux by increasing the frequency of swallowing alkaline saliva. With free reflux, this additional swallowed air seldom poses a problem, but when the lower esophageal sphincter is repaired, hyperflatulence tends to result. Treatment usually consists of simethicone as needed. If symptoms persist, referral to speech therapy for retraining to control the frequency of swallowed air may be helpful.

20. What is the probable cause of diarrhea seen after LARS?

This may be associated with traction injury to the vagus nerve or with the increase in gastric emptying seen after fundoplication. Treatment includes reassurance with antidiarrheal medication if needed.

21. What is the probable cause of nausea seen after LARS?

There may be some vagal nerve neurapraxia because nausea often is correlated with diarrhea. Nausea may be associated with duodenal gastric bile reflux. Sucralfate has been shown to provide some symptomatic relief.

22. Discuss the major reasons for conversion to an open procedure.

Inadequate visualization of the gastroesophageal region because of morbid obesity with fatty infiltration of the left lobe of the liver and significant adhesions from previous surgery are the two most common reasons for conversion. There have been reports of eliminating the problems with large livers by limiting the acceptable weight of patients undergoing surgery (maximum weight for men, 250 lb; women, 200 lb). The remaining large livers usually can be retracted adequately by the placement of two liver retractors side by side coming in from the right subcostal region. Although adhesions from previous surgery may be a formidable barrier to LARS, most surgeons attempt a laparoscopic approach, with the increased risk of conversion explained thoroughly to the patient preoperatively.

23. List the indications for partial fundoplication.
- Poor esophageal clearance because of esophageal motility abnormalities in association with GERD.
- Severe aerophagia, particularly in patients with daytime reflux associated with belching (acid belches).
- Insufficient gastric fundus to allow a loose total fundoplication (tubular stomach, previous gastrectomy).
- Physiologic inability to tolerate the side effects of total fundoplication.
- In association with a Heller esophagomyotomy.

24. What is a Toupet fundoplication?
Toupet, in 1963, described a posterior 270° partial fundoplication. The main differences from the Nissen fundoplication are as follows:
1. In the Toupet procedure, the edges of the stomach are attached to the anterior wall of the stomach, rather than to each other, leaving a space in between.
2. The wrap is fixed to the edges of the hiatus, which remains open.
Subsequent modifications, described by Guarner, include fixing the fundoplication to the under-surface of a closed hiatus. The Toupet fundoplication is the most common partial fundoplication constructed laparoscopically, and it is currently the operation of choice for patients with reflux and poor or absent esophageal peristalsis. Reports of reoperation for dysphagia with laparoscopic revision of a Nissen to a Toupet procedure have shown complete relief of symptoms with only a short postoperative recovery.

25. What is a Dor fundoplication?
Dor, in 1962, described an anterior 200° fundoplication. In principle, this operation is the reverse of a Toupet procedure, with the fundoplication covering the anterior aspect of the distal esophagus and fixed to the edges of the diaphragm. This is routinely used to perform an antireflux procedure after a myotomy of the distal esophagus. Its main advantage, under those circumstances, is the fact that the fundus of the stomach covers the exposed mucosa of the esophagus.

26. Describe the laparoscopic Hill repair.
The Hill repair involves plication of the lesser gastric curvature around the right side of the esophagus with an esophagogastropexy to the preaortic fascia. Intraoperative manometry is used to achieve a lower esophageal sphincter pressure between 20 and 30 mm Hg intraoperatively. The essential features of the repair consist of posterior closure of the hiatus, followed by secure anchoring of the so-called anterior and posterior phrenoesophageal bundles—the fibroareolar tissue surrounding the gastroesophageal junction, including the underlying seromuscular layer of the stomach—to the preaortic fascia with a series of four sutures. The exact placement of sutures is important, and when pulled downward and posteromedially to the preaortic fascia, the effect is that of a valvuloplasty, reestablishing all significant components of the antireflux barrier. With all repair sutures in place but not tied, the top two sutures are tied with a single half-hitch over a 28–36F dilator in the gastroesophageal junction. The circumferential pressure created by the repair can be altered by adjusting tension on the sutures, while measuring the effect manometrically, until the desired pressure is achieved.

27. List the potential advantages the laparoscopic Hill repair has over other LARS.
1. Because the fundus is not wrapped, division of the short gastric vessels is never required, making laparoscopic dissection simpler and safer.

2. The location of the suture placement is precise, with easily defined landmarks, a particular advantage with the limitations of two-dimensional vision during laparoscopic repair.

3. No sutures are placed in the wall of the esophagus, eliminating the risk of fistula formation.

4. The Hill repair is the only commonly performed antireflux procedure that anchors the gastroesophageal junction at its normal location securely, to a relatively immobile fixation point below the diaphragm, which may be important in restoring function to the distal esophagus in patients with abnormal motility.

5. The Hill repair is the only commonly performed antireflux procedure that allows the surgeon to monitor directly and modify the tightness of the repair based on suture tension. The final configuration comes closer to approximating normal anatomy than that of any other antireflux procedure.

28. When is an esophageal lengthening procedure indicated?

After extensive mediastinal esophageal mobilization, when it is not possible to deliver the gastroesophageal junction 2.5 cm below the hiatus. In most patients, mobilization of the esophagus allows 3 to 4 cm of the distal esophagus to lie comfortably within the peritoneal cavity. Some patients have a true short esophagus, however, an esophagus of inadequate length to descend completely into the abdominal cavity. This occasionally may be congenital, but it usually is acquired. Esophageal shortening is found more frequently in association with a gastroesophageal junction that is >5 cm above the hiatus on barium swallow, type III paraesophageal hiatal hernia, and esophageal stricture with or without Barrett's esophagus. Approximately 5–10% of these patients are not able to have the esophagus mobilized adequately to place the gastroesophageal junction within the abdominal cavity, necessitating an esophageal lengthening procedure.

29. How is a video-assisted Collis gastroplasty performed?
Transthoracic approach
- A sealed thoracic port is placed into the right chest at the fourth intercostal space in the anterior axillary line, and a pneumothorax using 10 mm Hg of carbon dioxide is created.
- A scope is inserted and advanced to the mediastinal pleura at the posteroinferior pulmonary sulcus.
- Once the proper trajectory is established, the scope is withdrawn, and an endoscopic linear stapler is inserted through the esophageal hiatus into the abdominal cavity, allowing the stapler to be placed parallel to the esophagus beginning at the angle of His. This provides 2.5–5.5 cm of neoesophagus, which is generally adequate to allow intraabdominal fundoplication.
- A chest tube is not routinely needed because the thoracic port is vented at the end of the procedure.

Laparoscopic approach
- An end-to-end anastomosis stapler is passed through a small skin incision to create a full-thickness hole through the stomach approximately 3 cm distal to the angle of His, adjacent to a dilator along the lesser curvature.
- A linear stapler is directed from the end-to-end anastomosis hole proximally along and to the left of the dilator to create a new angle of His.
- Complete or partial fundoplication can be added after a Collis gastroplasty.

30. What long-term complication is seen after Collis gastroplasty?

Increased distal esophageal acid and persistent esophagitis. Although most patients show significant improvement of symptoms after Collis gastroplasty and fundoplication, 50% show abnormal results on postoperative pH testing, 36% have evidence of esophagitis, and 50% have distal esophageal aperistalsis or hypoperistalsis that was not present preoperatively. The best explanation is the presence of functional gastric mucosa, with acid-secreting cells, in the neoesophagus proximal to the fundoplication, coupled with poor distal esophageal clearance. These findings mandate rigorous postoperative objective testing and use of medical acid suppression when neoesophageal acid production is documented.

CONTROVERSY

31. Should the short gastric vessels (SGV) routinely be divided during LARS?

Most agree that routine division of the SGV allows the fundus to be mobilized fully and have shown an improved outcome with regard to dysphagia and wrap disruption. Proponents of routine division believe that dividing the SGV enhances visualization of the high retrogastric space, which facilitates division of the gastropancreatic ligaments and posterior gastric vessels. The sites of insertion of the SGV also identify clearly the lateral border of the fundus, which is used for fundoplication. By dissecting along the fundus of the stomach, the left crus of the diaphragm becomes much more apparent, leading to a reduced rate of inadvertently dissecting into the side of the esophagus.

Some surgeons forego this additional step, believing that the construction of a loose wrap is more important than whether the SGV are divided and only selectively divide them when a loose wrap of the fundus cannot be constructed without division. A prospective, randomized trial showed no benefit to SGV division and an increase of about 40 minutes in operating time, resulting in increased expense and technical difficulty as well as adding the potential for intraoperative and postoperative hemorrhage that follows division of these vessels.

BIBLIOGRAPHY

1. Anvari M, Allen C: Laparoscopic Nissen fundoplication: Two-year comprehensive follow-up of a technique of minimal paraesophageal dissection. Ann Surg 227:25–32, 1998.
2. Aye RW, Hill LD, Kraemer SJM, Snopkowski P: Early results with the laparoscopic Hill repair. Am J Surg 167:542–546, 1994.
3. Aye RW, Mazza DE, Hill LD: Laparascopic Hill repair in patients with abnormal motility. Am J Surg 173:379–382, 1997.
4. Hinder RA, Klinler PJ, Perdikis G, Smith SL: Management of the failed antireflux operation. Surg Clin North Am 77:1083–1098, 1997.
5. Horgan S, Pellegrini CA: Surgical treatment of gastroesophageal reflux disease. Surg Clin North Am 77:1063–1082, 1997.
6. Hunter JG, Swanstrom L, Waring JP: Dysphagia after laparoscopic antireflux surgery the impact of operative technique. Ann Surg 224:51–57, 1996.
7. Hunter JG, Trus TL, Branum GD, et al: A physiologic approach to laparoscopic fundoplication for gastroesophageal reflux disease. Ann Surg 223:673–687, 1996.
8. Jobe BA, Horvath KD, Swanstrom LL: Postoperative function following laparoscopic Collis gastroplasty for shortened esophagus. Arch Surg 133:867–874, 1998.
9. Landreneau RJ, Wiechmann RJ, Hazelrigg SR, et al: Success of laparoscopic fundoplication for gastroesophageal reflux disease. Ann Thorac Surg 66:1886–93, 1998.
10. Laws HL, Clements RH, Swillie CM: A randomized, prospective comparison of the Nissen fundoplication versus the Toupet fundoplication for gastroesophageal reflux disease. Ann Surg 225:647–654, 1997.
11. Peters JH, DeMeester TR, Crookes P, et al: The treatment of gastroesophageal reflux disease with laparoscopic Nissen fundoplication prospective evaluation of 100 patients with "typical" symptoms. Ann Surg 228:40–50, 1998.
12. Richardson WS, Bowen JC: Minimally invasive esophageal surgery. Surg Clin North Am 78:795–803, 1998.
13. Richardson WS, Trus TL, Hunter JG: Laparoscopic antireflux surgery. Surg Clin North Am 76:437–450, 1996.
14. Schauer PR, Meyers WC, Pappas TN, et al: Mechanisms of gastric and esophageal perforations during laparoscopic Nissen fundoplication. Ann Surg 223:43–52, 1996.
15. Soper NJ: Laparoscopic management of hiatal hernia and gastroesophageal reflux. Curr Probl Surg 36:767–838, 1999.
16. Soper NJ, Dunnegan D: Anatomic fundoplication failure after laparoscopic antireflux surgery. Ann Surg 229:669–676, 1999.
17. Swanstrom L, Wayne R: Spectrum of gastrointestinal symptoms after laparoscopic fundoplication. Am J Surg 167:538–541, 1994.
18. Watson DI, Pike GK, Baigrie RJ, et al: Prospective double-blind randomized trial of laparoscopic Nissen fundoplication with division and without division of short gastric vessels. Ann Surg 226:642–652, 1997.

72. VIDEO-ASSISTED HELLER MYOTOMY

Paul C. Kerr, D.O.

1. What are the acceptable therapeutic options for achalasia?

Endoscopic balloon dilation, video-assisted extramucosal esophagomyotomy, and esophagomyotomy via left thoracotomy. Right-sided approaches, especially via video-assisted thoracic surgery (VATS), are best for lesions of the upper and mid-esophagus, because they allow exposure of the esophagus without interference by the aorta. For procedures involving the gastroesophageal junction, such as a myotomy or antireflux procedure, a left-sided approach should be used.

2. Which steps are required before beginning a surgical procedure for achalasia?

All of the following are necessary for an adequate and safe myotomy via standard thoracotomy or VATS approach: double-lumen endotracheal intubation, adequate one-lung anesthesia, and a left thoracotomy position. Having a dilator or endoscope in the esophagus aids in mobilizing the esophagus and identifying the mucosa of the esophagus as the muscle is divided.

3. Describe correct port placement for VATS myotomy.

Port placement is critical to ensure a successful VATS procedure. A port in the 7th intercostal space (ICS) in the midaxillary line is used for the video camera during VATS. Ports in the 8th ICS (anterior and posterior) are used for the instruments. A port in the 10th ICS is useful for retraction of the diaphragm and esophageal hiatus.

4. How are the layers of the esophagus divided in a Heller myotomy?

A successful Heller myotomy involves dividing all the muscle fibers of the esophagus, including both the outer longitudinal layer and the inner circular layer, without entering the mucosa of the esophagus.

5. Identify the proximal and distal landmarks used in performing a Heller myotomy.

Complete division of both layers of muscle is critical in performing a successful myotomy. The landmarks are the aortic arch proximally and distally, and the myotomy should extend onto the surface of the stomach 1 cm beyond the gastroesophageal junction.

BIBLIOGRAPHY

1. Anseimino M, Hinder RA, Filidi CJ, et al: Laparoscopic Heller cardiomyotomy and thoracoscopic esophageal long myotomy for the treatment of primary esophageal motor disorders. Surg Laparosc Endosc 3:437–441, 1953.
2. Cade RJ, Martin CJ: Thoracoscopic cardiomyotomy for achalasia. Aust J Surg 66:107–109, 1996.
3. Foley R, Brough W: Thoracoscopic cardiomyotomy for achalasia of the cardia: Early results. Ann R Coll Surg Engl 77:60–62, 1994.
4. Monson JRT, Darzi A, Carey PD, et al: Thoracoscopic Heller's cardiomyotomy: A new approach for achalasia. Surg Laparosc Endosc 4:6–8, 1994.
5. Pellegrini CA, Leichter R, Patti M, et al: Thoracoscopic esophagomyotomy: Initial experience with a new approach for the treatment of achalasia. Ann Surg 216:281–299, 1992.

73. VIDEO-ASSISTED REPAIR OF PARAESOPHAGEAL HERNIAS

Mohammad Pourshahmir, M.D., and Jeffrey Visco, M.D.

1. Describe the different types of hiatal hernias.

1. In type I or sliding hiatal hernia the gastroesophageal (GE) junction migrates through the esophageal hiatus into an intrathoracic location (see figure below).

2. In type II or true paraesophageal hernia the fundus of the stomach herniates into the mediastinum relative to a normal location of the GE junction (see figure below).

3. Type III is a combination of sliding and paraesophageal hernia in which the GE junction is displaced into the thorax as well as a hernia sac containing the fundus and body of the stomach.

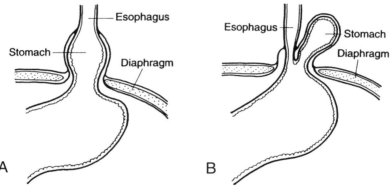

A, Sliding hiatal hernia. *B,* Paraesophageal hernia. (From Dorland's Illustrated Medical Dictionary, 28th ed. Philadelphia, W.B. Saunders, 1994, with permission.)

2. When is surgery indicated in the treatment of paraesophageal hernia?

Surgery in asymptomatic patients is controversial. The classic teaching was that elective surgery should be performed once the patient has been diagnosed with paraesophageal hernia due to the high morbidity and mortality associated with strangulation and necrosis; however, in 1993, Allen and colleagues demonstrated that asymptomatic patients could be followed safely over a long period of time. Symptomatic patients (those with postprandial pain, dysphagia, reflux, bleeding, or weight loss) or patients with chronic anemia should undergo an elective laparoscopic paraesophageal hernia repair. Another indication for surgery is a totally intrathoracic stomach due to the high risk of volvulus and strangulation.

3. Is a simultaneous anti-reflux procedure always necessary with paraesophageal hernia repair?

This is a controversial issue. Some centers routinely perform an anti-reflux procedure in conjunction with paraesophageal hernia repair. This decision is based on the fact that approximately 18% of the patients undergoing only anatomic repair without an anti-reflux procedure will experience reflux symptoms. Perkidis and Hinder routinely perform anti-reflux procedure (most often Nissen fundoplication) in conjunction with paraesophageal hernia repair, but Ferguson advocates simultaneous fundoplication based only on preoperative symptoms, pH monitoring, or endoscopic findings.

4. What are the advantages of laparoscopic versus open technique?
- Superior visibility of the hiatus, diaphragm, and the hernia sac
- Better pain control
- Decreased blood loss
- Faster recovery
- Shortened hospital stay
- Better cosmesis

5. What are some of the contraindications to laparoscopic repair of paraesophageal hernias?

Absolute contraindications include the inability to tolerate general anesthesia and uncorrectable coagulopathy. Relative contraindications include prior upper abdominal operations, severe obesity, foreshortened esophagus, and the presence of other intra-abdominal pathologies.

6. Describe the steps in paraesophageal hernia repair.
- Hernia reduction
- Excision of the hernia sac
- Crural repair
- Anti-reflux procedure (controversial)
- Gastropexy (optional)

7. Is gastrostomy performed routinely?

No, but it is helpful in preventing gastric volvulus and recurrent migration into the chest by anchoring the stomach against the anterior abdominal wall. This is especially helpful in the elderly, where it can also serve as means of decompression and nutritional support.

8. How is the patient positioned during laparoscopic paraesophageal hernia repair?

The procedure is done under general anesthesia in the lithotomy position with the patient's knees extended. Pneumatic pumps are applied to the lower extremities and the gastric contents are aspirated with a nasogastric tube. The surgeon stands between the legs with the assistants standing on either side of the patient. The patient is placed in reverse Trendelenburg position to provide maximal exposure to the esophageal hiatus.

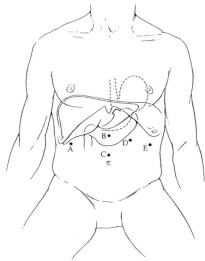

Port placement for laparoscopic repair. The port for the laparoscope is placed a few centimeters above the umbilicus. *A*, 10-mm port with fan retractor; *B*, 10-mm port with scissors; *C*, 10-mm camera port; *D*, 10-mm port with grasper; *E*, 10-mm port with babcock. (From Eubanks WS, Swanstrom LL, Soper NJ (eds): Mastery of Endoscopic and Laparoscopic Surgery. Philadelphia, Lippincott Williams & Wilkins, 1999, with permission.)

9. Describe the port placements for laparoscopic paraesophageal hernia repair.

CO_2 pneumoperitoneum is obtained using Veress needle through a vertical incision 2–3 cm above the umbilicus. Subsequently, a 10-mm port is placed through the same incision and the laparoscope is introduced (see figure above). A second 10-mm port is placed 3–4 cm below the xiphoid in the midline under direct camera visualization. Right and left subcostal 10-mm ports are placed along the midclavicular lines. The last 10-mm port is placed in the far-left lateral subcostal position. The right subcostal port is used for liver retraction. The subxiphoid and the left subcostal ports are used by the surgeon. The left-most lateral port is used for further retraction.

BIBLIOGRAPHY

1. Allen MS, Trastek VF, Deschamps C, Pairolero PC: Intrathoracic stomach: Presentation and results of operation. J Thorac Cardiovasc Surg 105:253–258, 1993.
2. Casabella F, Sinanan M, Horgan S, Pellegrini C: Systematic use of gastric fundoplication in laparoscopic repair of paraesophageal hernias. Am J Surg 171:485–489, 1996.
3. Edelman DS: Laparoscopic repair of paraesophageal hiatal hernia. In Cameron JL (ed): Current Surgical Therapy, 6th ed. St. Louis, Mosby, 1998, pp 1212–1216.
4. Ferguson MK: Paraesophageal hiatal hernia. In Cameron JL (ed): Current Surgical Therapy, 6th ed. St. Louis, Mosby, 1998, pp 51–54.
5. Perdikis G, Hinder R: Laparoscopic paraesophageal hernia repair. In Eubanks WS, Swanstrom LL, Soper NJ (eds): Mastery of Endoscopic and Laparoscopic Surgery. Philadelphia, Lippincott Williams & Wilkins, 2000, pp 165–173.
6. Soper N: Laparoscopic management of hiatal hernia and gastroesophageal reflux. Curr Probl Surg 36:791–833, 1999.
7. Willekes CL, Edoga JK, Frezza EE: Laparoscopic repair of paraesophageal hernia. Ann Surg 225:31–38, 1997.

74. FETAL THORACIC SURGERY

*Raffy L. Karamanoukian, M.D., Marco Ricci, M.D., Ph.D.,
and Hratch L. Karamanoukian, M.D.*

1. Which thoracic lesions are amenable to fetal surgical intervention?

Congenital diaphragmatic hernia (CDH), congenital cystic adenomatoid malformations (CCAM), and other lung lesions associated with nonimmune hydrops.

2. How is fetal CDH managed?

Harrison et al. have developed an algorithm for the management of fetal CDH. Fetuses who herniate late in gestation have a reasonable outlook with conventional management and are delivered safely in tertiary care centers with plans for surgical interventions after stabilization of the pulmonary hypertension. Fetuses with early herniation, mediastinal shift, or severe herniation of the liver may be candidates for fetal repair of the diaphragmatic defect after reduction of the herniated abdominal viscera. An extensive and elaborate series of animal studies in lambs has shown this to be a viable procedure with reversal of the pulmonary parenchymal and vascular abnormalities. A prospective NIH-funded trial in human fetuses is currently ongoing at the University of California, San Francisco.

3. What is an alternative fetal therapy for CDH?

Fetal lung development is accelerated by controlled tracheal obstruction in utero called "plug the lung until it grows" (PLUG). Originally attempted for fetuses deemed unsuitable for in utero reduction and diaphragmatic repair, the PLUG technique has been shown to be efficacious in both animal models and human fetuses with CDH. It reverses the pulmonary hypoplasia, reverses the surfactant deficiency, and reverses the pulmonary vascular abnormalities that are characteristic of the pathophysiology of CDH.

4. Are CCAMs amenable to fetal surgical intervention?

Large prenatally diagnosed CCAMs that cause physiologic derangements such as mediastinal shift, hypoplasia of the lungs, polyhydramnios, and cardiovascular compromise causing fetal hydrops and occasionally death are suitable for fetal surgical intervention. The most common cause for an unfavorable outcome is fetal hydrops. Fetal surgical lobectomy of the lung has been performed with good success with resolution of the hydrops, in utero growth of the remaining lung, and neonatal survival.

5. Is open fetal heart surgery possible?

Yes and no. The response of the fetus to extracorporeal circulatory support is currently being investigated at the Fetal Treatment Center at UCSF. It is conceivable that open fetal cardiac surgery with good survival will become feasible within the next 15 years.

BIBLIOGRAPHY

1. Adzick NS, Harrison MR, Crombleholme TM, et al: Fetal lung lesions: Management and outcome. Am J Obstet Gynecol 179:884–889, 1998.
2. Bruch SW, Adzick NS, Reiss R, Harrison MR: Prenatal therapy for pericardial teratomas. J Pediatr Surg 32:1113–1115, 1997.
3. Harrison MR, Adzick NS, Bullard KM, et al: Correction of congenital diaphragmatic hernia in utero. VII. A prospective trial. J Pediatr Surg 32:1637–1642, 1997.
4. Karamanoukian HL, O'Toole SJ, Holm BA, Glick PL: Making the most out of the least: New insights into congenital diaphragmatic hernia. Thorax 52:209–212, 1997.
5. Mychaliska GB, Bealer JF, Graf JL, et al: Operating on placental support: The ex utero intrapartum treatment method. J Pediatr Surg 32:227–230, 1997.

75. ROBOTICS-ASSISTED THORACIC SURGERY

Hratch L. Karamanoukian, M.D., Raffy L. Karamanoukian, M.D.,
and Jacob Bergsland, M.D.

1. What are the potential applications of robotics-assisted surgery in thoracic surgery?

In addition to endoscopic takedown of the left internal mammary artery (LIMA) in cardiac surgery using the AESOP voice-activated camera (Computer Motion Inc., Santa Barbara, CA), there are potential applications of this technology in thoracoscopic surgery. The LIMA takedown is facilitated by a surgeon-activated voice control system which moves the camera in the chest and facilitates takedown of the LIMA with great visualization and without the need for an assistant. It only responds to the voice signals given by the surgeon. The AESOP system has also been used for takedown of the right internal mammary artery (RIMA) through a left-sided approach.

Noncardiac applications of the AESOP system are only limited by the imagination. It has been used for diagnostic thoracoscopy, to provide camera assistance for wedge resection of the lung and pleura, and for drainage of loculated fluid collections in the chest. It has also been used for the thoracoscopic staging of non-small-cell lung cancer.

2. What are the applications of robotics in thoracic and cardiac surgery?

In addition to the AESOP system, the ZEUSS system (Computer Motion Inc., Santa Barbara, CA) provides two additional instrument arms for robotic surgery. The surgeon is able to operate these arms from a console with actual hand-held instruments whose motion is translated to reality at the operative field.

The ZEUSS system has been used in FDA-approved trials for anastomosis of the LIMA to the left anterior descending artery (LAD) on cardiopulmonary bypass. This has been shown to be successful in more than 100 cases, with promise for widespread application in favorable patients with single-vessel disease limited to the left anterior descending artery. More recently, the ZEUSS system was used to bypass the LAD using the LIMA on the beating heart in London, Ontario, Canada. This application is currently under investigation and pending FDA approval. Additional applications include use of the ZEUSS system in mitral valve repair and replacement surgery.

The ZEUSS system can be used to harvest the LIMA for less invasive coronary artery surgery. In thoracic surgery, the system can be used to perform thoracoscopic esophagectomy, repair of paraesophageal hernia, Heller myotomy, resection of benign esophageal tumors (muscular), resection of mediastinal tumors, mediastinal lymphadenectomy, and lung and pleural biopsy, among others.

BIBLIOGRAPHY

1. Falk V, Autschbach R, Krakor R, et al: Computer-enhanced mitral valve surgery: Toward a total endoscopic procedure. Semin Thorac Cardiovasc Surg 11:244–249, 1999.
2. Mohr FW, et al: Computer-enhanced "robotic" cardiac surgery: First clinical results in 100 patients. Presented at the 80th Annual Meeting of the American Association for Thoracic Surgery, Toronto, Ontario, Canada, 2000.

INDEX

Page numbers in **boldface type** indicate complete chapters.